Transforming Nursing Education

Susan Dandridge Bosher, PhD, MA, is an Associate Professor in the English Department and Director of English as a Second Language (ESL) at the College of St. Catherine in St. Paul, Minnesota, USA. She completed her MA in Teaching English to Speakers of Other Languages (TESOL) from Columbia University, Teachers College, in New York and her doctorate in Second Languages and Cultures Education from the University of Minnesota. She has taught ESL in higher education since 1984 and has also taught in Germany and Turkey. From 1999–2002, she served as ESL expert for a federal grant to recruit and retain multicultural and economically disadvantaged students in nursing. She developed and has been teaching an English for nursing course since 2000. She has recently completed the first of two ESL for nursing textbooks, *English for Nursing, Academic Skills,* and is working on the second textbook, *English for Nursing, Clinical Skills.*

Margaret Dexheimer Pharris, PhD, RN, MPH, FAAN, is an Associate Professor at the College of St. Catherine (CSC), St. Paul, Minnesota, USA. She completed her BSN, MSN, MPH, PhD, and 2-year Adolescent Health Fellowship at the University of Minnesota. Dr. Pharris teaches an "Inclusivity in Nursing Practice" course for advanced practice nurses with LaVonne Moore, RN, MA, CNP, MS, CNM, and an "Inclusivity in Nursing Education" course for nursing education graduate students. In 2001, she worked with CSC and NorthPoint Health & Wellness Center to establish a National Community Center of Excellence in Women's Health (CCOE) at NorthPoint, where she chairs the quality assurance committee of the Board of Directors. From 2001–2007 she coordinated the CSC-NorthPoint community-based collaborative action research (CBCAR) process and grants. In CBCAR, community members determine the research question, are actively involved in the research process and data analysis, and direct the actions that arise from the community-based research. CBCAR research findings in North Minneapolis have demonstrated the negative effects of racism on health and well-being and have informed this book.

Transforming Nursing Education

The Culturally Inclusive Environment

SUSAN DANDRIDGE BOSHER, PhD, MA

MARGARET DEXHEIMER PHARRIS, PhD, RN, MPH, FAAN

Editors

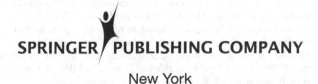

New York

Springer Publishing Company, LLC
11 West 42nd Street
New York, NY 10036
www.springerpub.com

Acquisitions Editor: Allan Graubard
Production Editor: Julia Rosen
Cover design: Joanne E. Honigman
Cover graphic design: Lyla Amini
Composition: Apex CoVantage, LLC

08 09 10 11/ 5 4 3 2 1

Library of Congress Cataloging-in-Publication Data

Transforming nursing education : the culturally inclusive environment / Susan Dandridge Bosher, Margaret Dexheimer Pharris, editors.
p. ; cm.
Includes bibliographical references and index.
ISBN 978-0-8261-2558-3 (alk. paper)
1. Nursing—Study and teaching. 2. Transcultural nursing. 3. Cultural diversity. I. Bosher, Susan Dandridge. II. Pharris, Margaret Dexheimer.
[DNLM: 1. Education, Nursing—organization & administration. 2. Cultural Diversity. 3. Emigrants and Immigrants. 4. Minority Groups. 5. Prejudice. 6. Transcultural Nursing. WY 18 T7716 2008]

RT73.T65 2008
610.73—dc22 2008024565

Printed in Canada by Transcontinental.

This book is dedicated to all nursing students and faculty who have felt marginalized or devalued in the nursing education system because of their race, culture, ethnicity, or language. May this work help create a system where they and those who follow are in the center; their contribution to the profession is vital so that health and healing can be an equal possibility for all. This book is also dedicated to the many nurse educators and leaders from countries around the world who have worked tirelessly to create a culturally inclusive environment in their institutions.

Contents

Contributors

Joyce Veda Abel, RNC, MA, CNP, LICSW, is an Assistant Professor of Nursing and the creator and Director of the Skills and Approaches to Grade Excellence (SAGE) Program for associate- and baccalaureate-degree nursing students at the College of St. Catherine in Minneapolis and St. Paul, Minnesota, USA. She earned a baccalaureate degree from SUNY at Buffalo, a master's in social work from the University of Chicago, and certification as an adult nurse practitioner at the College of St. Catherine. Her private practice is dedicated to people with a history of both trauma and ongoing illness. She has been awarded recognition by the Minnesota Department of Health for her health promotion programs.

Judith A. Andersen, MSN, RN, is the Nursing Director of the Workforce Improvement With International Nurses (WIN) Program at Clackamas Community College in Clackamas, Oregon, USA, and principal developer of its nursing curriculum. She serves as the Northwest Regional Director of the International Bilingual Nurses Alliance (IBNA), a coalition of similar programs in the United States, and participates on several other community boards of directors. Judith was formerly Program Director of the Clackamas Community College Nursing Department. She has held nursing faculty positions at the community college and university level since 1973. Judith was instrumental in organizing the Oregon–Mexico Health Professionals Exchanges that have been ongoing since 1989 and has led annual student cultural exchanges to Mexico and Central America.

Martha Baker, PhD, RN, CNE, APRN-BC, is currently a Professor of Nursing and Director of the BSN program at Southwest Baptist University in Springfield, Missouri, USA. Her primary clinical experience has been in critical care units both as a staff nurse and as a clinical specialist. She has been active in other professional organizations, including the Missouri Nurses Association, American Association of Critical Care Nurses, and Sigma Theta Tau. Dr. Baker is currently the President of the National Alaska Native American Indian Nurses Association (NANAINA) and is on the board of directors of the National Coalition of Ethnic Minority Nurses Association. She has worked on several national projects, including: *Pathways to Leadership: Native American Nurse Leadership Project* and the *Women's Best Practice Primary Care for Heart Disease* and has published in the area of Native American Health.

Susan Ellen Campbell, PhD, RN, is a Professor of Nursing at the College of St. Catherine in St. Paul, Minnesota, USA. She earned her PhD in nursing sciences from the University of Minnesota. She is a native-born Minnesotan and the mother of five children. Her life story is becoming more diverse as both of her sons-in-law are from South America. Her grandchildren are Hispanic and are being raised bilingual. Concurrent with the broadening of her family context, she has transitioned from being a "content expert" to a "story teller." Through the use of story she creates a context for students to engage and reflect on new learning related to the practice of nursing. Currently, she is refining the use of story as a learning tool for teaching thinking and reflective skills related to central concepts in pathophysiology, pharmacology, and medical-surgical nursing interventions.

Lorrie R. Davis-Dick, MSN, RN, BC, is a Clinical Assistant Professor in Mental Health Nursing at her alma mater, North Carolina A&T State University School of Nursing in Greensboro, North Carolina, USA, and is preparing to begin doctoral studies in nursing. She has 8 years of experience in Psychiatric Mental Health Nursing with The Guilford Center, the Nurse-Family Partnership Program, the Moses Cone Hospital Behavioral Health Center, Alcohol and Drug Services, and as a Control/Intervention Research Nurse with the UNC-Chapel Hill School of Nursing's *Reducing Depressive Symptoms in Head Start Mothers Project.* She is certified by ANCC in Psychiatric Mental Health Nursing and has earned more than 20 academic and professional honors and appointments since 2000. Ms. Davis-Dick's outlook for her future in nursing includes becoming a leader in nursing education and continuing to reflect her spirit of mentorship in nursing through her personal motto, "Learn, Mentor, and Empower Nurses of the 21st Century."

Lucy Epp, BA, BEd, CAE, MEd, is a researcher and test developer at Red River College in Winnipeg, Manitoba, Canada. She has been the lead researcher in the analysis of the English language demands of the nursing profession across Canada and the development of the Canadian English Language Benchmark Assessment for Nurses (CELBAN). She has taught ESL/EFL for over 20 years and has also developed ESL curriculum, needs assessments, and language proficiency assessments. For the past 8 years, she has been involved in a wide range of applications of the Canadian Language Benchmarks, including benchmarking college programs, assessment tools, and occupations.

Susan Gross Forneris, PhD, RN, is an Assistant Professor at the College of St. Catherine in St. Paul, Minnesota, USA. She earned her BA in Nursing from the College of St. Scholastica in Duluth, Minnesota, and her PhD in Nursing from the University of Minnesota. Balancing roles, she is married and the mother of one son. Sue's journey within nursing education has been examining the relationship between how we come to know, the impact of context, and improved critical thinking in practice. Reflection is an integral part of this relationship. Through the use of story and reflection, she offers students and practicing clinicians the opportunity to enhance their critical thinking as they come to know and understand the thinking behind the story.

William W. Frank, MS, is a Project Coordinator and full-time faculty member with Customized Training & Development Services at Clackamas Community College near Portland, Oregon, USA, bringing organizational development, education, and training services to business and industry in the Pacific Northwest. He was the initial Program Coordinator for Workforce Improvement With International Nurses (WIN) from 2003 to 2007. Since 1989, he has been a certified facilitator, trainer, and curriculum developer in the areas of leadership, team development, and communication. William received his Master of Science degree in Psychology from Eastern Washington University and his Bachelor of Science from the University of California, Los Angeles.

Donna Hill-Cill, DNP, MSN, RN, FNP, is the Director of Continuing Education at the University of Medicine and Dentistry of New Jersey, School of Nursing (UMDNJ-SN) in Newark, New Jersey, USA. She earned her BSN from the University of North Florida, MS from Columbia University, and DNP from UMDNJ-SN. She has worked as adjunct faculty, education specialist, nursing director, and nurse manager. She was honored with the Humanism in Health Care Award in 2007 from the Healthcare Foundation of New Jersey. Most important is Donna's vision for minority nurses. Her vision is that all nurses learn to trust in themselves, understand their educational needs, and excel to their greatest potential.

Vicki P. Hines-Martin, PhD, RN, is an Associate Professor at the University of Louisville School of Nursing. She earned her BSN and MA (Ed) at Spalding University in Louisville, Kentucky, USA; MSN in Adult Psychiatric Nursing (CNS) from the University of Cincinnati, Ohio; and PhD in Nursing from the University of Kentucky, Lexington. She has worked as a staff nurse, clinical nurse specialist, nurse manager, and educator. Her honors include being named an American Nurses Foundation (ANF) Scholar and an ANA Ethnic and Racial Minority Fellowship Fellow. Dr. Hines-Martin's research has focused on mental health and health disparities with funding from ANF, the National Institute of Nursing Research (NINR), and the National Institute of Diabetes and Digestive and Kidney Diseases (NIDDK).

Virginia Hussin, MEd (TESOL), has taught ESL in Australia and abroad, including China, for 25 years. She has also worked in staff development and curriculum design. For 10 years Virginia taught ESL in the School of Nursing at Flinders University, and for the past 9 years she has worked as a Learning Adviser at the University of South Australia in Adelaide, specialising in teaching ESL Health Sciences students, including Nursing, Physiotherapy, and Pharmacy students. She is currently working on her doctoral dissertation titled: "Interlanguage Pragmatics and the Negotiation of Meaning in Pharmacy Simulations."

Judy Jacoby, RN, MSN, is a member of the Montana Little Shell Tribe of Chippewa. She is currently teaching nursing at Salish Kootenai College in Pablo, Montana, USA on the Flathead Reservation. Judy received her undergraduate education from Montana State University–Northern in Havre. She received her Master's degree in nursing with a certificate of Health Administration from the University of North

Dakota in Grand Forks, where she was a participant in the Recruitment/Retention of American Indians Into Nursing (RAIN) program and was named a Hartford Scholar in 2004. Her areas of interest and research are health care for American Indian elders, access to health care, and public health and rural nursing.

Susan P. Kossman, RN, PhD, is an Assistant Professor at Mennonite College of Nursing, Illinois State University, Normal, Illinois, USA, where she teaches online and classroom-based courses in the undergraduate, Master's, and doctoral programs. She was a National Library of Medicine (NLM) Biomedical Informatics Postdoctoral Fellow at the University of Wisconsin-Madison from 2005 to 2008. Her current research focuses on informatics applications to enhance community-based chronic care management and innovative uses of information and communication technology in nursing education. Dr. Kossman is involved in efforts to increase student competence in informatics and cultural content and to address the needs of nontraditional and minority students in nursing.

Catherine Lewis, BA, BEd, PBCE, CAE, has worked in the field of ESL for 18 years, teaching and developing curriculum at all levels of ESL, from beginner to advanced. She holds a degree in education and post-baccalaureate certification (pre-Master's) in Teaching English as a Second Language (TESL). She has used the Canadian Language Benchmarks (CLB) since 2000 for teaching, curriculum design, evaluation, and test development, working primarily with adult ESL learners. In 2002, she joined the project team with the principal researcher Lucy Epp at Red River College's Language Training Centre in Winnipeg, Manitoba, Canada to assist with *Phase II, the Development of the Canadian English Language Benchmark Assessment for Nurses (CELBAN)*. In 2004, she co-authored a "how-to" manual *Developing an Occupation-Specific Language Assessment Tool Using the Canadian Language Benchmarks—A Guide for Trades and Professional Organizations*. In 2006, she codeveloped versions 2 and 3 of CELBAN, and in 2007, she codeveloped two versions of the *Institutional CELBAN* to be used by educational institutions working with internationally educated nurses across Canada.

Stuart Nairn, PhD, MA, RGN, is a lecturer at the University of Nottingham in the United Kingdom. His main research interests are emergency care, the science and practice of cardiopulmonary resuscitation, race and culture, narrative knowledge, media representations of health and health care workers, and social policy. He is currently exploring philosophical ideas about structure and agency in relation to nursing research, realist approaches to knowledge, and discourse analysis.

Lee Anne Nichols, PhD, RN, is an Associate and tenured Professor in Community Health Nursing at the University of Tulsa School of Nursing in Oklahoma, USA. Dr. Nichols is a tribal citizen of Cherokee Nation. She received her PhD in clinical nursing research from the University of Arizona College of Nursing. She completed a 2-year postdoctoral fellowship in developmental disability research at the University of Alabama at Birmingham Civitan International Research Center. Dr. Nichols has worked in collaboration with several Indian tribes in the Southeastern part of the United States, published several articles, and presented her work nationally and internationally. Her research is with American Indian families with children who have developmental disabilities. Currently, she is refining her conceptual model *The Pattern of American Indians: Harmony Ethos* for use with American Indian families. Dr. Nichols has developed an American Indian nurse leadership curriculum in collaboration with a team of Indian nurse leaders, Arizona State University, and the Indian Health Service. She has also served as a consultant to nursing programs regarding the recruitment and retention of American Indian nursing students and is an active member of the National Alaska Native American Indian Nursing Association (NANAINA).

Katrina H. Norvell, MBA, is a full-time, fixed-term instructional/research faculty member at Portland State University (PSU) in Oregon, USA. Ms. Norvell holds a Master of Business Administration degree from PSU and a bachelor's degree in journalism from the University of Central Florida. She is currently a doctoral candidate in the Public Administration and Policy PhD Program at PSU, preparing her dissertation on community-based scholarship in the field of public administration. Grants from Northwest Health Foundation have provided her with research opportunities regarding community-based nursing education and nurse workforce capacity issues. Her interest in community engagement is also enhanced through her teaching, which includes a number of graduate and undergraduate courses in PSU's School of Community Health and the Hatfield School of Government.

Alona H. Pack, RN, BSN, MA, is Project Director for the Initiative for Nursing Workforce Diversity (INDE) Program at the University of Louisville School of Nursing in Kentucky, USA, where she is also a clinical instructor in maternal child health assessment and an academic counselor for ethnic minority nursing students. Ms. Pack received her BSN from Spalding University in Louisville and a Master of Arts in Health Services Management from Webster University in Louisville. Her practice specialty areas include home health (clinical, management, and consulting), medical surgical nursing, and critical care.

Carmen Ramirez, PhD, RN, is the Director of the Latino Nursing Career Opportunity Program and Adjunct Assistant Professor at the Catholic University of America, School of Nursing, Washington, DC, USA. She received her BSN from the University of Texas, Austin; completed the MSN and Pediatric Nurse Practitioner program at the University of California, San Francisco; and received her PhD from the University of Oregon, Eugene, College of Education. Dr. Ramirez has taught nursing and worked in the Latino community throughout her nursing career. She has held positions as varied as setting up well-child clinics in migrant labor camps to being the Executive Director of the Mayor's Office on Latino Affairs, Washington, DC. Professional appointments include community and hospital boards and serving as president of the DC chapter of the National Association of Hispanic Nurses. Dr. Ramirez has been awarded a Distinguished Public Service Award by the District of Columbia and was recently recognized for outstanding contributions through her work at an inner city high school.

Gloria R. Smith, BSN, MPH, PhD, FAAN, FRCN, is retired Vice President of Health Programs, W. K. Kellogg Foundation in Battle Creek, Michigan, USA. Dr. Smith has a long history in nursing education as both a tenured faculty member and leader. She has served as Dean at Wayne State University and the University of Oklahoma schools of nursing. She was the Director of the Michigan Department of Public Health. She has long been an advocate for an inclusive environment and has a record of accomplishment in creating opportunities for disenfranchised minorities in nursing and public health. She has a distinguished record in nursing and health; in 2007 she was named an American Academy of Nursing Living Legend.

Barbara Jones Warren, PhD, APRN, BC, is an Associate Clinical Professor at The Ohio State University, College of Nursing in Columbus, Ohio, USA. In addition, she is a National Institute of Mental Health Racial/Ethnic Minority Fellow and Postdoctoral Fellow; she received the 2005 American Psychiatric Nurses Association Excellence in Leadership Award and the 2006 and 2007 Influential Leader Who's Who in Black Columbus Award. She has extensive experience in psychiatric mental health nursing and has published numerous articles and book chapters on practice, theoretical, and research issues regarding depression in African American women, cultural competence, and public mental health perspectives. Dr. Warren is considered a national expert and consultant in the area of cultural competence and mood disorders, and she has a private practice in which she provides counseling and psychotherapy services.

Avonne Yang, BSN, RN, is an ethnic Hmong refugee from the Southeast Asian country of Laos. Her professional nursing experiences include clinical practice, education, and research. She was inducted into Sigma Theta Tau International Honor Society of Nursing and received the President's Medal from her university in California and the Army Nurse Corps Spirit of Nursing Award from the Army Nurse Corps in connection with the U.S. National Student Nurses Association for leadership excellence. She served as Director of the Community Health Nursing Student Internship Program from 2004–2006 at the College of St. Catherine, St. Paul, Minnesota, USA, which provided leadership development and mentorship for nursing students from underrepresented ethnic minorities. Ms. Yang was a principal investigator in a community-based collaborative action research project examining the experience of Hmong women living with diabetes. She is an awardee of the State of North Carolina's prestigious Nurse Educators of Tomorrow program and is currently a graduate nursing student at the University of North Carolina at Charlotte.

Foreword

I have often thought that no other career during my lifetime could have offered the promise of respect, fulfillment, acceptance, and opportunity for me as an individual—race, gender, and religion notwithstanding—as has nursing. Like so many other minority persons in pursuit of the American dream, of a good life, the sentiments espoused in the words of philosophical statements issued on behalf of the profession by the college of nursing I attended struck a chord. After initial contact with the school of nursing, I was convinced that I had found a niche, a place that would foster my personal development and ambitions and from which I could satisfy my drive to help my own family and community. Later, inspiration from my basic nursing program broadened my vision to include contributing to societal improvements. After 53 years in the field, I can look back and say that I was correct on all counts—I consider myself one of the "lucky ones." All of the stars had come into alignment: personal drive; strong family support; solid basic education; strong basic nursing program; committed senior leadership in the school; strong faculty advocates and mentors; financial support; community support; high expectations from self, family, community, and faculty; and supplemental enrichment experiences.

Over the years, there have been many like me: "lucky ones." But far too many have not been lucky; they have not fulfilled their dreams to become nurses. This nation, indeed this world, can ill afford this waste of human capital when there is an urgent and dire need for nurses worldwide. This book is about the challenges of increasing the minority presence in nursing programs, overcoming barriers, and utilizing the vast reservoir of available knowledge and experience to convert luck into anticipated outcomes for minority and culturally different students. This book is about capitalizing on diversity and difference, on maximizing human potential. It is about increasing understanding about "the others" who look different and inspiring and guiding them to fulfill their aspirations to nurture, heal, and assist people to cope with threats to health.

Transforming Nursing Education: The Culturally Inclusive Environment is timely; it is a response to the urgent need and demand for increased graduation of well-prepared nurses to practice, manage, and lead in nursing and help to sustain and improve the quality of health care delivery. Trend data and studies describe a shortage of qualified nurses and project acute shortages into the near and distant future. Many current studies recommend, in fact urge, aggressive approaches for attracting minorities into nursing as a significant means for meeting supply requirements. Support for increasing minority enrollments in schools of nursing is not new; there has been support provided by governments and private philanthropy for such initiatives for decades. The support has been more significant in some periods than others. Funding agencies have shifted priorities as other pressing demands arise and compete for dwindling resources. By now, however, we in nursing should be experts in minority recruitment, retention, and graduation; there has been more than sufficient investment by government and private philanthropy to develop and test models for minority recruitment and retention. Various incentives have been offered to encourage programs to increase minority enrollments. Research outcomes and lessons learned have been disseminated through workshops, conferences, publications, and networking under the rubric of one label after another: minority recruitment, cultural inclusion, cultural pluralism, multicultural education, and transcultural nursing, to include a few. Nursing has pioneered in the areas of minority recruitment and retention, multicultural education, and transcultural nursing; thus, it is puzzling that we still have urgent need for this book. Yet, we do! What happens to all of that information developed through years of experience, reading, debate, demonstration, and discussion? What limits the transformation from knowledge to structural change?

The authors in this book attempt to overcome the beast that poses the major barrier by giving it its proper name: *racism.* No single volume could ever be sufficient to explore the topic of racism; however, the opening section of this book succeeds in providing definition, context, and stimulation for further exploration in the matter of race and racism and its impact on nursing education. I learned a very valuable lesson in attending the 1993 *UN World Conference Against Racism, Discrimination and Xenophobia (WCAR)* held in Durban, South Africa. People from across the world attended—people of all races, cultures, religions, sexual identities, and physical and mental abilities—many of whom sought to divert or broaden the focus from simply race and racism in order to direct attention to the pain associated with their particular source of disaffection. *Science* has proven that race has no biological reality; yet, for people who are victims of racism, prejudice, and discrimination, the social reality of being defined as "the other" is deeply experienced nevertheless. The pain is very real; the suffering is the same; and the outcomes result in inequities.

This book is targeted to nursing faculty, nursing education administrators, and graduate nursing students. The material is organized into four major sections so that one is guided from essential background information that helps set a context to case stories to methods and techniques and finally to programs that model structural change. This book contains insights, perspectives, and successful approaches drawn from the experiences of nurses from different races, cultures, and ethnicities. The case stories are poignant and powerful in their careful telling; the aspiration, bewilderment, disappointment, and finally joy and pride are revealed as the writers describe their personal journeys. The book offers an opportunity to examine the impact of discrimination on minority nursing students. It will teach some and reinforce for others that discrimination causes pain and humiliation. Some of the individuals who have suffered discrimination share how they have used their knowledge and experiences to develop approaches to eliminate or minimize similar experiences for other students who follow. Each chapter is followed by a set of questions to guide and provoke discussion that can lead to further understanding and growth.

I consider myself an experienced traveler on the journey of minority inclusion; yet, the book has raised some questions that I want to answer for myself and some that I plan to explore further with others. I have never accepted the idea that a nurse or any other health care provider can adequately and safely care for me if that person has to objectify me in order to carry out his or her responsibilities, that is, has to see me as an object rather than as a person. How can such an individual live up to the philosophy and ethics of nursing? What are the mechanisms that allow alienation yet permit "caring"? Nursing is caring *about* and caring *for* people. Does one wrap one's self in techniques and automatic functions? Are there separate codes for caring if the recipient is "the other"? Similarly, are there separate codes for teaching if the student is "the other"? I admit that I have been taught math and chemistry adequately by persons who have discriminated against me and have even been served food by persons who were admitted racists. None of these people had professed to be committed to a profession that pledged to respect and *care* for me. Because of these questions, I found myself wishing for more case stories from nonminority peers to give us more perspective and insights of a journey in coping with and managing White prejudice and bias toward "the other." In addition, it would have been equally instructive had the minority nurse case stories been reflective of their own capacity to discriminate against "the other," as well as how they have supported and been supported by "the others" who are different from themselves. Perhaps future collections of essays could further explore these manifestations of discriminatory attitudes and practices in nursing.

This book takes a step forward in uncovering the mystery that shrouds some of the ineffectiveness in securing and maintaining adequate minority enrollments. The point is made that more effective minority enrollment cannot be achieved in a vacuum; it requires an environment that is supportive and welcoming for all students. Properties of a welcoming environment are identified and underscored in *Transforming Nursing Education: The Culturally Inclusive Environment.* Faculty must believe their role is to teach, encourage, and assist all admitted students to achieve success and understand that teaching is more than facilitating students who are able to navigate solo. An environment for learning should be created in which assistance for student progression, such as tutoring, is customized and made available to those who require it; there should be little need to label students. It takes a great deal of courage and commitment by individuals and collective faculty to examine and be critical of a culture in which they are heavily invested.

Transformed nursing education is needed for a lot of reasons; creating a culturally inclusive environment is just one of them. To date, the profession has resisted by making small and often cosmetic changes, creating our own jigsaw puzzle. Transforming nursing education to a culturally inclusive enterprise requires determination and shared leadership from the collective. Administrators, faculty members, and staff alike must have a shared vision and be committed to the expressed goal of inclusion. There must be willingness to learn more about people who are different from oneself and to face one's own prejudices or antipathies. Discussions on race, racism, xenophobia, and discrimination are likely to be thorny. They should be supported by knowledge drawn from research and scholarship as well as from the lived experience. The school of nursing must be engaged in constant struggle to avoid sanctions against members who express divergent views and unpopular opinions. Vocabulary becomes critical in engaging one another because words can become loaded in some circumstances. Drawing on published knowledge, facts, theories, and analysis may facilitate achieving the more objective environment that is essential for discussion. *Transforming Nursing Education: The Culturally Inclusive Environment* could be a valuable tool for schools that are embarking on a course to create an inclusive environment or are seeking to improve on what has already begun. The book provides data, analytical frameworks, definitions, and lines of reasoning that can be used as points of common reference. The case stories that have been included are illuminating; their use will permit discussions of real experiences that can serve as surrogates until group members feel secure enough to relate and share their own stories. Emotions are attached to beliefs; shedding long-held beliefs takes time and is often difficult. Discussions clearly will benefit from research and scholarship; however, positive change also requires self-disclosure of beliefs, insights, fears, curiosity, opinions, and ignorance about race, culture, and difference.

This book provides rationale and support for undertaking the journey to achieve true transformation in nursing education. Along the way, readers will learn a great deal about themselves as well as learn more about how to create a dynamic, inclusive, and challenging learning environment that remains true to the purpose of graduating highly qualified nurses to meet the needs of a diverse multiracial, multicultural, multilingual society.

Gloria R. Smith, RN, MPH, PhD, FAAN, FRCN
Battle Creek, MI

Preface

Nursing texts that address cultural diversity have focused on studying and understanding the values, beliefs, and practices of clients from different cultures in an effort to create a more culturally competent workforce. It is also well documented that a diverse nursing profession is the most effective way to meet the needs of an increasingly diverse population; there has also been an obvious increase in minority and immigrant students in nursing programs. However, there has been little emphasis on implementing structural changes in nursing education to create a culturally inclusive environment that is welcoming and supportive of all students and faculty. Compared to the nursing practice workforce, the nursing education workforce is even less representative of the general population and has often been perceived by minority and immigrant students as nonsupportive and at times hostile. Our research and the work of many others point to a pressing need to diversify nursing education as well as engage in a process that dismantles discriminatory practices and reconfigures nursing education and health care delivery systems that currently disproportionately represent a privileged White[1] norm.

Rather than focus on different cultures, as if they were static and monolithic, this text turns the lens around to look at the culture of nursing education itself from the perspectives and experiences of minority and immigrant students and faculty. Through the stories that are told and the programs and initiatives that are described, the various chapters in this anthology address the urgent need for nurse educators, nurse administrators, and graduate students in nursing education to reconceptualize and redesign their pedagogical and programmatic approaches to more effectively recruit, engage, educate, and graduate nurses from underrepresented groups in the profession. This book focuses intentionally on the experiences of minority, indigenous, and immigrant students in predominantly White countries and the structural changes needed to facilitate their success. We believe that conversations about racism are the most difficult to enter into and that often, to avoid the discomfort of those conversations, the definition of diversity is broadened without examining the reason why. Because that discomfort is necessary for transformation to take place at both the personal and institutional levels, we chose to narrow our focus so that we could delve deeply into identifying and addressing barriers faced by minority, indigenous, and immigrant students. We hope that subsequent anthologies will broaden the discussion of diversity and, thus, of inclusivity.

Increased diversity in the nursing workforce will help reduce health care disparities and provide higher quality care for the increasingly diverse populations in countries such as the United States, the United Kingdom, Canada, Australia, and New Zealand. In these countries the faculty and administration of schools of nursing are overwhelmingly White because of the history of colonization in or by these countries and the subsequent concentration of power and economic advantage in the White population. In addition to ethnic minority and indigenous groups that have been traditionally underrepresented in nursing, rapidly increasing migration from war-torn and resource-poor countries to resource-rich countries has intensified the urgent need to reshape nursing education to better meet the needs of immigrant nursing students. With the majority of nurses close to retirement age and considering the impending nursing shortage, real and meaningful systemic change seems more within our grasp than ever before. It is our hope that this book will begin a much needed dialogue about systemic transformation and the shape it might take.

This book is not meant to be a cookbook approach to structural change but rather a stimulus for thought-provoking dialogue that will lead to concrete actions from an antiracist perspective, actions that are specific to the reality of nursing education in different cultural contexts. Ideally, the stories in each chapter will allow readers to appreciate the personal dimension of students' aspirations and struggles. The questions at the end of each chapter are designed to spark dialogue and insight into ways faculty, administrators, and graduate nursing students can look within themselves and come to terms with their own racialized experiences and perspectives to create the structural changes necessary for all students to be successful. We recognize that these are challenging questions and that the issues they raise are not conclusive. We trust that readers will engage in respectful dialogue with one another, move beyond assumptions and stereotypes, and be transformed in the process. Change happens within the context of carefully listening to one another's stories and engaging in open and safe dialogue; it is our desire that this anthology will contribute in meaningful ways to that process.

Part I, "Understanding Inclusivity in the Current Nursing Culture," addresses the issue of racism in nursing education from both personal and institutional perspectives. In "Inclusivity: Attending to Who Is in the Center," Margaret Dexheimer Pharris defines institutionalized, personally mediated, internalized, and colorblind racism and explicates how they permeate nursing education and practice and thus place nurses at odds with core tenets of nursing practice—such as caring, health, justice, and equal treatment. She explores the historical roots of racism and provides strategies for nurse educators to help all students identify and address racism within themselves and in practice settings. She proposes that when Whiteness is taken out of the center of the nursing education environment, everyone excels to a greater degree and becomes more vibrant and healthy. In "The Power of Nurse Educators: Welcoming and Unwelcoming Behaviors," Susan P. Kossman gives concrete examples from her research with students and faculty of how racism manifests itself in unwelcoming behaviors; she also offers examples of welcoming behaviors that could mitigate the effects of or possibly dismantle racism in nursing-education culture. Her concept map, located in the middle of the chapter, provides a model for creating an inclusive nursing-education environment. Stuart Nairn's chapter, "Addressing Race and Culture in Nurse Education," delineates how race is constructed and reproduced through discursive practices in society as well as in nursing. He challenges nurse educators to expand multicultural or transcultural approaches in nursing by addressing power relations and embracing an antiracism approach. In "Minority Nurses: A Story of Resilience and Perseverance," Donna Hill-Cill offers stories and lessons learned from nursing students whose lives have been affected by racism in nursing education and practice. Through her own practice as a nurse educator she models ways in which faculty can reach out and mentor students from diverse cultural backgrounds.

Part II, "Pedagogical Innovations in Nursing Education," addresses ways in which faculty and administrators can effect change in curriculum and pedagogy, as well as in the structural and support systems that create the broader context of nursing education. In "Coming Home to Nursing Education for a Hmong Student, Hmong Nurse, and Hmong Nurse Educator," Avonne Yang describes the essential ways in which minority faculty contribute to the successful outcomes of minority students in nursing programs. She raises issues of concern about unequal demands and added stress placed on minority faculty and describes actions that administrators can take to justly compensate minority faculty. Yang also describes how narrative pedagogy and the theory of health as expanding consciousness allowed her to reconcile differences between her Hmong culture and the culture of nursing. Susan Gross Forneris and Susan Ellen Campbell, in their chapter "Journeying Beyond Traditional Lecture: Using Stories to Create Context for Critical Thinking," discuss the role of stories in a contextual reflective case-based teaching approach to help students reflect critically on the biased assumptions they bring to clinical experiences. Similar to Yang, Forneris and Campbell use narrative pedagogy as well as guided reflection to help students learn to unpack their values and beliefs and take the perspective of "the other." In "INDE Project: Developing a Cultural Curriculum Within Social and Environmental Contexts," Vicki P. Hines-Martin and Alona H. Pack describe a 3-year federally funded project—Initiative for Nursing Diversity Excellence (INDE)—to increase recruitment, retention, and graduation of African American students in nursing. Various INDE initiatives include: academic and peer-mentoring support; stipends; early exposure to and academic preparation for nursing at the secondary level; and cultural awareness, sensitivity, and competence training for all nursing students and faculty with regard to client care and for faculty with regard to teaching and supporting minority students through the educational process. Barbara Jones Warren, in "Teaching the Fluid Process of Cultural Competence at the Graduate Level: A Constructionist Approach," describes materials and techniques that she developed for a graduate-level course on cultural competence. This course uses transformative learning theory and a constructionist approach to cultural competence, which emphasizes the dynamic and fluid nature of culture. Warren also describes her use of literature about health care challenges as a means of encouraging transformative, reflective learning. Lee Anne Nichols and Martha Baker, in their chapter "Pathways to Leadership: Developing a Culturally Competent Leadership Curriculum for American Indian Nurses," describe a curriculum—Pathways to Leadership—that was developed to educate and inspire American Indian nurses to assume leadership roles in tribal health programs. The curriculum consists of nine modules, six of which focus on general nurse leadership and three on leadership and nursing in the American Indian community. Their discussion of leadership within the American Indian community, in particular the focus on "who one is" rather than "what one does," counters traditional notions of what constitutes effective leadership.

Part III, "Assessment Practices: Leveling the Playing Field," describes initiatives that challenge traditional ways of assessing students by recognizing that structural change must also address bias in the ways in which students are assessed and their progression in nursing programs determined. In "The Role of Intentional Caring in Ameliorating Incapacitating Test Anxiety," Joyce Veda Abel describes an innovative program in test anxiety management (STAMP) for nursing students with test anxiety who are in danger of failing. The program consists of four components: intentional caring, cognitive restructuring, calming techniques, and test-taking skills. Students who have participated in the program have experienced significant reductions in test anxiety and have gone on to graduate from their programs and pass the nursing licensure exam. Susan Dandridge Bosher, in her chapter "Removing Language as a Barrier to Success on Multiple-Choice Nursing Exams," challenges nursing faculty to take a critical look at their multiple-choice tests, not only for lack of clarity but also for unnecessary linguistic complexity, both of which can hinder students' ability to demonstrate their nursing knowledge. Principles of good test-item construction are discussed as well as principles of linguistic modification, a process by which the reading load of test items is reduced without compromising the questions' content and integrity. In the chapter, "Innovation in Language Proficiency Assessment: The Canadian English Language Benchmark Assessment for Nurses (CELBAN)," Lucy Epp and Catherine Lewis describe the development of an occupation-specific English-language assessment for immigrant nurses seeking to reenter the nursing field in Canada. The test development process involved stakeholders and a wide range of expert consultants and included an analysis of target language use, pilot testing with the target population, and rigorous measures of reliability and validity. Such a test offers a more valid measure of immigrant nurses' language proficiency in nursing contexts than the general academic and occupational English-language proficiency tests that are traditionally used.

Part IV, "Programs That Model Structural Change," describes various programs that model ways in which to effect structural change in nursing education. In "Latino Nursing Career Opportunity Program: A Project Designed to Increase the Number of Latino Nurses," Carmen Ramirez describes a program at the Catholic University of America (CUA) to increase the number of Latino nurses, the most underrepresented group among registered nurses in the United States. The program consists of a pre-entry nursing program for students in grades 7–12, including a summer camp and other activities during the academic year to increase the visibility of nursing as a career; a comprehensive retention program for Latino nursing students at CUA; and a faculty development program to enhance skills in mentoring, advising, and teaching Latino and other minority students. Judy Jacoby, in her chapter "Barriers to Success: American Indian Students in Nursing," describes the Recruitment/Retention of American Indians Into Nursing (RAIN) program at the University of North Dakota, the barriers to success that Native Americans have traditionally faced in their education, and the ways in which the RAIN program honors and incorporates Native American cultural traditions to facilitate the success of Native American nursing students. In "It Takes a Village to Raise a Nurse," Lorrie R. Davis-Dick describes a mentoring program—Empowering Nursing Students in the Carolinas (ENSC)—designed to decrease the attrition rate of minority nursing students in baccalaureate-degree nursing programs. Her personal story illuminates the important role that mentors play in the educational journey of minority students. Virginia Hussin, in her chapter "Facilitating Success for ESL Nursing Students in the Clinical Setting: Models of Learning Support," describes five levels of a learning support program that were implemented at the University of South Australia to facilitate the success of English as a Second Language (ESL) students in their clinical placements: professional development of staff; workshops for students prior to and following their placements; individual consultations with students; on-site supervision of "at risk" students; and provision of Web-based learning support materials. In "Workforce Improvement With International Nurses (WIN): Immigrant Nurses WIN Road to Licensure," William W. Frank, Judith A. Andersen, and Katrina Norvell describe a program in Oregon to identify and prepare work-ready immigrant nurses to reenter the workforce. The program—Workforce Improvement With International Nurses (WIN)—includes: assistance with the credential review and licensure application process, courses in advanced communication and medical terminology, a Nursing Transition Program (NTP) focusing on developing critical thinking and evidence-based practice, and supervised clinical and hospital internships.

Throughout the past 3 years this book has broadened its focus from educating culturally and linguistically diverse nursing students to the culture of nursing education and its exclusionary practices. A primary influence on this evolution has been the result of a community-based collaborative action research project in North Minneapolis, a multiethnic inner-city neighborhood. This project, which was funded by the College of St. Catherine, identified racism as the major barrier to health for people of color. These findings served as a catalyst for us to expand the focus of the anthology to look within the culture of nursing education for parallel issues that affect the success of minority, indigenous, and immigrant students. Creating this book has been a unique and exciting journey for us, one that has been deeply inspirational not only for the way in which the book evolved over time to focus on broader truths that needed to be told but also for the truths that were revealed to us by the contributing authors. In addition, while many of the authors are published scholars in their field, others are emerging scholars who are just now realizing their power and potential to effect change within nursing education. It has been a privilege to work with all of them, to encourage their personal and professional voices to emerge, and to bear witness to the many layers of stories they have to share.

Susan Dandridge Bosher and Margaret Dexheimer Pharris
St. Paul, Minnesota, U.S.A.
March 21, 2008 (On the occasion of Nauroz—Persian New Year—symbolizing the coming of Spring and new beginnings!)

NOTE

1. White is capitalized throughout this book not to denote "race," which has no biological basis, but rather to call readers' attention to Whiteness as a sociological construct that has marginalized people of color and created exclusionary practices in educational institutions and professions. Because Whiteness is assumed to be the norm, it is too often not named. It is that unexamined assumption of White-as-the-norm that we hope to challenge by naming and capitalizing White.

Acknowledgments

We are grateful to the College of St. Catherine for its generous support of this work through two Carol Easley Denny Awards for excellence in research and scholarship, a Faculty Research and Scholarly Activities grant, and funding for a student editorial intern through the Centers of Excellence Assistantship Mentoring Program. We are also grateful to our many colleagues at the College who value and role-model ways in which to create a welcoming and supportive educational environment; their commitment to structural change has motivated and energized us. We have also been truly inspired by the contributing authors to this anthology, whose personal stories, passion, commitment, and professional expertise have illuminated the path toward creating a culturally inclusive nursing education environment. In addition, it is a great honor to be able to include the wisdom of Dr. Gloria Smith in the foreword to this book; her example has inspired thousands of nurses around the world.

We are grateful to Springer Publishing for its commitment to this book and particularly to our Acquisitions Editor, Allan Graubard. His guidance helped us realize the dialogic possibilities of the text for systemic transformation. His enthusiasm for this project and his support encouraged us in our work. We are also grateful to Katherine Tengco, Assistant Editor at Springer Publishing, for her prompt and clear technical guidance and to Julia Rosen from Apex CoVantage for her expertise in the production phase of the book.

Many thanks, too, to Kathryn-Ann Geis, our wonderful editorial assistant from the College of St. Catherine, for her extraordinary editorial skills, keen knowledge of copyright laws and procedures, and careful attention to detail.

PART I

Understanding Inclusivity in the Current Nursing Culture

1 Inclusivity: Attending to Who Is in the Center

MARGARET DEXHEIMER PHARRIS

It had been a full day of classes, and I was eager to leave my office and head for home. As I straightened from packing my computer bag, I noticed one of the junior students hesitantly looking in from the side of my open door. "Angelleen" was a student who had stood out among an impressive cohort of peers in those first few weeks of the semester for her insightful comments and critical analysis of course content, to say nothing of the confident manner in which she spoke up in the auditorium. I welcomed her into my office. As she settled into a stuffed armchair, I took note of the slight flushing of her dark-brown cheeks. Angelleen hesitated briefly and then said, "Dr. Pharris, with all due respect, the content in our class is really, REALLY important, but I don't want to hear it from a WHITE professor!" I was well aware that there were several layers to Angelleen's discomfort and concern.

That week in class, the students were assigned to go to the library and watch the video series *Race: The Power of an Illusion* (Adelman, 2003), which dispels the myth of a biological basis for "race," describes how the concept of "race" was invented and used for the economic advancement of a select group of people, and details how the institutionalization of racism into U.S. culture brought about significant economic and social disparities. The video series helps students understand that "race" is a sociological construct and that racism is a significant health threat for people of color and, thus, of central concern to nursing. The students were also assigned to read "White Privilege: Unpacking the Invisible Knapsack" (McIntosh, 1990), to understand the myriad unearned social and economic advantages that White people enjoy every day, and "Levels of Racism: A Theoretical Framework and a Gardener's Tale" (Jones, 2000). Jones explains that "race" is not a biological construct, and she presents a framework for understanding racism at three levels: "institutionalized, personally mediated, and internalized" (p. 1212). Institutionalized racism, also termed *systemic* racism, is defined by Jones as:

> differential access to the goods, services, and opportunities of society by race. Institutionalized racism is normative, sometimes legalized, and often manifests as inherited disadvantage. It is structural, having been codified in our institutions of custom, practice, and law, so there need not be an identifiable perpetrator. Indeed, institutionalized racism is often evident as inaction in the face of need. (p. 1212)

Institutionalized racism is the reason for "race" being highly correlated with poverty, stress, and environmental exposures, all of which lead to poor health outcomes. In the nursing education system, examples of institutionalized racism include consciously or unconsciously steering students of color into technical or practical nursing programs while at the same time steering White students toward professional and graduate nursing programs. Institutionalized racism is at work when there are more White people on college and university boards of directors, administrative teams, and in faculty and student bodies than there are in the communities they serve—when the percentage of Black and Brown people increases as you move down the widening hierarchical pyramid of academia from the board of directors to the community served at the base. To envision this, draw a pyramid of your institution, and for each level, use existing data to record the percentage of people of color; if there is not proportionality from the bottom to the top, dialogue and action are needed. Institutionalized racism is at play.

Personally mediated racism is defined by Jones (2000) as "prejudice and discrimination, where prejudice means differential assumptions about the abilities, motives, and intentions of others according to their race, and discrimination means differential actions toward others according to their race" (p. 1212). This is how most people conceptualize racism. Personally mediated racism can be conscious or unconscious and can be typified by what we do and do not do. For example, a Pakeha

(White) professor assumes that a Maori student might need extra help in a course, failing to realize that this student has the highest grades in her nursing class. If the professor realizes his assumption, he at least becomes aware that he has breathed in the pollutants of racism and has some work to do. Another example is a White professor consistently interrupting a colleague of color when she or he speaks or restating what was said. At our best, we recognize this and bring it to the attention of our White colleagues to encourage them and hold them accountable for change. Personally mediated racism is one of the building blocks of institutionalized racism. There is an aspect of internalized superiority to this dynamic, which mirrors internalized racism, the next level of racism.

Internalized racism is manifest when people from stigmatized "races" begin to believe the negative messages about their intrinsic value and abilities. They stop believing in themselves and in people who look like them (Jones, 2000). Internalized racism "involves accepting limitations to one's own full humanity, including one's spectrum of dreams, one's right to self-determination, and one's range of allowable self-expression" (p. 1213). Internalized racism is exemplified when faculty of color more readily accept the input and opinions of White colleagues over colleagues who look like them or when a student of color second-guesses her answers on an exam or her ability to do a clinical procedure in spite of having thoroughly studied for the task at hand. Internalized racism can be diminished through a process of critical examination (Ellis & Pharris, 2007).

To help the undergraduate nursing class Angelleen was enrolled in understand how these types of racism work together and how to deal with them as professional nurses, the course faculty used several role-plays and case scenarios. The scenario we worked on the day that Angelleen came to my office involved the students assuming the role of the nurse manager of a busy hospital unit on a day when two nurses had called in sick, several new admissions were anticipated, and a float nurse had been requested. The nurse manager witnesses the charge nurse's response to the arrival of a Native American woman who says she was sent from her unit to help out. The charge nurse rolls her eyes and states, "Oh no! I asked for a *nurse,* not a *nursing assistant!*" The Native American woman, speaking in a soft, calm voice, informs the charge nurse that she *is* a professional nurse *and* a graduate student in nursing.

After reviewing the scenario, students are encouraged to discern how they, as the nurse manager, would attend to and support the float nurse; what kind of conversation they would have with the charge nurse;

and what actions they would consider taking to assure a healthy climate in their unit. The first level of analysis usually involves seeing personally mediated racism on the part of the charge nurse—"She's racist! She just *assumed* that the Native American nurse was a nursing assistant!" When asked why the charge nurse might have made that assumption, the students query what the charge nurse's previous experience might have been with Native Americans, but then as they dig deeper, they begin to question what the racial make-up of the staff is in the hospital—from the people who clean to the people in the board room. Thinking that the float nurse was a nursing assistant may be a logical error in an institution where the majority of Native American employees work as nursing assistants or in other support staff roles, rather than as professional nurses—an example of institutionalized racism. The next level of analysis involves having the students work in small groups to develop a plan to systemically identify and address institutionalized racism on the unit. Students might choose to measure patient outcomes by "race," collect data related to recruitment and retention of nurses of color, conduct confidential surveys of patients and staff to listen to their experiences, and so forth.

The final level of analysis is to have students write down the "race" she or he envisioned the charge nurse and nurse manager to be when the scenario was first read. Even though the "race" of the charge nurse and the nurse manager was not noted when the scenario was presented, the students' answers usually involve some assumptions and resultant self-insight. This opens the door for further dialogue and understanding of the dynamics of institutionalized racism, internalized racism (on the part of the charge nurse in the scenario if she is a person of color, or on the part of the students of color if they envisioned the charge nurse and nurse manager as White), and internalized supremacy or privilege (on the part of White students if they envisioned the charge nurse and nurse manager as White). White professors can role-model and encourage White students to take leadership in identifying and addressing situations involving racism and taking the lead to enact change at the systems level. This is not to say that faculty of color cannot or are not doing this work or are not doing it very well. They can and are. They experience greater emotional and promotional costs. Because White people are the beneficiaries of White privilege—whether they want it or realize it or not—they are morally obligated to take the lead. White faculty can and should teach students that dismantling racism is an essential nursing intervention for health. This important work is often a new concept for White students, most of whom have not spent a great deal of time thinking about racism or their responsibility to identify and address it. The overwhelming Whiteness of the nursing culture, if not critiqued, perpetuates this blindness (Gustafson, 2007).

Students need to realize that in predominantly White countries racism is woven through the daily experience of everyone, whether it is consciously realized or not, and not only does it weaken the social fabric for all people, it is a significant health concern. An African American nurse participant in a study by Giddings (2005) demonstrates this when she states:

> I'll shave down and survive in their world and as soon as 5:00 comes, I unshave and get into my world where I am my own self. So I show two faces. That's why we [African Americans] are so hypertensive. It's because we have to deal in two worlds. White folks don't. It's their world. They operate the same way in their work world, their home, and in their environment. For us it's like wearing "two hats." I become another person when I walk out my door. (p. 309)

Many studies have shown that the failure to recognize and name racism is harmful to the health of people of color (Institute of Medicine, 2002; Krieger, 1990, 2003; Williams, Neighbors, & Jackson, 2003).

The good news is that racism is a social structure, and social structures can be changed. Nurses are uniquely situated to take leadership in making this change. The first step is identifying and naming the source of the problem, which is not always easy, particularly for those who do not have the critical vision to see it. Racism has been cleverly buried in every corner of our culture; it is the warp over which the myriad threads of economic advantage have been woven.

Psychologist Beverly Daniel Tatum (1997) describes racism as being like smog—sometimes it is thick and sometimes invisible. We don't describe ourselves as smog-breathers, but we are—all of us. This means that people of color are at danger for internalizing a false sense of inferiority, while White people assume a false sense of superiority—neither is real, and this distorted sense of reality can only be broken by critical attention to the history of racism and the purpose it has served around the world. This is essential nursing knowledge.

Angelleen's concerns were more local and immediate. As a first-year nursing student, she was concerned about how she would deal with racism as a Black professional nurse when the nursing profession is overwhelmingly and disproportionately White. How had this come to be?

How much harder would she have to work than her White counterparts to succeed in the profession? Would she be safe? If White nurses cannot see the dynamics of racism at play in health care encounters, are patients of color safe in their care? Angelleen had walked into my office and brought up the fact that she didn't want to hear about racism from a *White* professor, and she obviously wanted to talk about this, but she also needed mentors and guides who looked like her. We explored and made professional connections for her to have more people to talk with about these important professional issues. I told her that my research and scholarly work have shown that racism is a major health concern and that because racism was created by White people, I, as a White person, felt compelled to take leadership in addressing it, but I am also very attentive to discerning when to step aside and when to build coalitions. Many strong and amazing leaders have risen up from racialized groups to shine a light on the path toward health, yet there is much work to be done by *all* of us. We both expressed concern that even though empirical evidence suggests that racial inequalities are not improving and perhaps even worsening, there is an increasing trend not to talk about racism—the whole *"we've dealt with this—racism no longer exists—it's time to move on"* mentality. Because this dynamic can be distorting and disorienting, Angelleen decided to begin attending the Black Nurses Association meetings where she could network and anchor herself in a supportive community of nurse leaders. Having a circle of support gives nurses the strength and wisdom needed to do the important work of creating healthier systems and maintaining their own personal health and well being.

Angelleen and I had a long talk that day and have had many long-distance phone conversations and e-mail exchanges in the years since, during which she has successfully completed graduate school and has risen to leadership in a demanding work environment. I have continued to explore how we can switch the focus of our telescopic lens on diversity to turn it back on ourselves in academia—on the nursing education system and its White culture—to make the necessary structural and relational changes for a truly inclusive environment.

Nurse scholars have led the way by constructing theoretical models for culturally competent care (Campinha-Bacote, 2003; Giger & Davidhizar 2004; Leininger, 2001; Purnell & Paulanka, 2003). This first wave of scholarly work showed us what knowledge and sensitivities were needed for us to be able to best care for our patients and their families. They gave us a mirror that reflected our own "otherness" as we viewed "the other." A second wave of scholarly work warned us of the danger that our diversity efforts may not only exacerbate differences and divisions but also strengthen the privileged White normative structure of nursing as long as it is at the center (Allen, 2006; Alleyne, Papadopoulos, & Tilki, 1994; Hassouneh, 2006; Markey & Tilki, 2007; Nairn, Hardy, Parumal, & Williams, 2004; Vaughan, 1997).

Hassouneh (2006) makes a strong case for antiracist pedagogy being an essential aspect of nursing curricula. Similarly, Irihapeti Ramsden (2000, 2002), who proposed the model of cultural safety for New Zealand, suggests that nurses must attend to the power relations in nursing and health service delivery and that they need to be more concerned with *life chances* than *life styles* as the underlying causes of health disparities. Collectively, nurses from around the world have the ingredients needed to make nursing rise from cultural diversity to cultural safety and inclusion. Allen (2006) warns that we cannot simply "add colour and stir" (p. 66)—it is not enough to add diversity courses or to add faculty of color, but rather we must remove White culture as the main ingredient *and* as the bowl in which we do the mixing. The remainder of this chapter will present some concepts that you as a reader might find helpful as you look inside yourself to discern what actions you could bring to the mix. Pay attention to the insights that arise within you as you read this text—those internal insights is the text for you to study most diligently.

WAKING UP TO THE PERVASIVE EXISTENCE OF RACISM

Several years ago, I was asked to join a local health center in its effort to establish a center of excellence in women's health in the neighborhood where I live, which is predominantly African American but also Hmong, Latino, Vietnamese, American Indian, and European American. The health center staff needed a nurse with a PhD to help with the grant writing, and they asked me to develop a community-based action research program, which was a grant requirement. The grant was funded, so I recruited three brave nurse practitioner graduate students into the effort, telling them that they would not know what the topic of their thesis would be because defining the research question was up to the community. All I could promise them was a process of community engagement. They eagerly signed on. We joined with the health center staff to invite women representing 50 different organizations and places in the community where women gather to a Saturday morning meeting to identify the major barriers to health for women and girls of color in the neighborhood. We expected 10 to 15 women to show up, but 50 came. After 4 hours of small group dialogue, the women came back together and decided they needed another Saturday morning session—there was so much to talk about. Two weeks later, 65 women gathered. After another 4 hours of small group dialogue, the eight groups came back together, and each group reported that *racism* was the greatest barrier to health for women and girls of color. We spent a year listening to women's stories about the interplay of racism, health, and well-being (Amaikwu-Rushing et al., 2005).

In the small group I participated in that day, several Black women talked about not being touched by White providers during their health exams. One Black woman told of how her knee surgeon stood close to the door as he asked her to raise and bend her knee and tell him where and when it hurt. She said he did not touch her until it was time for the surgery. As each woman shared stories from her own experience and that of her family and friends, I listened with sadness to their accounts of receiving inadequate and unequal care and the fear these experiences engendered. I wondered to what extent my patients were carrying that same fear. After I left our Saturday morning dialogue, I headed to the local trauma center where I was scheduled to work in the emergency department (ED).

Upon arrival to the ED, I took report from an excellent White nurse. She and a very fine White physician had both been caring for two young women who just happened to arrive to the ED at the same time. Both were close to 20 years of age, and both presented with 9 out of 10 flank pain, indicative of kidney stones. After receiving report, I went to assess my patients. The first young woman, a White woman, was lying on an ED bed dressed in a patient gown and wrapped in a warm blanket. She had received a significant amount of morphine through an IV that was infusing into her left arm. The second young woman, a Black woman, was in a fetal position in the procto room, was still in her street clothes, and had received nothing for pain. In an instant it hit me that I might not have noticed this inequality had I not come directly from the dialogue about racism and health care. I wondered, how much more was *I* missing? These two women had the same physician and nurse—both of whom I had always respected. Was the nurse really "excellent" and was the physician really "fine?" How did this unequal treatment slip by them? How much unequal treatment slips by *me?* Am *I* a part of this? After reading the work on unconscious discrimination by Michelle van Ryn and colleagues (van Ryn & Burk, 2000; van Ryn & Fu, 2003), I realized that there was no way I could *not* be a part of the problem unless I did a lot of work to uncover and understand the dynamics of institutionalized racism in my clinical practice and in my work as a nurse educator.

Since that day, I have tried to make an increased effort to wake up to the dynamics of racism in the health care environment and in the education of health care professionals, particularly nurses. As a White person in the United States, I have been trained not to see racism in its myriad forms and manifestations in my life and in the lives of the patients and students with whom I work. I am not alone. The same thing has happened to light-skinned people in Canada, Australia, New Zealand, the United Kingdom, most of Europe, and much of Latin America—any country with a history of colonization and where the economy and social structure have been built on the genocide, enslavement, and exploitation of Black and Brown people. Nursing in these countries is part of the social fabric and hence has become White-controlled and defined. If we analyze how this has come to be, we will be able to create a healthier and more vibrant profession for all of us.

SANKOFA: LOOKING BACK TO MOVE FORWARD

In order to understand how racism is woven into the profession of nursing, we must first take an honest look at the collective history of the country in which we find ourselves. In order to understand why we are where we are, we must look back at where we have come from. When we look back at this history, we can disentangle ourselves from that which does not nurture the health of our students and the populations we serve. Ideally, this process becomes a source of decolonization and transformation. For example, a truthful look at the recorded history of nursing would take the profession back 2,000 and 1,000 years, respectively, before the time of Florence Nightingale. In 250 B.C. the first formal school of nursing was established for men in India (O'Lynn, 2007) and during the time of the Prophet Muhammad, Rufaidah bint Sa'ad established restorative and preventive nursing care for soldiers and the general population (Anionwu, 2006). (Rufaidah bint Sa'ad is also referred to in the nursing literature as Rufaida Al-Asalmiya, see for example, Aldossary, While, and Barriball [2008].) Engaging in a more expansive view of the history of nursing systems and leadership broadens perspectives of what nursing has and can be.

In outlining important principles of leadership, Bordas (2007) presents the image of Sankofa, the mythical West African bird that is always presented looking over its back toward the past. Sankofa invites us to learn from the wisdom and insights gained from an examination of our history. Sankofa reminds us that "our roots ground and nourish us, hold us firm when the winds of change howl, and offer perspective about what is lasting and significant" (Bordas, 2007, p. 28). In the Akan language of West Africa, the concept of Sankofa is translated to mean: "it is not taboo to go back and fetch what you forgot" (W.E.B. Dubois Learning Center, n.d.). Often the bird is symbolized with an egg in its mouth to represent the potential that can be birthed in the future from the process of looking back to the past.

In looking back from our various country perspectives, we find that the history of colonization changed our relationship with the earth from that of steward to subjugator, which "set the stage for an economic system that allowed the using up and abusing of natural and human resources" (Bordas, 2007, p. 34). In the process of looking back honestly, we acknowledge not only the violence and degradation, but we also uncover cultural treasures that can be invested to create a much richer and healthier future. Bordas (2007) states:

> When the past is reconstructed in the bright light of honesty—or at least when everyone's story is told—we can begin restructuring leadership from a Eurocentric form to one that's more diverse and inclusive. We can construct a new leadership covenant that reflects and respects the history and culture of all. (p. 32)

There is a certain excitement and exhilarating hope in the process of transforming our culture to one that is inclusive—where Whiteness is not the center, nor the norm. International nurses witnessed this quality of excitement and hope in London in 1999 during the centennial celebration of the International Council of Nurses. The vibrancy of the Democratic Nursing Organisation of South Africa (DENOSA) permeated the gathering. They presented an assertive, spirited collective of Black and White nurses whose positive energy drew everyone in. I sat down with several DENOSA members during a break and asked how they had come to such strong solidarity as a professional organization. They explained that it was only through the truth commission process that this was possible. The first step was to tell of the atrocities and to fully listen to the effects of apartheid. A Black nurse told me that she had returned to South Africa prior to the dismantling of apartheid after completing her professional nursing education in the United Kingdom. When she returned, she was supervised by a White nursing assistant who made more money than she did. It took a lot of honest dialogue to heal the wounds and repair the deep divisions. The values embraced by DENOSA are excellence and professionalism, humility, collectivism, solidarity, and unity; they are democratic, nonracial, and nonsexist (www.denosa.org.za). The warp of the fabric of nursing culture is much stronger if it is woven from our collective values in a way that reveals the truth.

As a quest for truth, when I was preparing to teach a graduate nursing theory course last fall, I began researching what became of the men and women of color who might have been among the established nurse theorists. I came across the story of Susie Walking Bear Yellowtail, who graduated from Boston City Hospital School of Nursing in 1923 to become the first Native American registered nurse. After graduating, she returned to the Crow Reservation to work for the Bureau of Indian Affairs Hospital where she soon realized that White surgeons were performing nonconsent sterilization surgeries on Crow women. By necessity, she spent the rest of her career educating the public on the abuses experienced by Native American people and advocating for improved health care service for Native Americans. Susie Walking Bear Yellowtail did not have the luxury of the reflective life of a theorist; she had to respond to the immediate and urgent needs of her community (Cohen, 1999).

Reviewing the works of Carnegie (1991, 2000), Davis (1999), Hine (1989), Robinson (2004), Seacole and Salih (1857/2005), Staupers (1961), and Washington (2006) gave me greater insight into the pressing social justice demands on the time and energy of nurse leaders of color and the discrimination they have battled on a daily basis. One example is that of Mary Grant Seacole, a Black Jamaican woman who, prior to the formation of schools of nursing in Jamaica, served in Panama and Cuba to help curb the spread of cholera and yellow fever epidemics and to care for those who fell sick. When the Crimean War broke out in 1853, Ms. Seacole petitioned to join the nurses being sent by the British government. She offered her vast knowledge of disease containment and treatment to aid in protecting soldiers in the British Army, many of whom were from Jamaica. In spite of having letters of support from British army physicians and the wife of the secretary of war, she was turned down because she was Black. Undeterred, Ms. Seacole financed her own way to make the 3,000-mile journey. Once there, she petitioned Florence Nightingale to join the Angel Band of military nurses, but Nightingale refused to give her a position. Seacole established Spring Hill, a lodging house with nutritious food and a place for the troops to come and heal on the outskirts of the battlefield. She brought knowledge of cures for dysentery and was cited by many military officers for her quick and thorough healing practices. Seacole worked tirelessly during the day at the lodging house, and then at nightfall, she headed to the battlefield to rescue and treat fallen soldiers. After the Crimean War ended, Seacole returned home, injured and economically poor, but rich in the satisfaction that she had made a difference in the lives of hundreds of soldiers (Carnegie, 2000; Robinson, 2004; Seacole & Salih, 1857/2005).

From the perspective of another island nation, New Zealand, nurse scholar Irihapeti Merenia Ramsden (2002) recounts how health disparities have risen for the indigenous people of New Zealand after the efflux of people from the United Kingdom in the 1830s. Ramsden points out that by the time she was born, slightly more than 100 years later, "the land had been largely stripped of native people, trees and birds" (p. 14). She draws on a report from a U.S. Fulbright research scholar, David Ausubel, who was in New Zealand from 1957–1958:

> One of the most surprising but also one of the most prevalent attitudes toward Maoris *[sic]* that I encountered in New Zealand was a feeling of complete and utter indifference about the welfare of the Maori people. Many persons hardly seemed aware that Maori persons existed and apparently cared even less . . . They took Maoris for granted as part of the general environment in much the same manner as they did telephone poles except for some vague awareness that the former were somewhat more of a tourist attraction. (Ausubel, as cited in Ramsden, 2002, p. 15)

Ramsden (2002) documents the difficulty of teaching about cultural safety and the power dynamics inherent in every nursing encounter when the nursing education environment does not recognize the history of marginalized people and encourages assimilation and denial of difference. Students and faculty in all countries repeatedly state in one way or the other, "I respect everyone" or "I care for everyone equally!" or "There's no racism here!" The fact is that marginalized groups of people see a different reality than people from the dominant culture.

Countless volumes could be filled with the painful stories of what students and faculty of color have suffered in predominantly White schools of nursing in New Zealand, Canada, Australia, the United States, the United Kingdom, and in other parts of the world. Hassouneh (2006) points out:

> Over the years, I have observed that many white faculty are comfortably oblivious to the realities of racism. In addition, faculty responses to anti-racist pedagogy suggest that many would like to stay that way. Efforts to raise issues related to racism and Eurocentrism in faculty meetings and other forums are usually not well received, and faculty of color who raise these issues are often ignored, discounted, and/or pathologized. (p. 260)

In addressing the ethics of diversity, Sorrell (2003) stresses the importance of people from the dominant culture listening in the "thin place" or the place where the natural and sacred worlds merge and where seen and unseen realities share common ground. She cautions against "benumbment" (para. 7), which is the failure to slow down and create the open space for intimate listening to the suffering of others. Rather, Sorrell asserts, we must work to hear, understand, and honor the entirety of the experience of marginalized people. It is in this open listening that potential for transformation and action arise.

One would think that schools of nursing would be places where no one is *benumbed,* where all faculty and students would feel known and appreciated for who they are, and where antiracism pedagogy would be embraced at the center of the curriculum. Yet, this is not the norm, although it could be. Many White faculty and administrators continue to believe that racism is a thing of the past and not an issue of central concern to the work they do. To understand why this is so, we turn to the work of sociologists who have studied the stratification of "races" in society and the purpose this serves.

COLOR-BLIND RACISM

If "race" was created to advance the economic gain of a privileged few, in other words, people who colonized and exploited the land, resources, and human labor of Black and Brown people, how can racism still be present in countries that have enacted strong civil rights legislation? Rosenberg (2004) asserts that a new racial consciousness is arising—one that avoids direct discourse centered on race, while safeguarding racial privilege. Bonilla-Silva (2006) has termed this new brand of racism *color-blind racism,* which he points out "otherizes softly" and involves "smiling face discrimination" (p. 3). In other words, the Latina applicant for a nursing faculty position is not hired, but she is treated very nicely as she is turned away in favor of a White candidate who is less qualified for the job but "would need less mentoring." In this situation, the mentoring that is most needed is likely the mentoring of the faculty on the search committee and the dean who made the hiring decision; yet, this is rarely recognized. Bonilla-Silva states that "the beauty of this new ideology is that it aids in the maintenance of White privilege without fanfare, without naming those who it subjects and those who it rewards" (pp. 3–4).

Moreover, there is an increasing triracial order emerging, which Bonilla-Silva (2006) labels as the "Whites," "Honorary Whites," and "Collective Blacks," stratified by skin color, with "the maintenance of systemic White privilege accomplished socially, economically, and politically through institutional, covert, and apparently nonracial practices" (p. 183). A smoke screen is created when a few people of color are invited into the "White" power structure; yet, the structure never changes the reality and suffering of the people at the bottom. Bonilla-Silva refers to this as the "Latin Americanization" of racial order in the United States and states that "this ideology, which is the norm all over Latin America, denies the salience of race, scorns those who talk about race, and increasingly proclaims that 'We are all Americans' " (p. 184). We need only to look back at the historical roots of this system, starting with the arrival of Hernán Cortés on the shores of Mesoamerica, who with his soldiers for two decades committed acts of genocide, violation, and enslavement before Pope Paul III finally proclaimed in 1537 that the indigenous people of the Americas do indeed have souls. By this time, a system was well in place to ensure the flow of gold, silver, cacao, and other riches to Europe, mined and harvested by an enslaved Brown indigenous people whose land and culture had been devastated. The Pope's decree had little effect; the new economic system was well in place, and the concept of "race" was developed to justify it. Over the centuries, the myth of race has been promoted by scientists and become part of our collective culture and consciousness (Graves, 2002).

As race relations have become globalized, color-blind racism has become prevalent in most Western nations. Markers of this new racial order include the refusal to measure "race," particularly as it relates to assessing for equal outcomes, intense denial of the existence of racism, smiling-face discrimination that is disorienting and dispiriting to its victims, and stratification of jobs from menial to managerial by skin tone. The effects of this ideology, if it is not recognized, challenged, and changed, will include increasing economic and health disparities by "race." The nature of color-blind racism is that it negates reality in favor of myth. In order to see reality, we need to be able to measure it. Accurate data are essential.

Nurses are in a position to bring light to healthy racial-identity development and the creation of sound social policy; nurse educators can lead the way. We can begin by listening, researching, recognizing the problem, educating ourselves on possible solutions, developing the space and means of carrying out bold conversations, and committing to change the nursing education environment based on the data we collect. We can do so in a way that names the agent that needs to be changed. For example, there is a difference between saying, "Immigrant students are more likely to be steered toward technical nursing programs than equally qualified native-born peers" and "Academic counselors are more likely to steer immigrant students toward technical programs than native-born students, whom they tend to steer toward professional degrees." We need active sentences with subjects as agents in our data reports, so that we can focus our interventions. We also need sound data that have been analyzed for all possible correlates. We can determine where change is needed and measure our progress through designing research projects that assess equal outcomes for students and faculty by "race" and ethnicity, which is necessary to ensure structural change.

LESSONS FROM THE EDUCATIONAL TRENCHES

So, there I am, trying to do some background reading for this chapter, and I had forgotten about lunch. I go into the cafeteria, buy lunch, and sit at one of the back tables facing the windows so as not to be distracted. I am one paragraph into my reading when a woman comes and asks if she can join me. I'm thinking, "Can't she see that I'm busy?" as I clear a space and put my work away, thinking that maybe there is something else I am to learn today. She introduces herself as a new faculty member in another discipline, having just completed graduate school at a prestigious university out East. I ask her how teaching is going for her and note that I am taking extra interest in her well-being because she is Black and we're in a historically White institution. An African American colleague whom I love and respect dearly—one of the most brilliant people I know—joins us for lunch. I'm pleased to have the distraction and the camaraderie, which is much more interesting than the great book I was reading, and I am glad that these two good women are connecting. My colleague had just come from being a guest speaker at a global search for justice course and recounted, "I feel like I came in at minus 10 and had to work my way up to zero with these students, just because I am a Black woman. The way they looked at me was like, 'show me that you have something to say that I don't know!' It is just so exhausting!"

Nurse administrators, particularly at historically White colleges and universities in predominantly White countries, need to realize the added burden and stress placed on faculty of color and compensate and support them accordingly. They also need to have a critical lens through which to analyze student evaluations. After coteaching four courses with Black colleagues, I have come to realize the extent to which my excellent student evaluations reflect the wave of White privilege I have been riding. This has been a painful realization, but the data are there. Even though the White colleagues I have taught with are excellent, my Black colleagues invest more intellectual and emotional energy into the course; yet, when I coteach a course with a Black colleague, we come out with lower student evaluations. For one course, it was the very same students I taught the semester before and from whom I had received outstanding evaluations. Color-blind racism is tenaciously and pervasively present, and it carries an institutional, personal, and internalized edge. One of the most painful realizations is that the lower evaluations are not only from White students or from students who do not have the capacity to critically analyze the dynamics. They are also from students of color and students who demonstrate critical thinking in other areas. To help students critically think about the dynamics of racism in clinical practice and in nursing education, we have developed courses for graduate nurse education students and graduate nurse practitioner and nurse leader students at the College of St. Catherine. These courses deal specifically with the dynamics of color-blind racism so that students don't carry it with them into the clinical or classroom setting.

In an *Inclusivity in Nursing Practice* course developed by LaVonne Moore, RN, MA, CNP, MS, CNM, and me, nurse practitioner students work to bring color-blind racism to the surface and determine a plan to create an inclusive nursing practice and health care environment. As concrete evidence of the existence of racism in the health care environment, we present an overview of racial and ethnic health disparities that persist after all social, age, and economic indicators have been held constant. Social and economic indicators are analyzed as concrete exemplars of racism in society. Readings, exercises, and films are used to bring racism to the conscious surface so that students can analyze the power dynamics and determine how to dismantle racism in its many forms in their personal and professional lives.

A tool we have found helpful in bringing racism to students' conscious awareness is a racial moments journal exercise that was developed by Dr. Terri Karis (in press). We ask students to keep a journal as they go about their day-to-day activities. When "race" comes to their awareness, whether through an interaction, thought, or feeling, they are to observe it and document it as soon as they get a chance. We instruct them not to change it or judge it, but rather to simply record: (a) what is the situation? (b) who is involved? (c) what are the thoughts, feelings and/or words spoken? and (d) as a reflection afterward, how do you understand what happened? What were your thoughts and feelings that came after the initial thoughts or feelings? We collect the journals and provide feedback twice during the semester. The students also reflect on the most significant things they learned about race and about themselves through the racial moments journal exercise (Karis, in press). In addition, we use Blackboard, a Web-based tool for dialogue outside of the classroom, for the students to post their synthesis of the readings and class content and to dialogue with one another. Even the most entrenched *"racism doesn't exist anymore"* belief-holders usually move along to a deeper understanding by the end of the course.

Research on the racial moments journal has demonstrated that students are willing to pay attention to race-related thoughts, feelings, and behaviors—even when it gets uncomfortable; they begin to develop conscious awareness of what was a previously unconscious racialized worldview; begin to understand themselves better and are more able to take on the perspective of *the other;* develop an understanding of how pervasive the White norm is and how it shapes their worldview; and apply the new information they have gained to life encounters (Karis, in press). By the end of our courses, we have found White students able to more comfortably take on the role of an ally and all students articulating how they can take leadership in changing the system so that it is more inclusive. Dr. Beverly Tatum (1994) describes the role of the White ally as being willing to:

> speak up against systems of oppression, and challenge other Whites to do the same. Teaching about racism needs to shift from an exploration of victims and victimizers to that of empowered people of color and their White

> allies, creating the possibility for working together as partners in the establishment of a more just society. (p. 474)

In summary, synthesizing the wisdom from the nursing literature with educational experience has led to an understanding of inclusivity in nursing education as evidenced by: classrooms, clinical conferences, and faculty meetings where students, faculty, and administrators openly talk about, identify, and address how to deal with racial discrimination and power differentials; curricular materials and processes that tell the truthful story of the creation and perpetuation of the concept of race and how it affects people's health; instructional and assessment materials that do not favor a White norm; a clearly stated and well-known process for reporting and addressing racial discrimination; an approach to knowledge that critiques its sources and employs multiple learning strategies; a commitment to engaging multiple perspectives and positions in democratic discourse and relationships; equal participation of students and faculty across racial and ethnic categories; and proportional demographic representation of the community at all levels, from the board of trustees to the administration, faculty, support staff, students, and environmental and promotional images of the university or college.

TURNING THE LENS AROUND: SYSTEM CHANGE

This chapter has explored various ways in which racism is manifest in the nursing education environment. It is important to understand the different kinds of racism, to know and teach the history and experiences of marginalized populations in your country and community, to have courageous and honest conversations about racism and how to teach students to dismantle it, and to work against color-blind racism in all of its forms. We need to find bold new ways to welcome students and faculty to the center of the educational community, even if that means that some of us must step aside. Most importantly, we need to dismantle the White hierarchical structure and replace it with a much stronger and more vibrant circular and collective model. This process will lead us to core tenets of nursing practice—caring, health, justice, and equal treatment—so that we can embrace them with renewed integrity.

At the College of St. Catherine, we have numerous programs to support students of color—from high school step-ahead programs and scholarships where high school students of color are mentored and welcomed into the educational environment and develop lasting collegial friendships—to the Community Health Nursing Student Internship Program where nursing students of color work with strong nurse leaders who look like them in leadership development positions, while serving as a role-model to encourage youth in the community to enter nursing as a profession. We have created Spanish, Somali, and Hmong language videos about college life so that students' families can understand the support our students need to succeed in college. While these and other programs are immensely important, the most important thing we can do is to analyze the college structure for institutionalized racism and work to change it—to talk about and change those spaces that continue to be White spaces, where White privilege thrives as if it were the natural order of things. Just as Juana Bordas (2007) promises, when we take Whiteness out of the center, we all excel to a greater degree, we all become more vibrant and healthy, and we all can reach a horizon of the human spirit not previously imagined. Our students deserve no less.

RECOMMENDATIONS FOR NURSE EDUCATORS

1. Listen across racial lines. Listen intently. Listen with your eyes, ears, mind, heart, and soul. Analyze the data that document disparities. Develop healthy, mutual relationships. If you are uncomfortable with or find yourself stereotyping a certain group of people, develop a meaningful relationship with people from that group. Think about who is around your dining room table during celebrations. Do they look like your colleagues, your students, and the community you serve? If not, reflect on why not, and think about how you can widen your circle.
2. Develop a process to review your curricula for cultural inclusion. You may want to analyze use of the Fair Representation of Diversity Content (FRDC) tool (Scisney-Matlock, McCloud, & Barnard, 2001) and the Byrne Guide (Byrne, Weddle, Davis, & McGinnis, 2003) as you design the process you will use.
3. Take part in antiracism education seminars and sessions.
4. Learn the history and listen to the experiences of students in your school of nursing.
5. Organize small study circles to meet and talk about how to dismantle racism in your educational environment.

6. Dialogue with colleagues about how you as a faculty talk about "race" and racism. What are you modeling for your students?
7. Discuss how you help students move through racialized encounters in the health care clinical setting and in the educational environment.
8. When students make stereotypical or discriminatory comments in class or clinical settings, do not be silent. Address the importance of not making generalizations or hurtful comments. If identifying and addressing the dynamics of racism are taught on day one as essential nursing knowledge, it will be natural for you and the students to embrace these as teachable moments. A democratic classroom can not exist without this practice.

RECOMMENDATIONS FOR NURSING EDUCATION ADMINISTRATORS

1. Routinely measure rates of student retention and graduation and employment, promotion, and tenure of faculty at your institution by "race" and ethnicity. Compare the demographic makeup of the community your school serves with the demographics of your student body, faculty, and administration. Dialogue and analysis for change are needed if your faculty and students do not represent the community you serve, if there are disparate rates of retention and graduation for students, or if there are disparate rates of employment, promotion, and tenure of faculty.
2. Assess whether faculty of color at your institution are being asked to speak at college events, serve on committees, and attend to students of color to a greater extent than White faculty and ensure that there is just compensation for this work. When faculty of color in predominantly White institutions are asked to take visible positions, this may be indicative of an administration that is more interested in aesthetic diversity than full diversity, and it leaves faculty members feeling valued mostly for the color of their skin, which means only a part of them is being accepted.
3. Assess how you can adequately support faculty to address students' needs to learn about racism and to work through racialized issues that arise in clinical and educational settings.
4. If you are White, consider how you are supporting faculty of color in your institution. Do you know the stresses they are

experiencing and the demands on their time? What are the power differentials that prevent them from coming to you? How are you removing those barriers? If you are a person of color, are you feeling additional pressure to succeed, and do you feel as though you cannot adequately support your faculty of color because of it? If so, how can you care for and advocate for yourself and your faculty? Where do you get your support?

QUESTIONS FOR DIALOGUE

1. What ideas or concepts did you find most meaningful in this chapter? Identify your insights and questions to bring to a dialogue with your colleagues.
2. List all the nursing leaders you know from nursing textbooks. What percent are White? Review your textbooks and other teaching materials for full inclusion. What messages might unconsciously be planted in students' minds? Dialogue with colleagues about how you could review your curricula for inclusivity. You may want to start by identifying evidence of inclusivity as listed at the end of the "Lessons from the Educational Trenches" section of this chapter.
3. The term *race* continues to be used despite the widespread acceptance that it is a biologically meaningless term. Why do you think this is the case? Provide examples from the nursing literature and your observations on how *race* is used or misused.
4. Dialogue with colleagues about how you might better introduce dismantling racism as a nursing health intervention. How do you teach students to identify racism and to deal with it when they experience it? Hold a dialogue for administration and faculty to identify what support is needed to better do this work and what policies and curricular changes you want to put in place.
5. How is color-blind racism manifested at your institution? Describe specific examples and dialogue with colleagues about what structural changes need to be made within your program.
6. At your institution, what hard data do you or could you collect to measure the need for structural change, such as: (a) equal recruitment, retention, and graduation of students; (b) differential treatment and experiences for faculty of color; and (c) other aspects of institutionalized racism? Be careful of excuses

and/or rationalizations that faculty and administrators often raise to minimize the experience of minorities and to avoid the need to address structural change—collect hard data to direct your structural change.

REFERENCES

Adelman, L. (Executive Producer). (2003). *Race: The power of an illusion, Episode I: The difference between us, Episode II: The story we tell, & Episode III: The house we live in* [Motion picture]. San Francisco: California Newsreel.

Aldossary, A., While, A., & Barnball, L. (2008). Health care and nursing in Saudi Arabia. *International Nursing Review, 55*, 125–128.

Allen, D. (2006). Whiteness and difference in nursing. *Nursing Philosophy, 7*(2), 65–78.

Alleyne, J., Papadopoulos, I., & Tilki, M. (1994). Antiracism within transcultural nurse education. *British Journal of Nursing, 3*(12), 635–637.

Amaikwu-Rushing, L., Fitzgerald, D., Wilson, C., Smith, K., Irwin, D., & Pharris, M. D. (2005, Feb.). Health, well being and racism. *Minnesota Medicine*, 28–31, 41.

Anionwu, E. (2006). Voices. *Nursing Standard, 20*(38), 31.

Bonilla-Silva, E. (2006). *Racism without racists* (2nd ed.). Lanham, MD: Rowman & Littlefield.

Bordas, J. (2007). *Salsa, soul, and spirit: Leadership for a multicultural age.* San Francisco: Berrett-Koehler.

Byrne, M. M., Weddle, C., Davis, E., & McGinnis, P. (2003). The Byrne guide for inclusionary cultural content. *Journal of Nursing Education, 42*(6), 277–281.

Campinha-Bacote, J. (2003). Many faces: Addressing diversity in health care. *Online Journal of Issues in Nursing, 8*(1), manuscript 2. Retrieved May 16, 2008, from http://www.nursingworld.org/ojin/topic20/tpc20_2.htm

Carnegie, M. E. (1991). *The path we tread: Blacks in nursing 1854–1990* (2nd ed.). New York: National League for Nursing Press.

Carnegie, M. E. (2000). *The path we tread: Blacks in nursing worldwide 1854–1994* (3rd ed.). Sudbury, MA: Jones and Bartlett.

Cohen, B. (1999). The 100 most influential Montanans of the century: Susan Walking Bear Yellowtail. "The Missoulian," Missoula, MT. Retrieved May 16, 2008, from http://www.missoulian.com/specials/100montanans/list/062.html

Davis, A. (1999). *Early Black American leaders in nursing: Architects for integration and equality.* Sudbury, MA: Jones and Bartlett.

Ellis, C., & Pharris, M. D. (2007). *Racism and how it affects our health: A curriculum guide for people who care about African American adolescents and their health.* St. Paul, MN: College of St. Catherine.

Giddings, L. (2005). Health disparities, social injustice, and the culture of nursing. *Nursing Research, 54*(5), 304–312.

Giger, J. N., & Davidhizar, R. E. (2004). *Transcultural nursing: Assessment and intervention* (4th ed.). St Louis: Mosby.

Graves, J. (2002). *The emperor's new clothes: Biological theories of race at the millennium.* New Brunswick, NJ: Rutgers University Press.

Gustafson, D. L. (2007). White on whiteness: Becoming radicalized about race. *Nursing Inquiry, 14*(2), 152–161.

Hassouneh, D. (2006). Anti-racist pedagogy: Challenges faced by faculty of color in predominantly white schools of nursing. *Journal of Nursing Education, 45*(7), 255–262.

Hine, D. C. (1989). *Black women in white.* Bloomington, IN: Indiana University Press.

Institute of Medicine (IOM), Committee on Understanding and Eliminating Racial and Ethnic Disparities in Health. (2002). *Unequal treatment: Confronting racial and ethnic disparities in health care.* Washington, DC: The National Academies Press.

Jones, C. P. (2000). Levels of racism: A theoretical framework and a gardener's tale. *American Journal of Public Health, 90*(8), 1212–1215.

Karis, T. A. (in press). The psychology of whiteness: Moving beyond separation to connection. In R. Osborne & P. Kriese (Eds.), *Global community: Global security.* Kenilworth, NJ: Rodopi.

Krieger, N. (1990). Racial and gender discrimination: Risk factors for high blood pressure. *Social Science and Medicine, 30*(12), 1273–1281.

Krieger, N. (2003). Does racism harm health? Did child abuse exist before 1962? On explicit questions, critical science, and current controversies: An ecosocial perspective. *American Journal of Public Health, 93*(2), 194–199.

Leininger, M. M. (2001). *Culture care diversity and universality: A theory of nursing.* Sudbury, MA: Jones and Bartlett.

Markey, K., & Tilki, M. (2007). Racism in nursing education: A reflective journey. *British Journal of Nursing, 16*(7), 390–393.

McIntosh, P. (1990). White privilege: Unpacking the invisible knapsack. *Independent School, 49*(2), 31–36.

Nairn, S., Hardy, C., Parumal, L., & Williams, G. A. (2004). Multicultural or anti-racist teaching in nurse education: A critical appraisal. *Nursing Education Today, 24,* 188–195.

O'Lynn, C. E. (2007). History of men in nursing: A review. In C. E. O'Lynn & R. E. Tranbarger (Eds.), *Men in nursing: History, challenges, and opportunities.* New York: Springer Publishing.

Purnell, L. D., & Paulanka, B. J. (2003). *Transcultural health care: A culturally competent approach* (2nd ed.). Philadelphia: F.A. Davis.

Ramsden, I. (2000). Defining cultural safety and transcultural nursing. *Kai Tiaki Nursing New Zealand, 6*(8), 4–5.

Ramsden, I. M. (2002). *Cultural safety and nursing education in Aotearoa and Te Walpounamu.* Unpublished doctoral dissertation. Wellington: Victoria University.

Robinson, J. (2004). *Mary Seacole: The most famous Black woman of the Victorian Age.* New York: Carroll & Graf.

Rosenberg, P. M. (2004). Color blindness in teacher education: An optical delusion. In M. Fine, L. Weis, L. Powell Pruitt, & A. Burns (Eds.), *Off white: Readings on power, privilege, and resistence* (2nd ed., pp. 257–272). New York: Routledge.

Scisney-Matlock, M., McCloud, P. K., & Barnard, R. M. (2001). Systematic assessment and evaluation of diversity content presented in classroom lectures: The FRDC tool. *Journal of Cultural Diversity, 8*(3), 85–93.

Seacole, M., & Salih, S. (Ed.). (1857/2005). *Wonderful adventures of Mrs. Seacole.* London: Penguin.

Sorrell, J. (2003). The ethics of diversity: A call for intimate listening in thin places. *Online Journal of Issues in Nursing.* Retrieved February 2, 2004, from http://www.nursingworld.org/ojin/ethicol/ethics_13.htm

Staupers, M. K. (1961). *No time for prejudice.* New York: Macmillan.

Tatum, B. D. (1994). Teaching White students about racism: The search for White allies and the restoration of hope. *Teachers College Record, 95,* 462–476.

Tatum, B. D. (1997). *Why are all the Black kids sitting together in the cafeteria? And other conversations about race.* New York: Basic Books.

van Ryn, M., & Burk, J. (2000). The effect of patient race and socioeconomic status on physicians' perceptions of patients. *Social Science and Medicine, 50*(6), 813–828.

van Ryn, M., & Fu, S. S. (2003). Paved with good intentions: Do public health and human service providers contribute to racial/ethnic disparities in health. *American Journal of Public Health, 93*(2), 248–255.

Vaughan, J. (1997). Is there really racism in nursing? *Journal of Nursing Education, 36*(3), 135–139.

Washington, H. A. (2006). *Medical apartheid.* New York: Harlem Moon Broadway.

W. E. B. Dubois Learning Center. (n.d.). *Sankofa.* Retrieved February 14, 2008, from http://www.duboislc.net/Sankofa/meaning.html

Williams, D. R., Neighbors, H. W., & Jackson, J. S. (2003). Racial/ethnic discrimination and health: Findings from community studies. *American Journal of Public Health, 93*(2), 200–208.

2

The Power of Nurse Educators: Welcoming and Unwelcoming Behaviors

SUSAN P. KOSSMAN

Our view of the world is filtered through a lens that is so much a part of who we are that we do not realize it is there. This lens reflects our deeply ingrained beliefs, shaped by socialization into our culture, as well as our personality and experience. Because this lens is invisible to us, we tend to assume others view the world in the same way. In reality, though, the lens through which we look affects our perception and interpretation of events; the same set of events appears different to a person looking through a different lens. I became aware of this phenomenon only a few years ago. I had been a nurse educator for 10 years at 2 colleges in Texas and Illinois. I noticed that many students who were older, male, or of a minority race had more academic difficulty in terms of lower nursing GPAs, more course failures, and higher program attrition. In both colleges, students entered the nursing program as Juniors with 60 hours of lower division work completed, largely in the sciences. These students had been successful in their first 2 years of college, but in the nursing program, they struggled and sometimes failed. It was painful to watch hopes and dreams die as students left the program. I wondered why these students had more difficulty in the nursing program than the

This study was partially supported by grants from Mennonite College of Nursing, Illinois State University, and the Xi Pi Chapter of Sigma Theta Tau International.

typical young, White, female nursing students; yet, I did nothing to find an answer.

Then one semester two things happened to make me aware of the lens through which I viewed the world and the limitations it imposed. The first one involved an older African American woman I'll call "Ada" who was in her first semester of our upper-division nursing program. She was a busy mother of several school-aged children as well as a full-time student who took on a leadership role at the college. Our program had a strict policy regarding exams: To receive an excused absence allowing the student to take the exam later, the student had to contact the course teacher before the exam began and schedule the retake within 48 hours. Ada missed an exam in the course I taught and left a message notifying me she was ill. During the next 2 days, I kept expecting her to call to schedule the retake; I grew more angry and frustrated as time passed. Finally she called, saying quietly, "You didn't call me back. I let you know I was sick. Why didn't you call back and let me know when to take the exam? I've been ready." The hurt in her voice surprised me; clearly, she felt I had let her down. I, on the other hand, felt she had let me down. In my view, a student should be assertive and take the initiative in contacting the instructor. After talking with her, I realized that, in her view, the student defers to the teacher. She viewed contacting me again as rude and instead patiently waited for me to contact her. This incident caused my perspective to shift a little; I realized there might be other ways of perceiving the same circumstances.

This shift in perspective widened later that semester during an elective course I took as a graduate student on social foundations of education. In the course, we addressed implications of the "Brown vs. Board of Education of Topeka" decision on African American students. My initial view that mandated integration was an unequivocally positive event because all students now had access to a better education system was tempered through an awareness of significant losses these students faced: a caring school environment, African American teachers and administrators, and a community-based center of activity. During this course, I became aware of the concept of structural racism and White privilege—hidden forms of prejudice built into social systems that privilege one group at the expense of another without any direct prejudicial action by an individual. I realized that I, as a White woman, had benefited from this invisible privilege all my life, though I had assumed that all my achievements were due solely to my own hard work. The lens through which I viewed the world shifted considerably as I became aware of hidden rules, expectations, and benefits that were afforded members of the dominant culture. I wondered if there was a dominant culture in nursing education and if some of the difficulty experienced by nursing students who were "other than" young, White, and female was due to being unaware of this culture's hidden rules and expectations. This led to my doctoral dissertation and the findings presented in this chapter.

The nursing profession faces two key problems: a shortage of nurses projected to become huge within a few years (Hecker, 2001) and a failure to reflect the diversity of the U.S. population, either in gender or race. One way to address both problems is to recruit and graduate more students who have been underrepresented in nursing: minority, male, and older students. An additional benefit to increasing these student groups would be to broaden the nursing profession's demographics, decreasing the overwhelming predominance of White women in this field (Barbee & Gibson, 2001; Spratley, Johnson, Sochalski, Fritz, & Spencer, 2000). Nurses are in a unique position to positively effect health care practices; yet, if they do not more closely resemble the U.S. population, they are at risk of being marginalized and ignored by the people they are trying to serve. Cultural sensitivity and awareness of diverse clients' worldviews are essential to appropriate holistic nursing care that affirms the worth and dignity of all clients. Increasing numbers of minority nurses can help address this concern.

Minority recruitment and retention efforts over the last 20 years have resulted in minimal change. In 2000, 4.9% of U.S. registered nurses were African American, 3.5% Asian American, 2% Hispanic, and less than 1% Native American (Spratley et al., 2000). Nursing students continue to be predominantly traditional age (18–23) White females, though racial and ethnic minority students in baccalaureate nursing programs are increasing and represented 24.1% of students nationally in 2005 (American Association of Colleges of Nursing [AACN], 2006). However, minority nursing students experience more academic difficulty and higher attrition rates than Whites (Miller, 1995), and traditional explanations such as poor academic preparation or lack of financial support do not adequately explain these differences. It may be more helpful to look at the problem from a different perspective—that of cultural fit. Does the culture of nursing education somehow favor traditional age White women?

The climate and culture of a school or institution of higher education affects how well students do academically. Nursing education culture may well reflect the values and norms of the largely White, female faculty pool. Lack of familiarity with this culture and its rules can lead to decreased academic success. An understanding of how welcoming or supportive nursing education's culture is perceived to be by nursing faculty and minority students will help nurse educators better understand the problems and barriers faced by these students and will hopefully lead to minimization of these barriers. Fewer barriers to minority students' success in nursing education could lead to increased diversity in nursing practitioners and educators, increased numbers of role models for underrepresented students, and improved health care delivery to ethnic/racial minority groups. This chapter reports findings and implications from a study of African American and White nursing students' and faculty members' perceptions of nursing education culture and its impact on minority student success. The findings give insight into the nursing education experience and suggest actions nurse educators can take to increase minority students' success.

MINORITY STUDENT PERSISTENCE IN NURSING PROGRAMS

The literature on culture and student persistence in higher education helps us understand the phenomenon of minority student persistence in nursing education. A brief review of relevant literature on student persistence in higher education, minority student persistence, cultural influences on minority students, and minority student persistence in nursing education follows.

Student Persistence in Higher Education

Student persistence in higher education has been extensively studied, especially persistence between the first and second years of college. Several student persistence theories or models have been proposed and tested (Astin, 1984; Cabrera, Nora, & Castaneda, 1993; Tinto, 1993). Although they vary in their emphasis, a common point is the idea of the higher education institution as a community (or collection of communities) into which the student attempts to fit. Persistence is strongly affected by the congruence of fit between student and institution in terms of underlying goals, values, and beliefs as well as the student's integration and participation in campus life (Astin, 1984; Cabrera et al., 1993; Tinto, 1993). Student attributes such as academic preparation, socioeconomic class, race, nationality, gender, age, and degree of financial and emotional support have been found to affect persistence (Astin, 1984; Tinto, 1993). Additionally, institutional variables such as urban or rural location, number of minority students and faculty, presence of academic and social support systems, and racial climate affect minority student persistence (Astin, 1984; Bourassa, 1991; Cabrera, Nora, Terenzini, Pascarella, & Hagedorn, 1999; Hurtado, 1994; McNairy, 1996; Tinto, 1993).

Numerous authors have explored minority students' difficulties at largely White higher education institutions. Miller (1995) notes that minority students face pressures from an unsupportive climate. He notes "the social context and attendant interpersonal relationships experienced in college tend to shape . . . academic performance . . . and blacks are much more likely to experience a favorable social context at a historically black college" (p. 365). Bourassa (1991) notes that students of color on White college campuses have greater social alienation and a higher dropout rate than White students. They experience anger, alienation, frustration, mistrust, and pressure to assimilate (especially when their numbers are small). McNairy (1996) and Kirkland (1998) comment on the culture shock minority students feel in largely White colleges, leading to feelings of inadequacy, emotional loss, and a self-protective denial that makes it difficult for them to seek academic or counseling help.

From the student perspective, persistence decisions are influenced by answers to the questions "Do I fit in here?" and "Do I belong here?" In a broad sense, these questions reflect issues of culture and climate. Their answers are influenced by the intersection of the students' culture with its underlying values, beliefs, and norms and the higher educational institution's as well as the specific discipline's culture. Additionally, they reflect the effect of the institution's climate on the student. Interactions with faculty and fellow students contribute to perceptions of the institution's climate and are important elements in students' persistence decisions (Astin, 1993; Campbell & Davis, 1996; Hurtado, 1994; Kirkland, 1998; Tinto, 1993). Studies have found that campus climates with racial discrimination negatively impact minority students' academic and social experiences and ultimately their persistence and success in college (Cabrera et al., 1999; Eimers & Pike, 1997; Nora & Cabrera, 1996).

Cultural Influences on Student Persistence in Higher Education

The culture and climate of a school or institution of higher education affect how well students do academically. Culture refers to shared, deeply held, and enduring values, beliefs, and ideologies that emphasize an organization's or group's uniqueness (Peterson & Spencer, 1990). Academic climate relates to common perceptions and attitudes that are more current and malleable than culture. It is the atmosphere or style of the institution and is linked to larger social phenomena such as political and sociological trends (Hurtado, Milem, Clayton-Pederson, & Allen, 1998; Peterson & Spencer, 1990). Nursing education culture is nested within the broader higher education and U.S. cultures and reflects values, beliefs, norms, and expectations from both of these cultures.

A group's culture is generally invisible to its members. Culture becomes most visible at the margins or boundaries, where interactions with other cultures occur and differences are noted (Ogbu & Simons, 1998; Tierney, 1991). In the United States, these interactions are typically between the dominant culture (which is largely a product of White, Protestant, European Americans) and minority group cultures. In U.S. nursing education, these interactions largely exist among nursing faculty (members of the nursing culture who are almost exclusively members of the dominant U.S. culture) and students (from various U.S. cultural groups who are learning nursing culture and becoming part of it).

Faculty–student interactions are important factors in college students' development and persistence. Additionally, in professional education programs, these interactions affect students' professional socialization, an acculturation process that requires identification with and internalization of the profession's values and norms, as well as acquisition of requisite knowledge and skills (DuToit, 1995). The extent to which students are successfully socialized may impact their persistence in professional programs (DuToit, 1995; Johnson, 1996). Faculty mentoring serves an especially important role in professional education where "it is recognized that part of what is learned . . . is socialization to the values, practices and attitudes of a discipline" (Johnson, 1996, p. 63).

Nursing faculty are overwhelmingly female members of the dominant White culture (Vaughan, 1997); they view the world through this lens coupled with the nursing culture lens. As members of the dominant White culture, they can be expected to agree with its major values, including individualism, democracy, and meritocracy. In nursing education, these values manifest as beliefs in autonomy, integrity, social justice (AACN, 1997), and equal opportunity for all students to succeed through individual effort. The idea of racial discrimination "is absolutely opposed to the image nurses have of themselves as caring professionals" (Jackson, 1993, p. 373); yet, racism is present in nursing as it is throughout society (Morris & Wykie, 1994; Vaughan, 1997). Tatum (1997) defines racism as a racially based system of advantage "involving cultural messages and institutional policies and practices as well as the beliefs and actions of individuals." It is a system of "prejudice plus power" (p. 7) that advantages Whites at the expense of people of color.

McIntosh (1995) notes that racism has "active forms that we can see and embedded forms that members of the dominant group are taught not to see . . . in invisible systems conferring racial dominance on (the white) group from birth" (p. 194). White privilege or "Whiteness" is a result of racism that is invisible to most Whites; its elements include unrecognized White privilege, belief in a meritocracy system—that everyone has the same chances in life—and lack of awareness of structural aspects of racism (McIntosh, 1995; McIntyre, 1997). Barbee (1993) and Jackson (1993) discuss covert forms of racism in nursing, including denial (avoiding discussions of racism through incorporation of race into "cultural diversity"), a color-blind perspective (ignoring racial/cultural differences), aversive racism (ambivalence between egalitarian beliefs and unacknowledged negative feelings about minorities), and a "blaming the victim" mindset. This covert, subtle racism may occur in nurse–client, nurse–nurse, or faculty–student interactions (Barbee, 1993) and leads to less understanding, acceptance, and support of minority nurses, clients, or students.

Minority Nursing Students

Studies of minority nursing students have findings that parallel more general studies of minority students in higher education. Various studies have identified personal and institutional issues affecting minority nursing students' success, categories consistent with the higher education student persistence literature. Personal issues include financial concerns, academic preparation for higher education, and support by family and friends. Financial concerns were identified by many researchers (Campbell & Davis, 1996; Jeffreys, 1998; Kirkland, 1998; Langston-Moss, 1997; Snyder & Bunkers, 1994; Villarruel, Canales, & Torres, 2001) as an influencing factor in choice of nursing program and/or a source of stress while enrolled. Issues related to academic performance concerned the difficulty of nursing programs (Kirkland, 1998; Snyder & Bunkers, 1994) and a need to change study habits (Langston-Moss, 1997), rather than poor academic preparation. Support from family and friends was widely identified as influencing minority nursing persistence, contributing to students' stress when it was absent and to their success when it was present (Jeffreys, 1998; Kirkland, 1998; Snyder & Bunkers, 1994; Villarruel et al., 2001).

Institutional influences include issues related to academic and social integration into the nursing program. Faculty–student interactions were identified by many as having an important influence on minority students, either as a source of support or of stress (Kirkland, 1998; Snyder & Bunkers, 1994; Villarruel et al., 2001; Watkins, 1997). Student interactions were also noted to be very influential in minority student success, with multiple authors noting a sense of marginalization or what Aiken (2001) called "the experience of being the Other" (p. 308) for African American students (Afrinson, 1999; Jordan, 1996; Kirkland, 1998) and for Hispanic students (Villarruel et al., 2001) in predominantly White nursing programs.

Only a few studies have looked at minority student persistence from a cultural perspective. Several studies identified the negative impact of a racially prejudiced academic climate on minority nursing students (among other barriers to success), noting descriptions of overt and covert racism from faculty and other nursing students in predominantly White programs (Afrinson, 1999; Aiken, 2001; Langston-Moss, 1997; Snyder & Bunkers, 1994; Villarruel et al., 2001). Snyder and Bunkers and Villarruel et al. found that Black and Hispanic students felt their culture's definitions of women's roles limited pursuit of nursing education, while Aiken found a cultural perception of nursing education as a means of increasing social mobility in the Black nursing students she interviewed. Yoder (1996) found that faculty varied widely in their cultural awareness and responsiveness to students from different ethnic cultures. Jordan (1996), in a phenomenological study of Black nursing students in a predominantly White program, noted students' perception of residing in a culture different from their own, but it was unclear if this difference was due to cultural conflicts with nursing education culture or to being a minority in a predominantly White educational setting.

The research literature tells us that minority student persistence in college and nursing programs is a complex, multifaceted issue influenced by academic culture and climate, faculty and student interactions, academic performance, support, and discrimination. Though several studies have looked at persistence from a cultural perspective, none have focused on nursing education culture and climate through the eyes of White and minority students and faculty. All students entering nursing programs encounter another culture and climate embedded within the larger university culture, setting up a possibility for cultural clashes. Little is known about minority students' perceptions of nursing education culture, its congruence with their ethnic culture, and the influence of cultural differences on students' experiences in nursing education. Additionally, though faculty interactions have been identified as an influence on persistence, research is lacking on how cultural differences influence these interactions and identification of specific faculty actions that facilitate or create barriers to success for minority students.

THE RESEARCH STUDY

The concept map and descriptions of the nursing student experience presented in this chapter are the results of a study designed to investigate minority persistence in nursing education from a cultural perspective by looking at the impact of higher education and nursing education culture and the role of nursing faculty on minority student success. Research questions addressed were: (a) What are student and faculty perceptions of how welcoming nursing education is to students, and are there differences in welcoming behaviors toward minority vs. majority race students? (b) What are barriers and facilitators to success for minority students, and which faculty practices inhibit or enhance success? and (c) What are minority students' perceptions of their fit with the nursing program in terms of underlying goals, values, and beliefs?

The study design used descriptive qualitative methodology with individual and focus group interviews. Four semistructured individual interviews, with two minority students and two White faculty members, were conducted to explore dimensions of the phenomena of interest (nursing education culture and its effect on minority students) and to determine the usefulness of the interview questions (see Appendix). Nine focus group interviews with nursing faculty and African American students followed to more fully elaborate the phenomena. A convenience sample of students and faculty were recruited from two predominantly White, public Midwestern universities and at regional and national conferences. Because the subject matter could be considered sensitive and perceptions could differ along race and role (student or faculty) dimensions, White and African American students were interviewed in monoracial focus groups; faculty were interviewed in mixed racial groups due to a lack of diversity. To protect confidentiality, aliases are used here in the reporting of data.

The sample consisted of 43 research participants: 29 students and 14 faculty. Student research participants were limited to prelicensure female senior nursing students to ensure adequate exposure to nursing education culture and climate and eliminated variability due to gender. White student participants (N = 8) were limited to 19- to 24-year-old women attending two predominantly White institutions to represent the typical nursing student in the United States. Minority students were African American women (N = 20) from four predominantly White and one predominantly Black institution. One Asian American student participated; the researcher was unable to solicit volunteer students from other minority groups. Of the 14 faculty participants, 11 were White, 2 were African American, and 1 was Indian. Demographic data are summarized in Table 2.1.

Interviews were audio taped and transcribed, and data analysis was concurrent with data collection. Interview data were coded using open

Table 2.1

STUDY PARTICIPANT DEMOGRAPHIC DATA

RACE	WHITE	BLACK	OTHER
Students (N = 29)	8	20	1
Age (yrs) Range	21–24	17–38	22
Mean	22	24	
GPA Range	2.9–3.75	2.5–3.7	missing
Mean	3.3	3.0	
Nurse Educators (N = 14)	11	2	1
Age (yrs) Range	40–59	52–62	58
Mean	50	57	
Years in Nursing Education			
Range	4–33	33–38	
Mean	17.6	35.5	30

coding techniques and N-Vivo software. Emerging codes and concepts influenced questions in later interviews, as clarification, validation, or refutation was sought. A data matrix was developed following guidelines from Miles and Huberman (1994) to allow analysis of the interview data along cultural (role and race) and geographic (location and minority presence) dimensions to identify similarities and differences in respondents' opinions.

RESULTS: THE NURSING EDUCATION EXPERIENCE

Analysis of concepts and themes identified in participants' comments led to formulation of a concept map, or holistic view of nursing education, described by students and faculty (Figure 2.1). An overview of the concept map is presented, followed by several findings about the nursing education experience.

Concept Map

The study participants described nursing education as a developmental process occurring within the context of a specific nursing education program. Faculty, administration, and students are key components of the program; they create the climate as well as embody nursing culture. Each of these three groups also contributes to a student feeling welcomed or not in nursing education. Nursing education culture is influenced by U.S. higher education and health care cultures. Participants described it as consisting of a set of values articulated by nurses and norms (typical behaviors), which are not always congruent with these values. Students learn nursing education values and norms from faculty, administrators, and more senior students. This learning is often accomplished through observation, as well as through explicit teaching in course content or program rules. Nursing education climate is influenced by the policies of a specific nursing education program as well as the personalities and attitudes of faculty, students, and staff in the program and college or university. The local community and current national concerns also influence climate.

All students' experience in nursing education occurs in two phases—*Belonging* and *Becoming a Nurse.* These phases are nonsequential; a student may not feel a sense of *Belonging* yet feel she or he is successfully *Becoming a Nurse. Belonging* relates to students' perception of their fit with nursing education culture and climate. It reflects how well

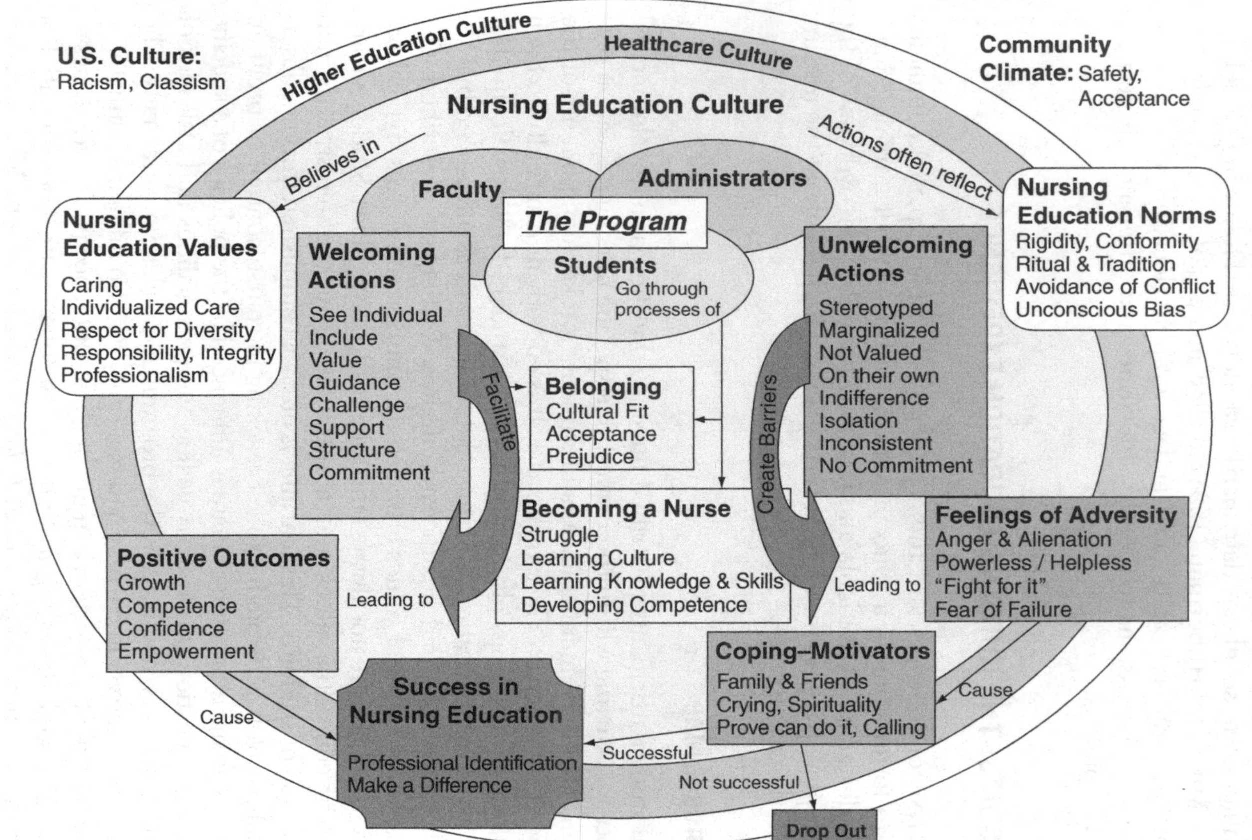

Figure 2.1 Welcoming and unwelcoming actions in nursing education culture.
© Susan Kossman, RN, PhD

the students feel their values, beliefs, and goals match those of nursing education and how comfortable students feel in the nursing education program, college/university, and community. Students' preconceived notions of nursing are generally limited to the concept of caring for others. The rest of nursing and nursing education's values and norms are learned as students progress in their programs. All students deal with cultural fit; however, minority students face additional issues related to this theme—nonacceptance, prejudice, and lack of racial understanding. Even if the cultural fit is good, students' sense of *Belonging* can be diminished in the presence of nonacceptance, prejudice, or poor racial understanding.

The theme *Becoming a Nurse* includes issues of struggle and stress in the nursing education program as well as learning and developing competence in the values, norms, knowledge, and skills of professional nursing. Students in general found nursing school to be very difficult academically, and many faced financial burdens causing additional stress. Social stresses, such as loneliness and lack of support, contribute to a sense of struggle as well. *Becoming a Nurse* also includes the developmental issue of professional socialization—learning the values, norms, knowledge, and skills inherent in nursing practice. Nursing requires learning a large volume of discipline-specific knowledge and skills, as well as developing higher-order critical thinking skills used less frequently in lower-division courses.

The nursing program engages in actions that affect student experiences. A welcoming or unwelcoming culture and climate are created by actions and interactions of students, faculty, and administrators within the program. If students feel welcomed in nursing education, the processes of *Belonging* and *Becoming a Nurse* are facilitated. Welcoming actions that support *Belonging* result in students feeling they are seen as individuals, included, and valued. Welcoming actions that support *Becoming a Nurse* are described as guiding, challenging, supporting, and demonstrating commitment to students. Additionally, clearly articulated program structure and rules support this process. A sense of feeling welcomed facilitates students' success in nursing education. It leads to positive outcomes such as growth, competence, confidence, and empowerment. These outcomes in turn lead to success in nursing education, exemplified by professional identification and a feeling students can make a contribution to nursing.

By contrast, students who do not feel welcomed in the program face additional barriers they must overcome in their processes of *Belonging* and *Becoming a Nurse.* Unwelcoming actions by any of the constituent groups (other students, faculty, or administrators) can lead to a sense of not feeling welcomed. Unwelcoming actions that create barriers to *Belonging* result in feelings of being stereotyped, marginalized, and not valued. Unwelcoming actions that create barriers to *Becoming a Nurse* are described as leaving students "on their own"; being indifferent, nonsupportive, and/or inconsistent; and lacking commitment to the students. These barriers cause feelings of adversity in students, such as anger, alienation, powerlessness/helplessness, feeling they have to "fight for it," and fear of failure. To overcome these feelings, students use coping strategies and motivators. Successful coping allows the student to succeed in nursing education while unsuccessful coping may lead to dropping out.

Both local climate issues and broader nursing culture issues affect welcoming and unwelcoming actions within the program. Local climate issues include attitudes of the people in the program regarding students, race, and rules of behavior. These vary among programs and within the same program over time. At a more entrenched, cultural level, nursing education's espoused values often conflict with the visible norms or typical behaviors of practitioners, creating a cultural conflict. For example, nursing education has a value of respecting diversity but norms of conformity and unconscious bias as well. Students may find nursing education's values to be congruent with their own but the norms and expectations to be less congruent. This conflict between stated values and typical behaviors that are incongruent with the values can have a negative impact on students' feelings of being welcomed, belonging, and becoming a nurse.

Study Findings

Several findings emerged from the data that have implications for nurse educators. In general, the study found that all students go through the same nonsequential processes of *Belonging* and *Becoming a Nurse* and that program actions (by faculty, students, administrators), as well as nursing culture (values and norms) and academic and community climates, affect both processes. More specific study findings are: (a) all students struggle with nursing education; (b) African American students have more difficulty due to pervasive prejudice and lack of acceptance; (c) welcoming actions help all students progress through the stages while unwelcoming actions create additional barriers that all students must overcome to succeed; (d) there is a conflict between nursing values and norms or typical behaviors, and when this is severe, all students suffer;

and (e) all students identify strongly with nursing values, which helps them overcome barriers to success. In the next section, these five findings are discussed more fully with illustrative quotes.

Finding 1: It's a Struggle

Nursing education is hard for all students. There were no racial, geographical, or role differences of opinion about this issue; everyone agreed. Nursing students struggle with difficult academic loads, have financial concerns, and find that friends and family do not understand the stress they face and thus are less supportive. Comments from two students, one Black and one White, respectively, illustrate this:

> At first I thought I'm struggling . . . but then I saw everybody was struggling . . . they just weren't expecting it to be as hard as it was.
>
> I look back and remember how I struggled . . . because I wasn't used to not getting good grades and not being confident . . . just such a shock at how stupid I felt because I thought I knew it!

Most students experience financial stress and need to work; again, this finding was consistent across geographic and race lines. A faculty member commented: "The students work anywhere from 8 to 30 hours per week." A Black student noted that she and fellow students are tired in class and teachers

> may look at that as being we're partying all the time. But I know I went to class from 8 A.M. to 4 P.M., then I work from 12 midnight to 6 in the morning. Then I have a 10:00 A.M. class.

Students also find that they have less social support for these stressors; friends and family do not realize the difficulties they face. A White student commented:

> No one can understand what it's like to be a nursing student. You know it's very frustrating to have it not understood by people on the outside. It's like they say: "Oh, it's so easy, they do nothing." I think they think we just do what the doctors tell us.

An African American student summed up multiple stressors she faces as a nursing student:

> You're dealing with being away from home, and you're trying to get adjusted. The minority students I know, we go to school, we work, we come from single parent homes. We have issues going on at home. We have issues with ourselves. There is so much. And sometimes that takes away from our schoolwork. There's so many outside factors.

Finding 2: It Is Harder for African Americans

In addition to the academic, financial, and support stressors consistently described by students, African American students faced additional barriers from prejudice and lack of acceptance.

Prejudice. Prejudice was pervasive; African American students in every focus group or individual interview described encounters with prejudice in school, clinical, or the community their school was in and sometimes in all three places. Students described acts of prejudice as subtle and committed unconsciously by fellow students, faculty, patients, and/or community members. The impact of prejudice, however, was far from subtle; students felt marginalized, and that affected their sense of *Belonging* in the nursing program.

Fellow Student Prejudice. African American students expressed anger and a sense of loss when they encountered prejudice from fellow students. It seemed to take them by surprise and leave them feeling diminished. Agape, the only minority student in her nursing class, described an encounter with several White students who asked if they could be her health assessment lab partners. "They were curious about my body, being an African American, and that threw me for a loop . . . I'm the same as you." Three Black students in a predominantly White program, who were interviewed together, described White students' reactions to them:

Wilma: It seems like a lot of the time, they're intimidated. Don't want to talk to you a lot.

Tina: Don't want to be in a group with you.

Angie: Don't want to sit near you during tests. They'll move all the way across the room on the first test, maybe just to see if you're going to look on their paper.

Another Black student tried to understand the prejudice; she explained that White classmates

> went to schools that might not have had a lot of Black people. So they don't know what to expect. So they'll kind of try to test you. Try to [test] you, doing things, saying things.

Lack of racial exposure and understanding goes both ways. A Black student in a predominantly Black nursing program said: "I have only a few White friends . . . what I know about White people is what I've seen on TV."

Faculty Prejudice. African American students identified the following faculty behaviors as examples of faculty prejudice: having lower expectations of minority students, stereotyping, expecting the student to be a spokesperson for her or his race, and discomfort with race talk. Students did not feel that faculty behaved in these ways intentionally, rather that they did so unconsciously. Examples of stereotyping and lower expectations from faculty members that African American students described include:

> Some people don't look at your intelligence or what you know or what you can do. They just look at color.
>
> You have to prove yourself, and I hate that . . . you have to prove yourself because less is expected.
>
> A lot of faculty, they see one Black student and they see them all . . . We've been here 2 years and they still can't tell the difference between us.

A sense of frustration and anger comes through in the quotes. These African American students feel they are neither seen nor valued as individuals.

Another subtle prejudicial behavior is to treat minority students as spokespersons for their race:

> Whenever the instructor is discussing something in the text referring to African Americans, I can just feel her eyes immediately go to me. [It makes me feel] different . . . negative. I feel like I'm supposed to be a spokesperson for my race. If instructors are talking about something that is more

> common with African Americans, they'll ask me in class if I agree, and I'll think . . . I'm not sure, I haven't experienced that.

Though the instructor's behavior seems innocent and was probably intended to increase cultural awareness, it objectifies and depersonalizes the minority student and leads to feelings of discomfort and embarrassment. Again, the student is not seen as an individual but as a representative of a group.

Community. When minority students encountered prejudice in the community, it often affected their sense of safety and security as well as their feeling of *Belonging*. One student said, "Everyone wants to be accepted. And no one wants to feel threatened. If I'm the only Black somewhere I have to stop and think, is it going to be OK? Is it safe?" Another minority student felt there was widespread prejudice in the community her school was in. "A lot of [minority students] feel intimidated by the police, and getting stopped and stuff like that. It's like the community is trying to keep it the way it is."

Minority students in these environments gravitated to each other:

> So it's just like, when you go someplace and you see another Black face you're like, "Oh here comes a Black person!" And you don't want to be like that, but it gives you a comfort level.

Black students reported coping with the prejudice and trying to get past it. One said: "As a minority student, you still face all these prejudices and all these hateful remarks and you come to live with it. What are you going to do? I can't change my color."

Overt Prejudice. Acts of overt prejudice were rare though frightening when they occur. A White administrator related the following story:

> A Caucasian female threatened a Black male nursing student. Threatened his life in front of the other students. She said, "I'm going to go to my car, get my gun and blow your little Black head off." Quote unquote. And the [other] students chose not to tell . . . He felt he would not get the attention. Which is a sad commentary on the school, maybe the university, certainly

> administration. But it hurt my heart to think that he didn't think I would give him the attention because of the discriminatory issues.

The administrator said she heard of the incident several weeks after it occurred from one of the students present, who was pressured by her mother to report the incident. Despite efforts to expel the instigator, she remained in the program and graduated a semester behind the others.

Lack of Acceptance. The vast majority of African American students interviewed said they did not feel a sense of welcome and belonging in their nursing programs, which made success more difficult. Of the 20 African American students interviewed, representing five nursing programs, the only students who felt welcomed in their program attended a predominantly Black community college. No Black students at predominantly White colleges or universities described their nursing programs as welcoming. A White faculty member described frustration with the climate at her school:

> There's not a welcoming climate among the traditional students that have come there, and I've been pretty appalled during the year at how isolated many of the minority students are and how they just stick together. And if there are enough of them, that's fine because they have a support group and they can help each other, but when they are just mainstreamed so to speak, they can get lost.

African American students also described frustration and impatience with not feeling welcomed. One student commented:

> I think people are just like, especially minority students, are like as soon as I graduate, I just can't wait to get back to a place where I am accepted. Where I can be with my own kind more, or I can be with people who aren't my own kind, but who have accepted that we live in an interracial or a biracial community where there are all different cultures, and they don't have a problem with it.

It is understandable, but unfortunate, that minority students would want to leave an unwelcoming environment after graduation. Their leaving represents a missed opportunity to increase racial diversity in the local community, school, and RN population.

Finding 3: Welcoming Actions Help and Unwelcoming Actions Hinder Success

A welcoming climate increases all students' success in nursing education. Welcoming actions are those that increase a student's sense of *Belonging* and help the process of *Becoming a Nurse.* Welcoming actions are needed from all three groups—faculty, students, and administrators—and from more than a few people in each group. Faculty and administrative actions influence the climate in the program and are very influential in students' professional development and socialization. However, students must also feel welcomed by their peers to feel a sense of *Belonging.*

Some programs are not welcoming to students in general. A White nursing instructor said her program "has almost evolved to a hostile environment. And we don't discriminate. We're kind of nasty to everybody." Black and White students interviewed at this nursing school agreed with her; none felt welcomed.

Of the five nursing programs African American student participants attended, only the predominantly African American program was perceived as welcoming. No African American student at a predominantly White program reported feeling welcomed even though they identified welcoming faculty or administrators. If minority students did not feel accepted by other students, they did not rate their program as welcoming.

Welcoming From Students. All students crave acceptance from their fellow students, a sense that "we're all in this together." Developmentally, this is appropriate; young adults are in Erikson's Intimacy vs. Isolation stage, and students are beginning their professional identification. They are eager to bond with other nursing students. White students take this acceptance for granted; none of the White students interviewed identified lack of acceptance as a problem. White students tend to assume that Black students in their program also feel accepted, as illustrated in this quote:

> It doesn't matter if you are Black or White or Hispanic or whatever you are, it's all about care and advocacy . . . I have never noticed a difference . . . We're all just the same people. We're all here to learn the same things. We're all here to do the same things. I've never seen anyone disrespected or treated differently because of their color . . . Everyone is disci-

> plined the same, everyone is treated the same. And it doesn't matter what race you are because everyone is here to do one thing. We're all here to learn how to be a good nurse.

However, an African American student in the same program clearly perceived problems. She described the difference between the predominantly African American nursing program she first attended and the predominantly White nursing program she was currently in:

> You did not have to deal with the stereotyping. It was more like a team effort, everyone trying to work together. We are all in this together. We are all trying to pass. We are all trying to become nurses. Not every man for himself. And especially if you were a minority student or an African American student, I'm really going to stay away from you. You didn't have to worry about that attitude there. We were all nursing students headed toward the same goal, and we were all going to work together and help each other.

This lack of acceptance left some African American students feeling disappointed and angry, as this student described:

> When I was a freshman or sophomore, it didn't bother me as much because I was dealing with people who were a different major and it didn't bother me because I knew I probably wouldn't see them again in my life. But when you think of nursing you think . . . it should be helping. I don't expect everyone to be best friends and we can dress up and do our hair alike. I don't want that. But you think you can work toward a common goal.

Welcoming From Faculty and Administrators. Welcoming actions by faculty and administrators include seeing students as individuals, valuing and reaching out to them, being committed to nursing education, and setting high expectations. In a welcoming environment, the student is known as an individual. All students mentioned the importance of being known by name and the acknowledgment of personal struggles and triumphs. An African American student at a predominantly White institution described feeling welcomed by a White faculty member:

> She made me her special case . . . she's shown her love for me by caring for me not just as a student but as a person. She is the only person I feel comfortable talking to . . . Anytime I just need a reason to keep turning in my papers, and to just keep doing, I go to her. And she's always there for me.

> She's always showing me my potential, and what she thought I would be. And although I sometimes try to present myself as a mean girl, she knows I'm just a loving, little, sweet girl inside who just has been through some hard things.

An African American student at a predominantly African American nursing school said:

> I feel love here . . . a sense of camaraderie and caring for us and with the instructors—they are all very approachable.

These quotes illustrate the students' sense of feeling important and valued by faculty.

Several faculty described valuing the enrichment minority students bring to their nursing programs. A White faculty member said:

> They bring a diversity to the school which should enrich it. So that you all become a little bit better because you have a better idea that people are different . . . what that difference is and how good that can be for a group.

Welcoming faculty are committed to student success, actively reach out to students, challenge them, and help them succeed. A White faculty member described reaching out to minority students:

> Part of the issue of trying to deal with diverse cultures is understanding that those cultures need to have an invitation to work with me . . . sometimes that invitation has to be personal, not just, "Here's my email, here's my phone number, here's my office hours."

Another White faculty member described the need to challenge students—setting high expectations, not "lowering the bar"—and to help all students meet these expectations. She emphasized the need to tailor her teaching, providing individualized rather than equal treatment:

> My role as a nursing faculty member is to promote growth and development. The students laugh when I say that, but they see what I'm talking about. I think that's basically why I can say you should mentor people differently. People have different needs, they're at different stages. So then it's OK not to do the same thing with everybody. . . . [Some] might need to have more help. [Others] might need to have less help. They might need to

> be sent someplace else. They might need to just know that they can come to your office and say, "I don't get it. Help me." . . . And I think in nursing, and particularly in nursing education, we get into this fairness issue. The philosophy of transcultural nursing is that you do *not* give the same nursing care to everyone because it is not appropriate, and I think the same is true for nursing education. Do not give the same nursing education to all people. Because they need different kinds of things . . . I'm not talking about changing a standard. I'm talking about different ways to help people meet the standard.

African American students emphasized the need for faculty to maintain the same high standard of expectations for all students, regardless of race. One said: "I don't want [a good grade] if I don't deserve it." Another did not want to be treated differently from White students, which contrasts with the faculty member's previous comments about individualizing teaching. The student said:

> Treat [Black students] the same as the White students. No different. Not even positive attention—that could be seen as negative too. It's that I'm a person with my own abilities. I don't have special needs because of my skin color—I don't need favors. Just treat me like a person and the same as other people.

Finding 4: Conflict Between Nursing's Values and Norms Decreases the Feeling of Being Welcomed

A fourth finding from the research is the existence of a conflict between nursing's values and norms. Study participants identified nursing values as caring, individualized approach, respect for diversity, service to others, responsibility, integrity, and professionalism. These values reflect professional nursing values identified by the American Association of Colleges of Nursing—altruism, autonomy, human dignity, integrity, and social justice (AACN, 1997). The value of professionalism reflects higher education expectations of assertiveness, critical thinking, and effective communication (Benjamin, 1996).

In addition to values, respondents identified norms—common patterns of behavior and rules (written or unwritten) reflecting expectations of students and clients; these included rigidity, need for control, conformity, ritual and tradition, avoidance of conflict, and unconscious bias. The norms reflect nursing, health care, and U.S. cultures. Rigidity, conformity, adherence to ritual and tradition, and avoidance of conflict match nursing norms identified by Barbee (1993) and DuToit (1995). They reflect historical patterns of nursing education that have been White culture dominant, rule driven, authority-and-control oriented, and hierarchical, with both women and students in subordinate roles (Bevis & Watson, 1989; Jackson, 1993). These norms are a result of "parochial attitudes engendered in the training schools [that] created rigidity in educational practices, small-mindedness in dictating the details of students' lives, and petty jealousies" (Baer, D'Antonio, Rinker, & Lynaugh, 2001, p. 5). In addition, the norm of unconscious bias reflects racism and unrecognized White privilege in U.S. society and nursing.

Faculty participants noted that norms conflicted with nursing values, sending a mixed message to students trying to learn nursing culture and creating barriers to *Belonging* and *Becoming a Nurse.* A White faculty member described the conflict between the value of respect for diversity and the norms of conformity, rigidity, and ritual and tradition:

> I'm not sure we're willing to open up our culture to be influenced by the minority and different ethnicities so much as we want them to accommodate to our culture . . . and that is what I think we desperately need—a change in our own culture of nursing education that I find very rigid . . . We're very set in our ways . . . There's a lot of ritual in our approach.

Norms of conformity and rigidity also conflict with values of caring and professionalism, which include attributes of critical thinking and assertiveness. This conflict is illustrated in quotes from two White faculty members that center on students' nursing care plans:

> Nursing faculty expect that everyone's care plans look alike. You write a nursing diagnosis like this and you write a goal like this, and that's what's right . . . I'm not sure the nursing profession, faculty, have a very wide margin of what's acceptable . . . We're still telling [students] where to jump, when to jump, and how to jump. And I'm not sure that's good for diversity.

A second quote illustrates rigidity in what a faculty member considers appropriate and a lack of willingness in this faculty member to accept a different viewpoint:

> A student wrote her care plan with a totally different focus and view from what I wanted. I guess it was her cultural view. I had problems with it, and

> she said, "But it's correct—these are the patient's needs," and I said, "Yes, I can see it that way . . . but this way [my way] is better." She asked why she had to do it my way. I used an art analogy. "If you're studying painting with Cezanne, you'll end up painting like Cezanne rather than like Monet." Right now she was hearing "paint like Cezanne" and when she graduated, she could choose to paint any way she wanted. She said she couldn't wait to graduate.

The desire for conformity and narrow concept of acceptability illustrated in these two quotes counters the critical thinking and assertiveness that nursing faculty try to engender in nursing students.

Another conflict is between the values of caring and respect for diversity with the norm of unconscious bias. A minority student said:

> I got frustrated because I was experiencing all these . . . mixed messages, this prejudice . . . so one message is "we're open and caring, we believe in the dignity of all people"—if they look like me.

Conflicts between actions reflecting values and actions reflecting norms create a tension within nursing education culture that influences nursing students' perceptions of a program being welcoming. The amount of conflict between values and norms differs between programs and reflects the individuals in the program and the local academic and community climate. Minority students in predominantly White nursing programs feel less welcomed than White students, due to prejudice and marginalization. In nursing programs where the values-norms conflict is extreme, race fades to the background; the program is perceived to be unwelcoming to all students. Black and White students in a very unwelcoming program described feelings of powerlessness and hopelessness that were so extreme, the students felt trapped—imprisoned. Here are comments from two White students who were interviewed together:

Erin: "I think [feeling powerless] has a lot to do with the way we're treated. It makes us discouraged."

Jane: "We get to a point where we're [wondering], 'Why am I even doing this?' "

Erin: "I know. I was at that point today. I was thinking in class, 'This is a total option for me to be sitting here right now' . . . I feel like I'm more in prison . . . I don't feel like we have much option anymore."

Jane: "I feel really incomplete."

Finding 5: Identification With Values

The nursing students interviewed felt a strong fit with nursing values. This identification reflects their ideals about nursing and sustains them through difficulties in the program. African American students commented that the values of caring, respect for diversity, and service reflect Christian tenets that are central to their lives. "I heard that every day at home from my Great-Grandma and at church." Values of responsibility, integrity, and professionalism reflect values in higher education the African American students were familiar with and had internalized as college students. This congruence between personal and professional values helped minority students cope with unwelcoming programs by remaining focused on their goal of becoming a nurse. They were able to differentiate nursing from the nursing program, as reflected in the comment: "I love it [nursing]—but not here." For these students, academic and social integration into the nursing program seemed to be less important influences on persistence than their connection with nursing values.

The strong identification with nursing values enhanced minority students' professional identity and shaped their plans to "make a difference" as nurses—both attributes of success in nursing education. An African American student said she wanted to "be that kind of nurse [who makes positive change]. I want to get out there and really make a difference." Several African American students also wanted to make a difference through combating prejudice. Many felt they were teaching White students and faculty to challenge negative stereotypes about African Americans. One African American student said: "I take on the role of informing others. I teach them how to act and how not to . . . so they'll become better people. It's a personal choice I make." Another African American student said her White classmates "felt that we've taught them a lot they didn't know about Black people . . . to see us differently and our culture differently." An African American faculty member highlighted the power of actions in helping to make a difference:

> And don't forget role modeling. So often people think that minority people cannot achieve and cannot do well and are not interested in being professionals. And we change that image, don't we? . . . We change the image that many people have of us.

This strong and sustaining link between nursing and personal values helps minority students find meaning in their experience of *Becoming a Nurse.* A woman who was the only African American student in her nursing program expressed this as follows:

> I feel that nursing is my calling from God and all these experiences are making me better and stronger. It's God's way of testing me, and leading me into the area where I can help.

IMPLICATIONS AND RECOMMENDATIONS FOR NURSE EDUCATORS

The findings of this descriptive, qualitative study shed light on the experience of nursing education, in particular, facilitators and barriers students encounter in their journey to become nurses and the effect race has on the experience. However, these findings cannot be generalized beyond the young African American, Asian, and White women students and the faculty members who contributed to the study. More research is needed to fully understand this phenomenon and to determine if other members of other underrepresented groups in nursing—students from other racial/ethnic groups, men, older students—experience similar challenges. Despite these limitations, the study has implications for nursing education practice and policy and highlights the importance of nurse educators in minority student success.

Implications for practice include: acknowledgment of the powerful effect welcoming faculty, administrators, and White classmates have on minority students; the pervasive and destructive nature of prejudice; and the sense of struggle all nursing students experience. Faculty and administrators could use these findings to redesign the teaching–learning environment in their nursing programs. Consideration of actions students described as welcoming and unwelcoming could lead to development of effective strategies that would address strengths and deficiencies in individual nursing programs. Reflective practice would allow identification of unconscious acts demonstrating nursing norms of conformity, rigidity, and adherence to ritual and tradition. A heightened sensitivity to prejudice could lead to monitoring for evidence of subtle, covert bias as well as overt racist actions. Increased awareness of the unconscious privilege of Whiteness and the European American cultural framework from which most nursing educators operate could increase sensitivity to their own cultural expectations, as well as openness to other cultural views. Nurse educators, both faculty and administrators, could reach out to minority students and play an active role in their success. They could watch for marginalization by White students and work with White students to increase minority student acceptance. They could also monitor the university and community climate for prejudice and be active in effecting change.

Nurse educators could rethink some of the traditional ways of teaching nursing. Care plans, a traditional teaching strategy to increase student preparation for clinical patient care, were cited frequently by faculty and students as problematic. Students spend long hours preparing the night before clinical, leaving them feeling tired and stressed during the clinical learning experience. The amount of knowledge to master and the teaching practices that reinforce a faculty–student power hierarchy contribute to students' struggle in nursing education. Consideration could be given to developing teaching strategies that are supportive, collaborative, and interactive while maintaining academic rigor and depth.

Policy implications are aimed at the program level. Administrators could create a "milieu for change" by setting policy that maintains program emphasis on nursing values, modeling these values, and providing transition, training, and support programs for faculty and students. Transition programs for all students entering nursing could be very helpful. Such programs could serve as an introduction to nursing education, making nursing values and expectations for value-driven conduct explicit. They could also be an opportunity for students to identify similarities and differences in cultural and ethnic viewpoints and serve as a forum for consideration of issues of social justice and their impact on nursing and health care. Finally, development of formal support structures in terms of financial aid, scholarships, and minority nurse support groups would be very helpful to minority nursing student success.

Creating a safe and supportive climate for minority students is essential; a White administrator described this as:

> Creating that culture of comfort that when you can go someplace and have a like face, you can be more comfortable than when you're the only one that is like you . . . you want to be sure you're in a safe environment. And that was some great effort we had from our college as a whole to make sure that if we are recruiting minority students, we are bringing them into a safe, accepting environment. That is more than just a matter of putting those statistics down, because everyone expects us to have them. But are we providing the support that would allow them to have success?

Nurse administrators need to provide courageous leadership to accomplish these changes in policy. A minority administrator emphasized the need to "stand in the gap" between actual and ideal practices and model the nursing values she wants to see in others. A White faculty member said: "We need to be freed up from the tyranny of whatever is keeping us in these old models [based on conformity, rigidity, and reliance on ritual and tradition]." Administrators can help break the bonds to the old models. Change may be incremental, but even small changes can have a large impact.

CONCLUSION

Current practices are not solving the problems nursing faces in increasing the number of minority nurses. This study indicates that nursing education culture influences all students' success. Student participants felt a good cultural "fit" with nursing education's values but not with the norms. Actions reflecting nursing values are perceived as welcoming and facilitate nursing student success, while actions that reflect norms are perceived as unwelcoming, especially to minority students, and create additional barriers students must overcome to be successful.

The study's findings indicate that nurse educators and fellow students play a central role in minority nursing students' success or failure. The educator role is powerful with broad and far-reaching effects. Educators can facilitate student success or create barriers through unconscious acts as well as purposeful ones. For minority students, the presence of even one welcoming nurse educator who affirms their individuality and includes and values them may make the difference between success and failure. It does not appear to be enough for nurse educators to *say* they believe in values of caring, respect for diversity, and individualized, culturally sensitive care; they must also *model* these values. Failure to do so—maintenance of the current status quo—is not a benign act. It leads to creation of barriers to minority students' education and increases their sense of isolation and struggle. An increase in barriers could limit minority students' graduation rates, and the nursing profession's ability to become more diverse.

Nurse educators face a choice: to align their actions with nursing's values and support students through nursing education or to continue the status quo. An old adage from the 1960s is pertinent still: "If you are not part of the solution, you are part of the problem." Modeling nursing education's values and creating a welcoming environment for all nursing students can be part of the solution to today's nursing shortage and lack of diversity.

QUESTIONS FOR DIALOGUE

1. What ideas or concepts did you find most meaningful in this chapter? Identify your insights and questions to bring to a dialogue with your colleagues.
2. What values attracted you to the profession of nursing? To what extent do you feel these values are carried out in nursing practice and education on a day-to-day basis? What values do you see as most compromised? What work do you see needs to happen in nursing education to model the values that nursing professes?
3. Identify practices in your program that reflect the unwelcoming nursing norms of "rigidity, need for control, conformity, ritual and tradition, avoidance of conflict, and unconscious bias." How can these practices be transformed? What specific steps can you take to move your nursing education program from a norm-driven to a nursing values–driven environment?
4. Identify the welcoming behaviors in your nursing program. What does your program offer in the way of an orientation to welcome new students, meet nursing faculty, and create a sense of belonging? Throughout the year are there opportunities for students to gather and reconnect with each other and with faculty to reinforce a sense of community and caring?
5. How does your program assess whether students feel welcomed or not? What suggestions do you have for creating opportunities for students to safely share their experiences and concerns without fear of retribution?
6. If students experience unwelcoming actions, what does your program have in place to validate and address students' concerns? What suggestions do you have for addressing institutionalized, personally mediated, and internalized racism in your program?

APPENDIX

SAMPLE INTERVIEW QUESTIONS

Faculty Questions

1. Please tell me about yourself. How long have you been in nursing? Nursing education? Where have you taught besides here? Please tell me about the program here . . . number of students . . . how many are minority students?

2. Can you tell me how you would define the culture of nursing?
3. Could you describe the culture of nursing education at this institution?
4. Could you describe key beliefs and expectations nursing faculty at this institution have about nursing students?
5. How is the nursing culture passed on to new students? New faculty?
6. How would you characterize an ideal student here?
7. How would you characterize a student who does poorly here?
8. How open do you feel the nursing education culture here is to students in general? To minority nursing students?
9. What, if any, cultural differences are you aware of with students from minority groups?
10. What, if any, unique qualities do minority students bring to nursing?
11. Could you tell me about a situation you may have observed or been a part of when a student might have been treated differently based on their race?
12. Can you give me some ideas about different problems minority students might face that young, middle-class, White women students wouldn't?
13. How might a minority student get help with these problems?
14. What can nursing faculty do to help minority students succeed in nursing?

Student Questions

1. Tell me about the nursing school here . . . how many students? How many are men? African American? Hispanic? Asian? How about the faculty?
2. How would you describe the culture, or values, beliefs, and expectations of the nursing school here?
3. How did you learn these values, beliefs, and expectations?
4. In what ways are these different than what you expected from nursing?
5. Can you tell me how open or welcoming the nursing school you attend is to you as a minority student?
6. Do you feel you have something unique to offer about yourself or your ethnic culture that will add to nursing as a profession? Do you feel faculty recognize or value these unique qualities?

7. Do you feel you face any barriers or specific problems that White women students do not face?
8. If you do face barriers, how do you usually resolve (cope with) them?
9. Could you tell me about a situation you may have observed or been a part of when a student might have been treated differently based on their race?
10. Are you comfortable talking with any faculty members about problems you encountered? If you spoke with faculty members, were you successful in addressing the problems?
11. Can you tell me if there is anyone in nursing school who is a role model or mentor to you? Tell me about this person.
12. Can you think of things nursing schools and/or faculty might do differently to create a more welcoming or supportive environment for minority students?

REFERENCES

Afrinson, J. (1999). Nursing students' perceptions regarding differences in the clinical learning experience that relate to minority-racial status. *Journal of the National Black Nurses Association, 10*(1), 56–67.

Aiken, L. C. (2001). Black women in nursing education completion programs: Issues affecting participation. *Adult Education Quarterly, 51*(4), 306–321.

American Association of Colleges of Nursing (AACN). (1997). *The essentials of baccalaureate education for professional nursing practice.* Washington, DC: Author.

American Association of Colleges of Nursing (AACN). (2006). *Advancing higher education in nursing: 2006 annual report.* Washington, DC: Author.

Astin, A. W. (1984, July). Student involvement: A developmental theory for higher education. *Journal of College Student Personnel,* 297–308.

Astin, A. W. (1993). *What matters in college: Four critical years revisited.* San Francisco: Jossey-Bass.

Baer, E. D., D'Antonio, P., Rinker, S., & Lynaugh, J. E. (2001). *Enduring issues in American nursing.* New York: Springer Publishing.

Barbee, E. L. (1993). Racism in U.S. nursing. *Medical Anthropology Quarterly, 7*(4), 346–362.

Barbee, E. L., & Gibson, S. E. (2001). Our dismal progress: The recruitment of non-whites into nursing. *Journal of Nursing Education, 40*(6), 243–244.

Benjamin, M. (1996). *Cultural diversity, educational equity and the transformation of higher education.* Westport, CT: Praeger.

Bevis, E. O., & Watson, J. (1989). *Toward a caring curriculum: A new pedagogy for nursing.* New York: National League for Nursing.

Bourassa, D. M. (1991, Winter). How White students and students of color organize and interact on campus. In J. C. Dalton (Ed.), *Racism on campus: Confronting racial bias through peer interventions. New directions for student services* (Vol. 56, pp. 13–23). San Francisco: Jossey-Bass.

Cabrera, A. F., Nora, A., & Castaneda, M. B. (1993). College persistence: Structural equations modeling test of an integrated model of student retention. *Journal of Higher Education, 64*(2), 123–139.

Cabrera, A. F., Nora, A., Terenzini, P. T., Pascarella, E., & Hagedorn, L. S. (1999). Campus racial climate and the adjustment of students to college: A comparison between White students and African American students. *Journal of Higher Education, 70*(2), 134–160.

Campbell, A. R., & Davis, S. M. (1996). Faculty commitment: Retaining minority nursing students in majority institutions. *Journal of Nursing Education, 35*(7), 298–303.

DuToit, D. (1995). A sociological analysis of the extent and influence of professional socialization on the development of a nursing identity among nursing students at two universities in Brisbane, Australia. *Journal of Advanced Nursing, 21*, 164–171.

Eimers, M. T., & Pike, G. R. (1997). Minority and nonminority adjustment to college: Differences or similarities? *Research in Higher Education, 38*(1), 77–97.

Hecker, D. C. (2001, November). *Occupational employment projections to 2010. Monthly Labor Review Online.* U.S. Bureau of Labor Statistics. Retrieved November 10, 2001, from http://www.bls.gov/opub/mlr/2001/11/art4full.pdf

Hurtado, S. (1994). The institutional climate for talented Latino students. *Research in Higher Education, 35*(1), 21–41.

Hurtado, S., Milem, J. F., Clayton-Pederson, A. R., & Allen, W. R. (1998). Enhancing campus climates for racial/ethnic diversity: Educational policy and practice. *The Review of Higher Education, 21*(3), 279–302.

Jackson, E. M. (1993). Whiting-out difference: Why U.S. nursing research fails Black families. *Medical Anthropology Quarterly, 7*(4), 363–385.

Jeffreys, M. R. (1998). Predicting nontraditional student retention and academic achievement. *Journal of Nursing Education, 23*(1), 42–48.

Johnson, I. H. (1996, Summer). Access and retention: Support programs for graduate and professional students. In I. H. Johnson & A. J. Ottens (Eds.), *Leveling the playing field: Promoting academic success for students of color. New directions for student services* (Vol. 74, pp. 53–67). San Francisco: Jossey-Bass.

Jordan, J. D. (1996). Rethinking race and attrition in nursing programs: A hermeneutic inquiry. *Journal of Professional Nursing, 12*(6), 382–390.

Kirkland, M. L. (1998). Stressors and coping strategies among successful female African American baccalaureate nursing students. *Journal of Nursing Education, 37*(1), 5–12.

Langston-Moss, R. (1997). Experiences and perceptions of Black American female nursing students attending predominantly White nursing programs. *Journal of the National Black Nurses Association, 9*(2), 21–30.

McIntosh, P. (1995). White privilege and male privilege: A personal account of coming to see correspondences through work in women's studies. In K. Rousmaniere (Ed.), *Readings in sociocultural studies in education* (2nd ed., pp. 189–195). New York: McGraw-Hill.

McIntyre, A. (1997). Constructing an image of a White teacher. *Teachers College Record, 98*(4), 652–681.

McNairy, F. G. (1996, Summer). The challenge for higher education: Retaining students of color. In I. H. Johnson & A. J. Ottens (Eds.), *Leveling the playing field: Promoting academic success for students of color. New directions for student services* (Vol. 74, pp. 3–14). San Francisco: Jossey-Bass.

Miles, M. B., & Huberman, M. (1994). *Qualitative data analysis: An expanded sourcebook.* Thousand Oaks, CA: Sage.

Miller, L. S. (1995). *An American imperative: Acceleration of minority educational advancement.* New Haven, CT: Yale University Press.

Morris, D. L., & Wykie, M. L. (1994). Minorities in nursing. In J. J. Fitzpatrick & J. Stevenson (Eds.), *Annual review of nursing research* (pp. 175–189). New York: Springer Publishing.

Nora, A., & Cabrera, A. F. (1996). The role of perceptions of prejudice and discrimination on the adjustment of minority students in college. *Journal of Higher Education, 67*(2), 119–148.

Ogbu, J. U., & Simons, H. D. (1998). Voluntary and involuntary minorities: A cultural-ecological theory of school performance with some implications for education. *Anthropology and Education Quarterly, 29*(2), 155–188.

Peterson, M. W., & Spencer, M. G. (1990). Understanding academic culture and climate. In W. G. Tierney (Ed.), *Assessing academic climates and cultures. New directions for institutional research* (Vol. 68, 3–18). San Francisco: Jossey-Bass.

Snyder, D. J., & Bunkers, S. J. (1994). Facilitators and barriers for minority students in Master's nursing programs. *Journal of Professional Nursing, 10*(3), 140–146.

Spratley, E., Johnson, A., Sochalski, J., Fritz, M., & Spencer, W. (2000). *The Registered Nurse population: Findings from the national sample survey of Registered Nurses March 2000.* Washington, DC: U.S. Dept of Health and Human Services, Health Resources and Services Administration, Bureau of Health Professions. Retrieved February 10, 2003, from http://bhpr.hrsa.gov/healthworkforce/rnsurvey/rnss1.html

Tatum, B. D. (1997). *Why are all the Black kids sitting together in the cafeteria?* New York: Basic Books.

Tierney, W. G. (1991). *Culture and ideology in higher education: Advancing a critical agenda.* New York: Praeger.

Tinto, V. (1993). *Leaving college* (2nd ed.). Chicago: University of Chicago Press.

Vaughan, J. (1997). Is there really racism in nursing? *Journal of Nursing Education, 36*(3), 135–139.

Villarruel, A. M., Canales, M., & Torres, S. (2001). Bridges and barriers: Educational mobility of Hispanic nurses. *Journal of Nursing Education, 40*(6), 245–251.

Watkins, M. P. (1997). Perceived impact of nursing faculty on the academic success of minority students. *ABNF Journal, 8*(6), 125–128.

Yoder, M. K. (1996). Instructional responses to ethnically diverse nursing students. *Journal of Nursing Education, 35*(7), 315–321.

3 Addressing Race and Culture in Nurse Education

STUART NAIRN

Along with some colleagues, I am currently researching how nurse academics in the United Kingdom manage issues around culture and diversity. After an interview with one of the participants, who happened to be from another country, I received an e-mail from her about an exchange she had observed between two British nurse educators. She kindly agreed to let me reproduce it as a vignette here:

> *Hi Stuart, by coincidence, a couple of hours after our interview I was sitting in the coffee room and gradually became aware of a discussion going on between several lecturers I had never seen before. One was saying that he had been leading a discussion . . . and the subject of immigrants came up and that things got very overheated. He said that he felt out of his depth, and quickly ended the discussion by saying that he didn't feel it was a good thing to be talking about in class. I was amazed, and felt this highlighted some of the points that emerged from our discussion.*
>
> *Just to be a bit reflective, I did not leap in and try to provide alternative perspectives, so obviously I must have felt a bit out of my depth as well . . . although in my defence, it would have been very unbritish to barge into a discussion with people that I don't know in order to disagree with them. . . . gets me thinking though, maybe in future I should barge in.*

It is easy to sympathise with the lecturer for avoiding the immigrant issue, but as the author of this e-mail suggests, addressing the issue has a moral imperative to it. Should we allow prejudiced views to go by, or should we risk intervening? Of course, it is not clear from the vignette what the cause of the dispute was. Nor is it clear what the disagreement was about or on what basis the lecturer decided to terminate the discussion. But the issue is worth "thinking through," and because it is clear that nurses have a responsibility to all patients, the heated exchange about immigrants suggests that discriminatory attitudes and the potential for discriminatory practice were clearly emerging in the discussion. Perhaps one of the key undercurrents of the exchange was racism, a term that was not mentioned. Feeling uncomfortable in this situation reflects a general unease among academics about tackling the subject of racism. It also suggests that the author of the e-mail is aware of something called British culture and is hesitant about moving into a conversation in which that person did not feel a part because she perceived such an act to be outside cultural norms in Britain.

In this chapter, I look at issues of race and culture in nurse education and argue for the importance of dealing with these issues in a more proactive way. However, I also argue that the subject is very difficult to deal with, not least because of the problems of using an appropriate language. I then look at the ways that racism is hidden within our everyday language and the consequent difficulties about even identifying the problem. Racism is not necessarily explicit, but as it is suppressed in official language, it emerges in other ways, usually by emphasising cultural differences. This provokes particular problems when trying to support culture as a legitimate part of a person's identity but also recognizes that it can be used as a means of isolating and differentiating people into deterministic categories. I then examine more explicitly the tensions between the terms *transcultural* or *multicultural* and *antiracist analyses.* Then I examine the way that culture can be essentialised in such a way that fails to address the problem of racism but reproduces it instead. I look at some possible educational strategies and make some brief comments on the problems of measuring the outcomes of such interventions.

RACE AND LANGUAGE

When discussing the issue of race, the academic, whose trade involves the use of language and who might be considered an expert in defining terms, is confronted by a set of problems that could keep the most rigorous linguist in work for a lifetime. It is difficult to use terms such as *race* without exploring the multiple ways in which the term is used and how it interpenetrates with other equally complex terms such as *ethnicity* and *culture.* There is a constant deferral of meaning as the terms ebb and flow between each other and then express themselves in the different languages of biology, sociology, anthropology, and policy discourse.

The problem is that the term *race* is biologically meaningless in the scientific sense. This is partly a product of biology's fraught relationship with racism culminating in the practice of racial hygiene in the Germany of the Nazi era. Indeed, Proctor (1988) has argued that the Nazi government elevated biological knowledge into state policy. Nonetheless, the term *race* continues to be used, but how it is used has changed. Williams (1997) examined how the social sciences used race in the 1960s and found that it was defined in terms of "major divisions of mankind" and "biologically considered varieties" and that race was based on "essentially physical characteristics" (p. 323). By the 1980s, the definitions of race had changed to "an unscientific term" or a "scientifically discredited term" with the emphasis clearly on "social-cultural-political" identification (Williams, 1997, p. 323).

The current consensus seems to be based on the view that race is biologically meaningless, a fictional entity, but that as a social and cultural construct it continues to plague and poison social relationships (Smedley & Smedley, 2005). For epidemiologists and clinicians, conceptualising human differences remains clinically useful in identifying at-risk groups. As Skinner (2007) points out, medical researchers focusing on differences in susceptibility to disease refer to ethnic differences rather than race. These differences in risk refer to genetic variations in populations, shared environment, and group identification. Some continue to use race as a category in identifying, for example, sickle cell disease but stress the social dimensions of the term rather than its biological roots (Bhopal, 2003). Sickle cell is not a product of some enduring racial distinctiveness but rather of the relationships between a person's genetic inheritance and environment. Sickle cell is found mainly in people descended from Africa, the Caribbean, the eastern Mediterranean, the Middle East, and Asia (Sickle Cell Society, 2004), and therefore, it makes sense for these characteristics to be noted in medical notes in patients who present with joint pain, for example. Nonetheless, this does not justify the term *race,* and yet, these characteristics become defined as racial dispositions. This illustrates the difficulties of finding a language that is precise enough for clinical purposes but that is not encumbered with assumptions about essential racial dispositions.

It seems that despite the best efforts to erase the term *race*, it continues to be used, and it could be argued that this recreates the racial categories that antiracists are attempting to challenge. Carter (2000), for example, dissects the term *race* into different properties. The problem is the cultural construct "race" or the "idea of race" rather than its actual underlying and nonexistent reality. For Carter, race is used by both those who promote racist ideologies *and* those who are challenging it. There is, therefore, a type of progressive "race-ism" whereby such bodies as the Commission for Racial Equality use the term to challenge discrimination and promote race equality. His point is that how the term is used and in what context are as important as the term itself. Nonetheless, Carter further argues that both those who use it in racist terms and those who use it for progressive purposes are equally incorrect to use the term *race* because both reproduce the idea that race actually exists when it clearly does not.

"I'm Not a Racist But . . . "

It is not simply the word *race* that causes problems but related terms, such as immigration, asylum seekers, and so on, and part of the problem for any teaching strategy to tackle racism is its inaccessibility. In other words, there are ways of being discriminatory without being explicit about it. Language is never neutral but is used in sophisticated ways by human beings, who adapt their use of language to their social circumstances (Bourdieu, 1991; Fairclough, 1995).

Nurse researchers have found these ways of using language particularly difficult to analyse as few people within the profession would openly admit to racist attitudes, simply because it would be considered unprofessional and contrary to nurses' code of conduct. For example, Eliason and Raheim (2000), in their study of undergraduate prenursing students, were unable to detect awareness of racial and ethnic oppression but were sceptical about these findings, suggesting that what they may have been measuring was people's inhibitions and awareness of "politically correct" attitudes.

Van Dijk (1992) argues that one of the critical characteristics about contemporary racism is denial. Ethnic and racial prejudice is reproduced in everyday conversation and texts; Van Dijk argues that: "Such discourse serves to express, convey, legitimate or indeed to conceal or deny such negative ethnic attitudes" (p. 88). Hence, apparently neutral words such as *minorities, immigrants,* and *refugees* are used in ways that emphasise negative representations. These values are expressed both in everyday interactions and at broader social and institutional levels. For Van Dijk, the denial of racism is a crucial discursive strategy given that:

> General norms and values, if not the law, prohibit (blatant) forms of ethnic prejudice and discrimination, and many if not most white group members are both aware of such social constraints and, up to a point, even share and acknowledge them . . . Therefore, even the most blatantly racist discourse in our data routinely features denials or at least mitigations of racism. Interestingly, we have found that precisely the more racist discourse tends to have disclaimers and other denials. This suggests that language users who say negative things about minorities are well aware of the fact that they may be understood as breaking the social norm of tolerance and acceptance. (p. 89)

His central point is that we should be wary of people who begin sentences with "I have nothing against Blacks, but . . . " The ubiquitous "but" is usually a prelude to some rant about the very people whom the person is supposedly not prejudiced toward, but they are likely to soften their discourse by using neutral descriptive language. What is happening is that the discourse is used as a way of denying an enduring attitude of racism, an attitude that is considered unacceptable, but then the discourse focuses on specific situations, such as demands on welfare, illegal immigration, and criminal activity to justify the person's apparently non-prejudiced opinions.

The problem is that what is said is not always what is meant. Trying to encapsulate this is highly problematic. For example, the term *immigrant* in the United Kingdom is a term largely restricted to the far right, such as the British National Party, which uses the term as a defining characteristic of individuals, whereas the centre-right uses broader, collective terms such as *immigration*, but they may use the term *illegal immigrant* when referring to a person's legal status (Charteris-Black, 2006). The term *immigrant* therefore automatically connotes certain negative associations independent of the individual with his or her own experience and skills. Furthermore, Charteris-Black identifies two metaphors in relation to immigration: firstly, a metaphor of natural disaster, such as "flooding" or "swamping" or "tidal waves," and secondly, a metaphor of containment relating to a build-up of pressure, such as the country is full and unable to meet the demands of immigrants, a metaphor which then broadens into concepts of the "Nation" and "security."

The central point about these discourses is that apparently neutral language is used to objectify these social groups, to remove their own personal stories and narratives, and to carve out a metaphor of order that is threatened by outsiders with their own incompatible cultures. These metaphors have predominantly negative connotations, but what they also suggest is that much of the criticisms are based on notions of "culture" rather than any explicit use of racist language (Carter, 2000).

The term *culture* is also saturated with problems and is used across the political spectrum. For example, the British National Party in their mission statement refers to themselves as the "Torch bearers of culture," a culture that they see as appropriate to the "indigenous peoples of these islands . . . which have been our homeland for millennia" (British National Party, 2007, para. 1). By setting up clear criteria between British culture and other cultures, *culture* here is seen as a deterministic structure, an essential feature of who the British are, and as central to their identity. Softer versions of this can be found in Huntington's (1996) book, *The Clash of Civilizations and the Remaking of the World Order*, where this differentiation between people is a cultural determinant of who we are and where differences between cultures are the root of conflict at the local, national, and international level.

Although writers such as Huntington might think of these descriptions as reflecting a cultural reality, their rigid view of culture is as likely to produce fear and conflict and therefore create that reality. An alternative view sees culture as a flexible, interactive product of complex human narratives. As Archer (1996) argues, cultures pre-exist us, but they do not determine how we live within them or make sense of them, only that we have to deal with them. Furthermore, cultures are not homogenous; they are complex and our relationship to them is not predetermined. We may or may not change them, but how we interact with them is affected by the cultures we are a part of and what resources we have to engage, reproduce, and resist them. For example, associating Islam with fundamentalism is a common error and fails to grapple with the diverse ways in which Muslims interact with their belief system (Sutton & Vertigans, 2005). Dress codes are often regarded in the West as a form of oppression for women, and they can be problematic and act as a means of enforcing patriarchal values. But the wearing of the veil is a context-specific activity and can also be a means of resisting predominant oppressive and discriminatory practices. For example, in France, where school children were banned from wearing the Muslim headscarf, people were asserting their identity by wearing the headscarf. According to Terray (2004), the banning of this practice reflected the political hysteria of the French polity in which the Muslim community is systematically segregated in "pockets of misery and unemployment, ghetto schools, educational failure, discrimination in the job and housing markets, workplace racism—and, finally, the retinue of violence that these phenomena provoke in their victims, especially the young" (p. 120). In other words, the concept of women's oppression is reconfigured by the French authorities in a way that produces negative views about the Muslim community as a whole and erases the underlying context in which that community lives and reacts to the predominant culture. This strategy fails to either improve the position of women or challenge racism. It simply reproduces a set of stereotypes about Muslims that fails to take into account the complex ways that women within these communities live and experience their own culture and the predominant French culture. As Tobin (2007) argues, Muslim women are highly reflective about their own situation and position within their own culture, but they also draw on that same culture as a source of personal strength and resistance, which does not neatly fit into the universalistic principles espoused in the West.

What this suggests is that culture is a complex construct that interacts with notions about race. Indeed, *culture* can sometimes become a substitute term for *racism* (Carter, 2000). This means that culture should be understood as a complex and flexible reality, not a rigid set of rules. Gilroy (2000) captures these characteristics in the definition of diaspora:

> The idea of diaspora offers a ready alternative to the stern discipline of primordial kinship and rooted belonging. It rejects the popular image of natural nations spontaneously endowed with self-consciousness, tidily composed of uniform families: those interchangeable collections of ordered bodies that express and reproduce absolutely distinctive cultures as well as perfectly formed heterosexual pairings. As an alternative to the metaphysics of "race," nation, and bounded culture coded into the body, diaspora is a concept that problematizes the cultural and historical mechanics of belonging. (p. 123)

When these characteristics are applied to culture, the result is that:

> The notion of culture oscillates between a rigid deterministic structure that shapes and forms our behaviour and which is a source of division and distrust, through to a malleable, ever-changing and flexible product of sociohistorical circumstances. A strong attachment to culture can be a source of personal strength and collective resistance to a dominant culture or as a medium for oppression, intolerance and bigotry. (Nairn, Hardy, Paramul, & Williams, 2004, p. 190)

MULTICULTURALISM AND ANTIRACISM IN NURSING

This tension between race and culture is reflected in the way that educational strategies have been discussed in the nursing literature. It is taken as a given that lack of cultural sensitivity is an important issue for nurses, and it is also widely acknowledged that racism exists within the health care systems, although to what extent remains unclear (Fearfull & Kamenou, 2007; Kyriakides & Virdee, 2003; Likupe, 2006; Xu, 2007). Tackling this problem is more complex than any specific educational strategy, but much of the debate has been about the relative strengths and merits of a multicultural and an antiracist approach.

In the United Kingdom, *multiculturalism* as a term emerged in the 1960s as a response to racial discrimination in relation to employment, housing, and so forth. Multiculturalism was seen by minority communities as a means to attain social justice and oppose racism. Bourne (2007) argues that multiculturalism then became appropriated by governments in a way that erases the struggle against racism but emphasises the need to address cultural sensitivities. Furthermore, "It ceased to be an outcome of struggle for equality from below, and became, instead, policy imposed from above. And as the antiracist component ebbed, multiculturalism degenerated into a competitive culturalism or ethnicism which set different groups against one another as they competed for hand-outs from office" (p. 3). The result, according to Bourne, is that minority groups are then blamed for the types of divisions that the policies that were promoted by government produced. Bourne is nonetheless committed to multiculturalism but sees antiracism as a central component of a multiculturalist strategy. To remove racism from the equation nullifies the progressive element of a multicultural policy and becomes a resource for cultural division and isolation.

For nurses, the concept of multiculturalism has much to offer but has often been utilised in a way that softens the antiracist ideas that underpin its political edge. Nonetheless, multicultural or transcultural approaches have played and continue to be an important aspect of nurse education. For example, beginning in the 1970s, Leininger argued that a humanistic approach to nursing should include knowledge about culture-specific and culture-universal care practices to identify the cultural needs of patients. By approaching care in this way, nurses are empowered to appreciate that illness is not culture free, but responsive to the cultural understandings of patients. Patients' understanding and coping strategies are therefore influenced by their values and beliefs, and the way nurses manage these issues requires an understanding and sensitivity to patients' cultural needs (Leininger, 1994). There have been considerable developments in this approach to nursing, as shown in the work of Yoder (1996); Bhui and Bhugra (1998); Bengiamin, Downey, and Heuer (1999); Shumate (2001); Pinikahana, Manias, and Happell (2003); and Narayanasamy and White (2005). The emphasis in this work is on addressing misconceptions due to cultural differences, for example, cultural variations in eye contact and time consciousness, and on developing general sensitivity to patients' cultural distinctiveness.

Multicultural nursing is then conceptualised as "a strategy of caring which takes into account, with sensitivity and consideration, the individual's culture, specific values, beliefs and practices" (Narayanasamy, 2002, p. 643). This has generated a focus on models and teaching strategies that concentrate on cultural sensitivity. For example, Narayanasamy has developed a comprehensive model, the ACCESS model, for transcultural nursing practice. Abrums and Leppa (2001) outline the contents of a course on culture that emphasises how everyone, including White, middle-class students, are part of and have a culture. It is not a term only to be applied to minorities or subordinate groups as a way of relativising those cultures against some social norm, but every culture has its own dynamics and content that is as historically formed as any other culture. Normality is thus challenged and ethnocentrism undermined within a broader paradigm where culture is addressed through multiple perspectives. It is acknowledged within this approach that nurses cannot be expected to have comprehensive knowledge about all the different cultures they are likely to interact with, or understand the nuances of all those cultures, or anticipate individuals' sensitivities regarding what is or is not appropriate within their culture. What is important, therefore, is to show respect for another's culture and negotiate care in a way that genuinely values that person's belief system in relation to the nursing care provided (Narayanasamy, 2002).

Some, though not all, of these nurse theorists mention racism, but whether it is mentioned or not, it is certainly implicit to a cultural approach that in some way racism will be undermined through a strategy of mutual cultural respect and sensitivity. But, as I have already argued, the consequences of a multicultural approach are not as clear cut because the term *culture* can just as easily be interpreted in racist ways that create divisions as in ways that promote mutual respect. In other words, the emphasis on difference is inherently problematic. One cannot automatically draw out antiracist implications from a multicultural approach (Papadopoulos & Alleyne, 1995).

ESSENTIALISING CULTURE, SOCIAL STRUCTURE, AND THE PROBLEM OF RACISM

The central criticism of a multicultural approach is that it fails to acknowledge that culture is a contested concept. Culley (2006) argues that nurses are comfortable with the term *culture* as an appropriate aspect of individualised nursing care but are reluctant to challenge racism, which is a broader and more contentious term. Culley is particularly critical of the idea that culture can be defined as a set of checklists and guides to practice, rather than the emphasis being placed on culture as relational with internal and external pressures constantly changing and reshaping the way that people live within cultures. By emphasising the cultural needs of clients in relation to diet, religious requirements, and so forth, culture simply becomes "the functional equivalent of race" (p. 146), and a deterministic approach to culture ends up doing the work of biological racism. Therefore, culture becomes essentialised as a set of defined characteristics, rather than acknowledging the ways that individuals interact with, reproduce, change, and critique their own cultures (Culley, 2006). While this may be pushing the argument too far, nonetheless Culley usefully explores the logical consequences of multiculturalism. What is reflected is an ongoing tension between notions of race and culture and how its discursive uses remain at the centre of the problem.

Furthermore, multicultural approaches are also identified with a central assumption that we live in a society that is fair and equitable in terms of opportunity, individual freedom, and autonomy (Gustafson, 2005), but this is primarily an assumption, or perhaps more an ideology, of neoliberalism that often fails to be realised in everyday experiences:

> But even if denying equal human worth has gone out of fashion in public discourse, that doesn't mean it has disappeared from social practice. Indeed, one might say that one of the particular obscenities of our own age is that, while enormous lip-service is paid to the *idea* of equal respect, that idea is systematically violated as a routine feature of the social world. (Callinicos, 2006, p. 235)

In short, laws and ethical codes are not enough to ensure social justice. These codes exist within current social and structural systems, which it is argued restrict the opportunity to exercise one's rights. For example, private health care may be a right, but it is primarily dependent on ability to pay. In the previous example about Muslim headscarves, the right to dress according to one's culture or religion is restricted by systematic oppression and discriminatory practices. Liberal principles of equality have been used to resist affirmative action programs for Aboriginal people in Australia (Augoustinos, Tuffin, & Every, 2005), and job interviews can be constructed in such a way as to undermine foreign-born ethnic minority candidates (Campbell & Roberts, 2007).

So, while there is no formal discrimination, there is strong evidence that power relations that exist within social structures can be used in ways that restrict and reproduce discrimination. This can have direct health consequences. Mortality rates in the United States are affected by income but also fundamentally by ethnicity. So, White people at similar income levels as African Americans have lower mortality rates. When this type of relationship occurs, there is usually an identifiable relationship to social status (Marmot, 2004; Wilkinson, 1996), but it has also been argued that health inequalities have a specifically racist dimension in relation to notions of disrespect (Kennedy, Kawachi, Lochner, Jones, & Prothrow-Stith, 1997). So the day-to-day experience of being disrespected, of being reminded of one's status through everyday interactions, has direct consequences on people's sense of self-esteem, and as Marmot (2004) has noted, this has direct consequences for one's life chances.

These arguments go beyond the multicultural approach with its emphasis on cultural knowledge. What this suggests, therefore, is that the central problem of racism is related to oppressive practices in which dominant and subordinate discourses retain a liberal ideology of equality while systematically undermining that discourse in social practices. As Hagey and MacKay (2000) point out, when examining nursing discourse: "In the hierarchical scheme of whiteness and otherness there is a continuum, of lesser and lesser privilege and more domination/subordination and exclusion from resources and power" (p. 50). Dominant discourses include an emphasis on whiteness, normality, freedom, and control, while subordinate ones include otherness, marginalisation, and restrictions. Tackling these issues requires a more explicit approach to the issue of racism than the notion of cultural knowledge. Drevdahl (2001) has put together a course that explicitly examines concepts of race, theories about race, policies about race, and research issues. The introduction of ideas about race can be difficult to insert into a nursing curriculum, not least because of the potential to generate conflict within the classroom setting, but if it is true that racism is a problem within the health care system, then responding to it is a necessary component of nurse education. The content of such teaching remains uncertain, but the literature suggests a broad range of approaches and subjects (see Table 3.1). The central recommendations relate to directly addressing racism, acknowledging and respecting cultural differences, and incorporating them into nursing practice. This should be done in a way that does not essentialise culture, but recognises that culture is dynamic, that individuals interact with their culture in very personal ways, and that other dimensions, such as class and gender, interact with culture in important ways.

Table 3.1

RECOMMENDATIONS FROM THE LITERATURE

Curriculum must identify White privilege/dominance.	Eliason (1998); Le Var (1998); Tayebi, Moore-Jazayeri, and Maynard (1998); Hagey and MacKay (2000)
Curriculum should identify racism and promote antiracist teaching. As part of this process it should also critique cultural essentialism.	Alleyne, Papadopoulus, and Tilki (1994); Papadopoulus and Alleyne (1995); Culley (1996); Le Var (1998); and Drevdahl (2001)
The issue of institutional racism and the consequences for health care provision should be integrated into the curriculum.	Eliason (1998), Le Var (1998), Foolchand (2000), and Drevdahl (2001)
Students should have training in culturally sensitive care and develop knowledge about cultural beliefs in relation to health and illness.	Baldwin and Nelms (1993), Alleyne et al. (1994), Papadopoulos and Alleyne (1995), Bhui and Bhugra (1998), Eliason (1998), Le Var (1998), Bengiamin et al. (1999), and Shumate (2001)
Policies and procedures should be in place for actual or perceived instances of racism to be addressed so that students can access appropriate support.	Anfinson (1999)
Mentor programme of support should be put in place specifically to support minority students.	Anfinson (1999)

(*Continued*)

Table 3.1 *Continued*

Workshops and seminars should be introduced for staff as well as students.	Anfinson (1999)
Curriculum should have a focus on improving cross-cultural communication skills.	Papadopoulos and Alleyne (1995) and Le Var (1998)
The subject of culture should be integrated into the curriculum as a core theme.	Le Var (1998) and Shumate (2001)
International exchanges of students should be encouraged and universities should develop links with overseas educational institutions.	Le Var (1998)
Numbers of Black nurses and Black applicants should be monitored so that recruitment strategies can be deployed.	Le Var (1998)
Involve students with people who have direct experience of racism. Invite outside speakers, etc.	Baldwin and Nelms (1993)
Encourage manufacturers to produce ethnically diverse manikins for resuscitation training.	Shumate (2001)
Critique nursing textbooks for racial bias.	Byrne (2001)

From "Multicultural or Anti-Racist Teaching in Nurse Education: A Critical Appraisal," by S. Nairn, C. Hardy, L. Paramul, & G. A. Williams, 2004, *Nurse Education Today, 24,* pp. 188–195. Reprinted with permission from Elsevier.

RECOMMENDATIONS FOR CHALLENGING RACISM

The recommendations in Table 3.1 come from a range of literature, but only a few of these authors have evaluated their work, usually through questioning the students who were exposed to their interventions and documenting which ones students responded to positively. These studies certainly enhance our understanding of the subject and provide useful pointers toward educational strategies within a nursing curriculum. However, in terms of outcome measures, none of these studies has really evaluated how effective these curriculum strategies have been in encouraging nurses to be culturally sensitive or in overcoming racist attitudes. An adequate evaluation must take into account the multiple contexts in which the problem arises, identify the specific influences of the intervention, and then identify realistic outcome measures (Pawson & Tilley, 1997).

However, as Narayanasamy and White (2005) argue, while there has been progress in developing educational strategies to promote cultural sensitivity and respect toward people of diverse ethnicities, they suggest that it will take "generations to reshape attitudes and behaviours" (p. 107). Any attempt at measuring interventions is highly problematic because educational interventions exist within a complex and ever-changing set of social, economic, and historical circumstances. Furthermore, as has been argued in this chapter, racism is often a concealed attitude resulting in denial. In fact, it often seems that people who make racist comments are often unaware of the implications of what they are saying and are genuinely perplexed by charges of racism. This makes the problem of measurement very difficult, to the point where some researchers question their own results, seeing them as reflecting attitudes of political correctness and a consciousness of stigma rather than representing real beliefs and attitudes (Eliason & Raheim, 2000).

Given the multiple contexts in which students experience the world and the variety of educational interventions employed by nurse educators, and then the difficulty of analysing outcomes from these interventions in anything other than very local contexts, it is always going to be difficult to determine what has and has not been effective in challenging racism and promoting cultural sensitivity. Furthermore, changing attitudes and practice in areas such as culture will always come up against what is essentially a conflict over values, and these are never stable and do not always develop in progressive ways. Only the most optimistic academic could believe that educational interventions on their own would be an effective means of overcoming oppressive practices, but such interventions are nonetheless an integral part of nursing education based on the moral belief and ethical obligation to deliver high-quality care to all patients, regardless of their ethnic background.

There are sound and compelling reasons for including antiracist and multicultural strategies in nurse education, including the need to reinforce the professionalism of nursing, provide culturally sensitive care, and identify and then challenge instances of racism. Multicultural approaches should be a central component of nurse education, but these approaches also have important limitations because they have the potential to reproduce cultural essentialism. Antiracist approaches are not antithetical to multicultural approaches and, indeed, are essential to them. As Bourne (2007) has pointed out, the undermining of multiculturalism is precisely because its antiracist component has been neutralised into a benign discourse of egalitarianism in which power relations are neutralised within a discourse of cultural difference. Also, while codes and policies that emphasise equality are a ubiquitous feature of the current political climate, their efficacy is undermined by structural inequality and cultural values that reproduce dominant and subordinate discourses. Educational interventions have the potential to empower students to address these issues in their own practice and identify areas where cultural values are disrespected so that care can be both sensitive to culture and yet also identify and challenge racism. Such a strategy is modest in that it acknowledges the reality of factors outside educators' control, where racism exists within a changing and contested cultural value system, but also argues that nurses have a moral duty to recognise the cultural needs of patients and to challenge racism both within themselves and in others and thus positively contribute to a broader cultural context of tolerance and difference.

QUESTIONS FOR DIALOGUE

1. What ideas or concepts did you find most meaningful in this chapter? Identify your insights and questions to bring to a dialogue with your colleagues.
2. Nairn states that racism "is not necessarily explicit, but . . . it emerges in other ways, usually by emphasising cultural differences." Identify examples of this in nursing curricula and texts.
3. Why is emphasizing cultural differences a barrier to antiracist education? Consider why an antiracist education approach is essential in nursing education.
4. How does your program define and address cultural diversity in nursing? To what extent does your program challenge or promote essentialist notions of culture? Give specific examples.
5. What pedagogical strategies are in place in your program to help students and faculty identify and overcome racist attitudes in nursing?

6. Give specific examples of ways in which "apparently neutral words such as minorities, immigrants, and refugees" are used to "emphasise negative representations." Consider recent conversations, faculty meetings, news reports, and curricular materials as possible sources of examples.

REFERENCES

Abrums, M. E., & Leppa, C. (2001). Beyond cultural competence: Teaching about race, gender, class, and sexual orientation. *Journal of Nursing Education, 40*(6), 270–275.

Alleyne, J., Papadopoulos, I., & Tilki, M. (1994). Antiracism within transcultural nurse education. *British Journal of Nursing, 3*(12), 635–637.

Anfinson, J. (1999). Nursing students' perceptions regarding differences in the clinical learning experience that relate to minority-racial status. *Journal of National Black Nurses Association, 10*(1), 56–67.

Archer, M. (1996). *Culture and agency: The place of culture in social theory* (Rev. ed.). Cambridge: Cambridge University Press.

Augoustinos, M., Tuffin, K., & Every, D. (2005). New racism, meritocracy and individualism: Constraining affirmative action in education. *Discourse and Society, 16*(3), 315–340.

Baldwin, D., & Nelms, T. (1993). Difficult dialogues: Impact on nursing education curricula. *Journal of Professional Nursing, 9*(6), 343–346.

Bengiamin, M. I., Downey, W., & Heuer, L. J. (1999). Transcultural healthcare: A phenomenological study of an educational experience. *Journal of Cultural Diversity, 6*(2), 60–68.

Bhopal, R. (2003). *A contribution to discussion on a national electronic library on ethnicity and health.* Retrieved December 12, 2007, from http://www2.warwick.ac.uk/fac/med/research/csri/ethnicityhealth/aspects_diversity/bhopal.pdf

Bhui, K., & Bhugra, D. (1998). Training and supervision in effective cross-cultural mental health services. *Hospital Medicine, 59*(11), 861–865.

Bourdieu, P. (1991). *Language & symbolic power.* Cambridge: Polity Press.

Bourne, J. (2007, February). *In defence of multiculturalism.* Institute of Race Relations Briefing Paper No. 2. London: Institute of Race Relations.

British National Party. (2007). *The British National Party.* Retrieved November 11, 2007, from http://www.bnp.org.uk

Byrne, M. M. (2001). Uncovering racial bias in nursing fundamentals textbooks. *Nursing and Health Care Perspectives, 22*(6), 299–303.

Callinicos, A. (2006). *The resources of critique.* Cambridge: Polity Press.

Campbell, S., & Roberts, C. (2007). Migration, ethnicity and competing discourses in the job interview: Synthesizing the institutional and personal. *Discourse and Society, 18*(3), 243–271.

Carter, B. (2000). *Realism and racism: Concepts of race in sociological research.* London: Routledge.

Charteris-Black, J. (2006). Britain as a container: Immigration metaphors in the 2005 election campaign. *Discourse and Society, 17*(5), 563–581.

Culley, L. (1996). A critique of multiculturalism in health care: The challenge for nurse education. *Journal of Advanced Nursing, 23*(3), 564–570.

Culley, L. (2006). Transcending transculturalism? Race, ethnicity and healthcare. *Nursing Inquiry, 13*(2), 144–153.

Drevdahl, D. (2001). Teaching about race, racism, and health. *Journal of Nursing Education, 40*(6), 285–288.

Eliason, M. J. (1998). Correlates of prejudice in nursing students. *Journal of Nursing Education, 37*(1), 27–29.

Eliason, M. J., & Raheim, S. (2000). Experiences and comfort with culturally diverse groups in undergraduate pre-nursing students. *Journal of Nursing Education, 39*(4), 161–165.

Fairclough, N. (1995). *Critical discourse analysis: The critical study of language.* Harlow: Longman.

Fearfull, A., & Kamenou, N. (2007). Exploring the policy and research implications for the British National Health service and its customers. *Equal Opportunities International, 26*(4), 305–318.

Foolchand, M. K. (2000). The role of the Department of Health and other key institutions in the promotion of equal opportunities, multi-cultural and anti-racist issues in nurse education. *Nurse Education Today, 20,* 443–448.

Gilroy, P. (2000). *Between camps: Nations, cultures and the allure of race.* London: Allen Lane.

Gustafson, D. L. (2005). Transcultural nursing theory from a critical cultural perspective. *Advances in Nursing Science, 28*(1), 2–16.

Hagey, R., & MacKay, R. W. (2000). Qualitative research to identify racialist discourse: Towards equity in nursing curricula. *International Journal of Nursing Studies, 37,* 45–56.

Huntington, S. P. (1996). *The clash of civilizations and the remaking of the world order.* London: Simon & Schuster.

Kennedy, B. P., Kawachi, I., Lochner, M. S., Jones, C. & Prothrow-Stith, D. (1997). (Dis)respect and Black mortality. *Ethnicity and Disease, 7,* 207–214.

Kyriakides, C., & Virdee, S. (2003). Migrant labour, racism and the British National Health Service. *Ethnicity and Health, 8*(4), 283–305.

Leininger, M. (1994). *Transcultural nursing: Concepts, theories and practices.* Columbus, OH: Greyden Press.

Le Var, R.M.H. (1998). Improving educational preparation for transcultural healthcare. *Nurse Education Today, 18,* 519–533.

Likupe, G. (2006). Experiences of African nurses in the UK National Health Service: A literature review. *Journal of Clinical Nursing, 15,* 1213–1220.

Marmot, M. (2004). *Status syndrome: How your social standing directly affects your health and life expectancy.* London: Bloomsbury.

Nairn, S., Hardy, C., Paramul, L., & Williams, G. A. (2004). Multicultural or anti-racist teaching in nurse education: A critical appraisal. *Nurse Education Today, 24,* 188–195.

Narayanasamy, A. (2002). The ACCESS model: A transcultural nursing practice framework. *British Journal of Nursing, 11*(9), 643–650.

Narayanasamy, A., & White, E. (2005). A review of transcultural nursing. *Nurse Education Today, 25,* 102–111.

Papadopoulos, I., & Alleyne, J. (1995). The need for nursing and midwifery programmes of education to address the health care needs of minority ethnic groups. *Nurse Education Today, 15,* 140–144.

Pawson, R., & Tilley, N. (1997). *Realistic evaluation.* London: Sage.

Pinikahana, J., Manias, E., & Happell, B. (2003). Transcultural nursing in Australian nursing curricula. *Nursing and Health Sciences, 5,* 149–154.

Proctor, R. N. (1988). *Racial hygiene: Medicine under the Nazis.* Cambridge, MA: Harvard University Press.

Shumate, P. L. (2001). Cultural and ethnic diversity: Unique challenges in critical care education. *Critical Care Nursing Clinics of North America, 13*(1), 63–72.

Sickle Cell Society. (2004). *What is sickle cell anemia?* Retrieved November 21, 2007, from http://sicklecellsociety.org/education/sicklecell.htm

Skinner, D. (2007). Groundhog day? The strange case of sociology, race and 'science.' *Sociology, 41,* 931–943.

Smedley, A., & Smedley, B. D. (2005, January). Race as biology is fiction, racism as a social problem is real. *American Psychologist, 60*(1), 16–26.

Sutton, P., & Vertigans, S. (2005). *Resurgent Islam: A sociological approach.* Cambridge: Polity Press.

Tayebi, K., Moore-Jazayeri, M., & Maynard, T. (1998). From the borders: Reforming the curriculum for the at-risk student. *Journal of Cultural Diversity, 5*(3), 101–109.

Terray, T. (2004, March/April). Headscarf hysteria. *New Left Review, 26,* 118–127.

Tobin, T. W. (2007, Summer). On their own ground: Strategies of resistance for Sunni Muslim women. *Hypatia, 22*(3), 152–174.

Van Dijk, T. A. (1992). Discourse and the denial of racism. *Discourse and Society, 3*(1), 87–118.

Wilkinson, R. G. (1996). *Unhealthy societies: The afflictions of inequality.* London: Routledge.

Williams, D. R. (1997). Race and health: Basic questions, emerging directions. *Annals of Epidemiology, 7,* 322–333.

Xu, Y. (2007). Strangers in a strange land: A metasynthesis of lived experiences of immigrant Asian nurses working in Western countries. *Advances in Nursing Science, 30*(3), 246–265.

Yoder, M. K. (1996). Instructional responses to ethnically diverse nursing students. *Journal of Nursing Education, 35*(7), 315–321.

4

Minority Nurses: A Story of Resilience and Perseverance

DONNA HILL-CILL

BECOMING A NURSE: LESSONS LEARNED

As I walked into the elevator, I brushed off my new black suit, flipped out my mirror, and straightened my posture. I took another look inside my briefcase to assure myself that I had three copies of my résumé. I began to recite my years of employment history and how they related to teaching. I smiled as I remembered all of my jobs and experiences in nursing school. What a long road . . . look how far I have come. Am I ready to educate others?

Standing in the elevator, I began to recall my first class in nursing school. I had attended an LPN program in Orlando, Florida. I was 30 minutes early. There was only one other girl in the room; she smiled as I took my seat. I sat down waiting and wondering. Would I be able to handle the course work? Is this what I really want to do? I have made so many mistakes; will this be another one? By returning to school, it felt like my life was taking a dramatic turn overnight.

At the very lowest point of my life, 18 years old, pregnant, and without paternal support, I learned a habit that would help me throughout my years in nursing school and, most importantly, throughout life. This habit is called resilience.

Resilience

Searching for nursing schools had been disheartening; applying for grants, financial aid, and monies to attend school had also been difficult. Feeling down and low, I called multiple schools, ready to make the first step to a better life for me and my unborn child. Many calls resulted in disappointment: There were waiting lists, no scholarships, missed deadlines, and so forth. Each phone call and disappointment broke me down further. In life, when you're down, any negative comment can destroy you. I wanted to give up! But, to my surprise, each time I gave up and stopped calling, my spirit wouldn't allow me to forget about my dreams. So I would cry and call again. After a while I realized that I had to change my attitude because, if I didn't, I would become depressed. So, I made a conscious decision. Because I could not change the negative comments, I needed to change myself. How could I do that? I realized then that I could change the way I reacted to those comments.

It's like the old saying: "The only person you can change is yourself." I had to remember not to take it personally. I created an action plan to accomplish the change I needed to make. I created a visual copy of my goal, written very large and in bold. It read: "I AM GOING TO BE AN RN." Underneath the quote were the steps it would take to accomplish this goal. I took this piece of paper with me every time I made my calls, went to my interviews, or visited a school. Whenever I received a negative response, I looked at my visual, took a deep breath, said a quick prayer, and said out loud: "I am going to be an RN." In retrospect, I was verbally reinforcing myself. After a while, I didn't need the visual or the verbal reinforcement. It had become ingrained in me.

I can remember the first time I confronted an issue without my visual action plan. I started to make a call and, as the phone began to ring, I remembered I didn't have my paper. It was too late; someone had already answered on the other end. My initial response was fear of rejection, but then I remembered my goal; although it was not on the piece of paper, it was embedded in my mind. I became solid, secure, and ready for any response. I realized then that I had been building up my confidence, which in turn gave me the resilience I needed to succeed. So I continued to call, sometimes three or four times, until I received what I needed to accomplish my goals.

I snapped back into reality; what a daydream! I was still on the elevator and I had not even pressed the number of the floor. I pressed 5, and up I went. My stomach dropped from the instant jerk of the elevator, which reminded me of the anxiety I had felt as a student nurse in the LPN program. In this program, I was greeted by other minority students who looked like me. It was the very first time that I was in the majority in an academic setting. In addition to the importance of resilience, the other lesson I learned from this experience was validation.

Validation

Every clinical day, I would cling to my friend Marie, who had the confidence of a well-equipped army. She was a crutch for me. Marie had worked as a nurse's aide for years, so she was familiar with the hospital setting. Every clinical day for me was a challenge; although I did a good job, I often second-guessed things I did. This would cause me to take twice the time to accomplish a goal. I always felt more comfortable with someone at my side. Marie was always there for me, checking on me, and assuring me that I was all right.

One day, Marie said, "Donna, someone is going to say something about me always helping you."

Immediately tears came to my eyes, and I replied, "I know, but I am so scared and unsure of everything; it is all so overwhelming." Marie agreed but told me that I needed to gain confidence. It all made sense, but I figured I needed time to gain the confidence I needed. Then the day of dread occurred! One clinical day, my professor asked me to complete a task.

Nervous, I looked up at her at each step for validation. She nodded and said, "You know it, now do it! From now on, do your work independently."

In my evaluation, she wrote that I needed to work independently. She then put her pen down, took off her dark-rimmed glasses, looked me straight into the eyes, and said, "You have what it takes." My mind raced with thoughts of inadequacy, but my heart was full of joy. My professor saw in me something I wondered if I even possessed. I knew I had worked hard on the clinical unit, read my textbook, and gave 150%, but I didn't know if I "had what it takes." Those five words changed the way I perceived myself as a potential nurse and as a person.

My thoughts of inadequacy changed to thoughts of grandeur. Why did such a transformation occur? Because someone who I modeled myself after, my clinical professor, who was a confident, intelligent, and enthusiastic educator, saw in me what I thought I possessed but wasn't sure. Those were the words I needed to succeed. They gave me the edge to believe and feel that I was skilled and that I could practice safely and independently. So I began to walk taller, smile wider, and exude the confidence I needed because I had been validated.

Another jerk. The elevator stopped on the second floor, and the doors opened. A group of students screeched, "You going down?"

"Sorry, I am on my way up," I replied. The elevator doors closed as the students resumed their conversations. I giggled to myself, as I remembered the laughter on the pediatric unit at a hospital in Orlando. I was in the LPN to RN transition program. I had enrolled in this program almost 2 years after completing the LPN program. My friend Keri and I commuted in together as we lived in the same neighborhood. Keri was from Africa, and she was very intelligent. She had a prior degree in business and had returned to school for nursing. We spoke about many things—politics, history, and, of course, nursing. Keri's husband was a civil engineer at a *Fortune* 500 company; she went to school full time and concentrated on her studies.

The hospital was an excellent teaching facility that provided state-of-the-art specialty services for women and children. On any given day, the hospital was swamped with physical therapists, respiratory therapists, residents, nurses, and medical interns and externs. Keri and I received our assignments. I cared for a 2-year-old near-drown victim with brain stem injury. I was overwhelmed by his sad history and prognosis. Keri cared for an 18-month-old with acute exacerbation of asthma. The patient was awake and alert but needed frequent respiratory therapy treatment.

The day seemed to move slowly; at the end of clinical, the instructor asked Keri to stay behind. I waited, too, as it was Keri's turn to drive. I sat and waited for Keri as she spoke to our clinical instructor; every minute seemed like an hour. Finally, after 20 minutes, Keri walked toward me with her head down, carrying a yellow form, and handed me her keys. I took the keys and handed them back to Keri and began my spiel . . . that I do not drive others' vehicles. Then she raised her head, and I saw she had tears swelling in her eyes and rolling down her face . . . I took the keys back and got in the driver's seat.

As soon as we sat in the car, Keri began to cry from the heart, groaning and grasping the dashboard. I turned to her as she began to repeat, "I cannot believe this is happening to me."

"What is happening to you?" I asked.

She handed me the yellow form. I unfolded it and, in the center of the paper, read "Clinical Failure."

"What is this?" I asked. I knew that Keri held over a B average, she was an active participant in class, and she had no previous infractions in the clinical area.

Between the crying, Keri began to tell the story. Our instructor had walked into the room of Keri's patient and had seen the 18-month-old child in the crib with one side rail down.

"Wow!" I interrupted with a scream. "Nursing 101 tells you when it comes to patients, especially pediatrics, safety comes first." Keri looked up at me and continued her story. The instructor was appalled . . . pulled up the side rail and ran to Keri to tell her the findings. Keri informed the instructor that the side rails had been up and that the patient's mother had been in the room when she left the child. The instructor continued to scold Keri for the irresponsible act and told her she would address it after clinical. Keri was overwhelmed with sadness. How could she fight this, her word against what the instructor thought? Keri began to cry louder and harder, repeating the words, "I've worked so hard!"

I began to question myself: Didn't Keri's reputation of clinical and scholastic excellence account for, at the very least, the benefit of the doubt? Given that this facility caters to so many disciplines, couldn't it have been a resident, physical therapist, or the patient's mother who left the side rail down? Because the patient was safe, this was a first incident for Keri, and there was no proof that she had left the side rail down, I felt a clinical warning would have been much more appropriate. This would be one of many times that I would lose a colleague to a similar unjust situation.

Strength Against Adversity

Keri never filed an appeal, feeling as if she would not be heard. She wondered what made the instructor fail her. She felt the burden of adversity. She wondered if this unjust decision was due to her race; if she went in front of the dean (who was not a minority), would she win? If she won, would she be tainted throughout the program? These events happen far too often, and each time one is left to wonder if it is you or your race. As educators, we must bond together on the common ground of nursing that ties us together and concentrate on being strong, fierce nurses. We must learn to draw strength from each other's race and look past judging and try to understand. By doing this, we may find we are more alike than we once thought.

Keri chose to persevere by enrolling in a different nursing program.

Perseverance

"Bing," the elevator rang. I finally arrived on the fifth floor. The walls were gleaming with freshly colored yellow paint. I stepped off the elevator and passed a room. I was looking for Room 525. My anxiety began to rise as I approached the room and saw two women smiling at me. I walked toward them; they extended their hands as they recited their names, "Hi, I am Karen," and she pointed to her office mate, "This is Annie." I shook their hands as they offered me a seat. The office was small; it held two medium-size desks that were artfully decorated with family photographs and clever quotes. The walls were covered with professionally framed certifications, diplomas, and the one that caught my eye—the award from the international honor society for nursing, "Sigma Theta Tau."

Holding a high GPA, I had awaited an invitation in undergraduate school to Sigma Theta Tau. I had worked hard, belonged to many organizations, and even worked with one of the major research teams on campus. I was a model student and was excited that invitations were finally going out. I checked my mailbox at least twice daily, until I realized I had been skipped over. Confused, I went to my counselor to assure that I met the requirements for invitation; she assured me that I was a top candidate. I spoke to nonminority classmates who held lower GPAs than myself and were in no organizations, yet, they had received invitations to join Sigma Theta Tau.

I went to the Dean for an explanation but to no avail. Her explanation was vague and nonspecific; she didn't empathize with my situation. I didn't understand how this could have happened. There was only one explanation I could ascertain: selection was determined on a subjective basis, and bias can overshadow justice. I was saddened but not defeated.

Two years later, in graduate school, I was checking my correspondence, and there was my invitation to Sigma Theta Tau! My heart lit up with pride. I didn't even know induction time was near. I had honestly forgotten about my hope to be a part of such a prestigious organization. The only thing that chimed in my head over and over was:

> "What is for you cannot be against you."
>
> —Donna Hill-Cill

I refocused my attention on Karen and Annie as the interview began. "So, Donna, it's great you could make it on such short notice," Karen said with a smile. She paused, shifted her head to the left slightly, leaned toward me, and with her blue eyes gazed at my face. She exhaled and with extreme sincerity, she said, "We're so glad you're here." In response, I smiled and relaxed slightly in my chair.

I understood then that they had been waiting for more than an educator; they were waiting for "a role model." I reached into my briefcase and handed them two crisp copies of my résumé. They smiled as they showed me their photocopied version of the résumé I had e-mailed to them with my online application. The interview went well, and within one month I was educating student nurses in the RN program for clinical pediatrics.

BECOMING A NURSE EDUCATOR: LESSONS LEARNED

In my career as a nurse educator, I have learned many lessons on how nursing faculty can support minority students toward professional success and personal well-being. The next five vignettes pertain to lessons I have found to be essential for student learning: teaching accountability, confronting the adversity of racism, recognizing talent and promoting self-efficacy, being a mentor, and understanding cultural and social dynamics.

Lesson One: Teaching Accountability

When I received my first position as a nurse educator, I reviewed about 50 journals, 10 pediatric textbooks, and my notes. I purchased pediatric pocket guides and, of course, a brand new penlight. I was prepared for my first clinical day with eight students at a premier hospital in the heart of Newark, New Jersey. I was ready for the challenge. I called the dean of the nursing school that morning, as clinical was not until 5:30 P.M., to ensure that the students would be meeting me in the lobby of the hospital. I wore a soft, pink sweater with my pearl necklace, earrings, black tapered slacks, sleek black socks, and comfortable black loafers. I had a freshly starched lab coat with my name and credentials on my left pocket. My braids were neatly pulled back in a black clip. I looked in the mirror and smiled; I was ready for work. "Who would have thought," I said to myself, "that I would be educating others?"

> "Being subtle, at times, can bring about the greatest changes."
>
> —Donna Hill-Cill

As I walked into the lobby, I immediately noticed two students; I walked over to them and greeted them with a smile. I introduced myself and told them to wait. It was still very early, so I would check the room for preconference. I went and set up the room. I returned 15 minutes later to see seven of the eight students in the lobby. I walked over to them and introduced myself. There was one male and five females; some students much older than I. I led them into the room, and as they sat down, I excused myself to look one last time for the missing student.

There she was: a tall, thin, dark-skinned girl with shoulder-length hair, asking security for information. At this point the student was over 30 minutes late. I approached her, greeting her as her clinical professor. She smiled with relief. I then asked, "Why are you late?" (Rule #1: Accountability.) As she explained about the traffic, I listened intently. Immediately, my demeanor changed. I wiped my smile off, stepped closer toward her, raised my eyebrows, and with the most serious tone I said, "My job is to teach you nursing; one aspect of this profession is timeliness. YOU MUST be on time!" I stepped back and stated with a smile, "Now, let's join your peers." This student had a very successful semester, and most importantly, she was never late again.

As I stood in front of the room, reviewing the syllabus, I saw eyes of pride. I was now that clinical instructor I once admired: confident, intelligent, and soon to be an enthusiastic educator. I saw the inner glow of minority students as they watched my every move, wrote down my every word, and laughed at my every joke. I knew then that I was where I needed to be. As educators, we often want to ensure that our students are learning the theoretical and clinical components necessary to learn. But what I have noticed is that some of the greatest learning techniques have nothing to do with theory but involve self-efficacy and validation of one's self-worth and a greater understanding of oneself. Seeing me as a minority educator in front of the class made the minority students realize they could "make it," too. They experienced an increased sense of self-efficacy. This validation also involves recognizing the students' talents, telling them their strengths each step of the way to ensure they reach their goal, and coaching them on how to move through experiences of discrimination and racism.

Lesson Two: Confronting the Adversity of Racism

"The ground is no place for a champion."

—Mohammed Ali

Sheena

Sheena stood five feet tall, with copper skin, long, dark black hair that was shielded by her head scarf, a kind smile, and laugh lines that highlighted her 50-plus years of life. Sheena is Indian and Muslim from South America. This was her second attempt to complete a nursing program after having transferred from a community college where she held a borderline GPA. Sheena's magic was not in her grades; it was in her warm smile and gentle touch. She was in my clinical group for her first upper-division course, Nursing Fundamentals. Her first 3 days of clinical were a success; she completed her assigned tasks of bathing her patients, giving meds, explaining the disease process, and implementing her plan of care. All the patients were satisfied, and so was I. The fourth clinical day was here, and I gave Sheena her assignment: "Sheena, this will be an easy day for you. You are assigned to Mrs. Davis in 205B; she is a 56-year-old White female, status post-appendectomy." We discussed her plan of care for the patient and expected outcomes.

After an hour had passed, Sheena approached me. Her eyes were saddened, and she appeared exhausted and uncertain of herself. She said, "The patient is requesting not to have a student." At times there are patients who don't want students, but this patient had previously agreed to take a student when asked by the staff. I wondered what could have happened. I decided to speak with the patient to do "damage control." I needed to be sure that the student hadn't done anything wrong. As I walked toward the room, the primary nurse stopped me in my tracks. "Donna, the patient doesn't want *that* student; she said the student smells like curry." I stopped and gasped as I realized that this was more than not wanting a student. I turned back and asked Sheena what happened. Sheena told me that when she was in the patient's room reviewing her vitals on the clip chart, the patient had questioned why she was reading her chart and demanded that Sheena put the chart down.

The answer was evident here: racism. How should I respond to this event? I was hurt and offended, and I empathized with my student. I never told Sheena the patient's comment about her smelling of curry. That comment was extremely inappropriate and furthermore was not true.

I could see in Sheena's eyes that she was disappointed. She assured me that she had taken all the correct steps in engaging with and caring for her patient, and from her past clinical performance, I believed her. Also, her patient never complained to the nurse about any negative interaction or care.

I was now ready to speak with the patient to ensure that I wasn't making any assumptions. I knocked and waited for my cue to enter. I greeted the patient by her surname and introduced myself. I started by saying, "My goal is to assure that the student took the correct measures in providing you the best care; can you tell me if this is so?"

The patient appeared aloof and stated very flatly, "I just do not want a student." I thanked the patient for her time and asked if there was anything I could get for her before I left. She exhaled and stated, "No." I walked out of the room, my assessment having been confirmed; this patient was biased against the student.

I motioned for Sheena to follow me into another room to speak. We spoke about diversity, and as we spoke, two other minority students who were aware of the situation asked to join us. My first goal was to reassure Sheena that she was not at fault; she was a victim of a racist or culturally biased incident. My second goal was to release Sheena from ownership of another person's misguided notion toward people of different cultures.

My final and most important goal was to assist Sheena and the other students present to deal with these situations in a professional manner. I guaranteed them only one thing: that this type of incident WOULD happen at least once again in the future.

"Seek first to understand, then to be understood."

—Stephen Covey (1998)

Some people may doubt you or have negative feelings toward you because you are different from them. That person could be your patient. First line strategy is to educate. Educate your patient about what you are doing and why; educate them of their diagnosis, medications, and plan of care. This strategy will dispel myths about incompetence. Some may argue that one should not have to prove oneself. I believe one of the best ways to combat ignorance is education.

Second line strategy is to shower the person with kindness; this is a strategy I learned from my mother who is a registered nurse and a Christian. This strategy involves constantly checking on your patients to ask if there is anything else you can do for them. Do things for them that you would do for all of your patients despite their negative behavior. And most importantly, keep reminding yourself, "This is not about me, I am a professional nurse."

After a while, they will look at you without seeing just the color of your skin and see you as they should: as a person. Hopefully through the first strategy of education, they will see that you are competent, and that will dispel myths of incapability. Your kindness will hopefully allow them to look inside themselves and see themselves for who they are. If that doesn't occur, one should seek the last strategy.

The last and most difficult strategy is confrontation, not directly but indirectly. If a patient makes a racist or otherwise inappropriate comment, ask them in an unassuming tone: "What do you mean by that?" Don't move and be silent. This is a strong and powerful question if asked correctly. Sometimes people are not aware of their own prejudice or bias . . . this is a friendly reminder, one that forces them to explain their behavior.

As a nurse, I have used these strategies, and they have worked for me for over 11 years. In only one incident did I need a reassignment, and only on a few occasions did I need to resort to strategy three.

Lesson Three: Recognizing Talent and Promoting Self-Efficacy

"Our crown has been there already, now pick up the crown and wear it."
—Oprah Winfrey

Sky Blue

In her mid-20s, Sky Blue stood 5'9" tall with shoulder-length, thick, black hair. She wore glasses and a big bright smile. Her demeanor was always cheerful and filled with spunk. She is Dominican, of African descent. She came to the nursing program after obtaining a bachelor's degree in exercise physiology. Sky's grades were a B average before entering upper division. Now, in her first nursing fundamentals course, she faced challenges to keep her grades up; however, clinically her skills were excellent. As I watched Sky interact with her patient, look in the chart, and speak with the primary nurse, I stopped her and said, "Sky, you have what it takes; you think like a nurse."

As an educator, I often utilize a technique I call "blind student–student mentorship." I partner a weak clinical student with a stronger clinical student, without the students realizing why. I utilized Sky in these partnerships as the stronger clinical student; the other student always benefited a great deal from their interaction.

Unfortunately, Sky's theory grades were low, so she failed the course. Sad for Sky, I had a talk with her. To my surprise, she was very optimistic, not discouraged, and had already applied to another nursing program. She explained to me that in her sophomore year of college, her science professor had told her she could never be a doctor. Due to this comment, she then changed her major to exercise physiology. She told me how she regretted listening to him and how she would never allow that discouragement to prevail again.

Her explanation for her failure was simply that the school did not match with her learning style. What I admired most about Sky was her ability to stare defeat in the face and move forward with conviction. John Maxwell (2007) states in *Failing Forward: Turning Mistakes into Stepping Stones for Success* that achievers have one thing in common: the ability to bounce back after a failure.

I caught up with Sky 1 year later. Not only had she become an excellent academic student, but she was also a delegate for the student nursing association for her school and had been chosen for a state position as "Break Through to Nursing" director. In this role she recruited minority students, with a strong push on recruiting males into the profession.

In a blink, I had seen in Sky what was now unfolding—that she had talent and could make it. She has often told me she never forgot what I said, that she thought like a nurse. It truly made a difference. I remember the day I said it to her; she paused and smiled and thanked me. I told her to thank herself for her hard work and commitment to nursing.

It is our duty as educators to utilize and trust our "gut judgment." At times this knee-jerk response is different than the current picture that is painted for us—that a student is a failure because she or he has failed in academic coursework. We should see beyond that and recognize what is truly there. Many times, others paint the picture, or they plant seeds of doubt in our head. Negative words reinforce our already doubtful mind. As a minority, you are constantly proving yourself because history has it that we were less. Unfortunately, other cultures still view us that way today. So when you fail, many emotions surface. You ask yourself: "Am I really a failure? Can I be successful?" We must learn to trust our judgment, reinforce positive behavior, and build a layer of resistance to failure. We must feel at peace with what our gut is saying, and at that moment and only then, will we excel.

In his book *Blink,* Malcolm Gladwell (2005) speaks of adaptive unconsciousness and the power of thinking without thinking. He speaks about how this thinking often times is more reliable than our cognitive process. Embracing this power within me to think without thinking has allowed me to make better decisions and to respect my judgment calls, especially when working with students who might have been too easily written off in the past.

Lesson Four: Being a Mentor

"He ain't heavy, he's my brother."

—Men of Boys Town

Helga

Nursing research lab started at 8:30 A.M. every Tuesday and Thursday morning, and Helga was always the first student at her desk, which gave us a little one-on-one time to talk about nursing research. Helga was always smiling and attentive, and she asked many questions; her thirst for knowledge made her passion for nursing very clear.

Helga also talked to me about her long commute and how she would listen to music as a form of therapeutic relaxation. Her efforts of relaxation paid off as her fair skin glowed, demonstrating her youthful 22 years of life. At times she would speak to other students in her native tongue, Spanish, to get a better understanding of concepts.

During class, as I was helping her do a literature search on her topic of interest, Helga shared with me that she was a single parent and that at times she felt like she had the weight of the world on her and often wanted to give up.

I smiled at her as I told her those feelings were normal. I asked her what motivated her; she told me buying a home and being a role model to her son. I told her to cut out a picture of her dream home and imagine the colors of the walls, the rooms, the kitchen, and her son's face as she walks in from work. I winked at her and told her that as a single mom in the same program 12 years ago, that's what pulled me through. She smiled at me as she placed her focus back onto her computer. I was the face of her tomorrow; now she knew for sure she could achieve. Don't be afraid to share your story with others; many of us share the same struggles.

There have been many students who needed instructors to demonstrate the correct catheter size, IV solution, and dressing change technique, but there have been many more times that instructors have been needed to be mentors or to suggest mentorship to their students. Some minority students are the very first in their family to attend college, and they need mentorship in navigating the academic arena. Other students may have never dealt with other races or cultures and don't know or feel comfortable interacting with those outside their race or cultural community. In these situations, I do a one-on-one session or postclinical conference on appropriate communication and emphasize that slang and jargon are not the make-up of professional behavior. I also create practice sessions on communication. We strategize healing reactions and healthy coping mechanisms to situations involving racism and discrimination. We talk about community-building as students learn how to be allies to each other and to professional colleagues experiencing situations of racism and discrimination. The dialogue includes consideration of how to create a healthier work environment.

Lesson Five: Understanding Cultural and Social Dynamics

"We cannot become what we need to be, remaining what we are."
—Max De Pree (as cited in McNally, 1990)

Deborah

At 26 years, Deborah smiled with pride and excitement each clinical day. She was the first in her family to enroll in college. Hard work was nothing new for her; she held a high grade point average, was always prepared, and gave 100% effort in everything she did. She was the pride of her family. She once shared with the class a story told to her by her great-grandmother, who had been the daughter of a slave. Her great-grandmother told of her experience as a little girl, having to drink from different water fountains than Whites and to attend inferior schools. Deborah's great-grandmother was elated that her great-granddaughter was in college to be a nurse. The irony of Deborah's story began as she spoke of the death of her great-great-grandmother. Her death was one of great tragedy. She died hours after arriving at a distant hospital that served Blacks, which was over three hours away because the local hospital, which was five minutes away, did not treat her race. Deborah began to tear as she lifted her head and said, "The hospital she died in didn't have the latest equipment or supplies."

"How times have changed," I commented as I leaned forward to touch Deborah's hand. "It amazes me that in a person's lifetime, one can witness this drastic degree of change. Now you, a Black woman, are training to treat others in a hospital that caters to all races."

This also made me reflect on culture—that in Deborah's lifetime, she had known someone firsthand who had experienced legally sanctioned racism and segregation. How does this impact her life and the way she views the world? Also, if she is the first in her family to attend college, how well are her family members doing financially? Deborah's ancestors worked so hard to build this country, as did countless other enslaved African Americans; yet, their toil produced wealth for other people. The wealth that was generated has been passed down to the descendents of slave owners, not to the descendents of the people who toiled the most to generate it. There are burdens that African Americans carry and have carried for generations. I will share with you Deborah's story and how the burdens she carried impacted her educational career.

That day, Deborah entered the clinical area without her usual smile and cheer. She looked exhausted and was close to tears. She sat slumped in her chair with her lab coat hanging off one shoulder. I approached her after preclinical conference to see if everything was okay. She talked about the pressures of motherhood and marriage.

Having three children at an early age was very difficult, and now she was dealing with her husband's struggle to secure a good job with benefits. Her extended family was struggling with rent and keeping current with bills. They were constantly requesting help each month from her husband, who was already having difficulty staying current with their own bills.

She began to cry and express her thoughts of dropping out of school to assist her family financially. My heart sank, as I knew that most students who stopped school with the intention of finishing later do not return. I understood her concerns, which are common in her culture, but I also knew that: "We cannot become what we need to be, by remaining what we are" (Max De Pree, as cited in McNally, 1990).

I encouraged Deborah to stay in school and to remain strong. I told her that we need to run harder and stronger at the end of the race to win. I suggested she get a weekend job and assist her husband with his job search and work on his résumé. I referred her to the career placement program on campus and also suggested programs for her parents that would complement them financially.

Deborah remained in school and worked a part-time job, sometimes during the week, but mostly on weekends. Her grades declined and she lost her scholarship, and she had to obtain a student loan. However, she completed the program and became a registered nurse. At graduation, Deborah thanked me for my advice on that day 2 years prior. She said she envisioned herself in the same place in 3 years, and that motivated her. Now she looked forward to a lucrative career with higher financial rewards. I was proud of her.

KEYS TO EDUCATING THE MINORITY STUDENT: THE THEORY OF MULTIPLE INTELLIGENCES

There are many nursing theories and theories about teaching/learning strategies that I have incorporated into practice. One in particular is Howard Gardner's (1993) Theory of Multiple Intelligences. Dr. Gardner created this theory in 1983 after studying psychologists such as Piaget and Erikson. There are, according to Gardner, at least eight ways to demonstrate and tap into students' potential to learn. He describes the mind as a computer waiting to be turned on. It can be turned on by switching the channel or sparking an interest on the right intelligence marker. The eight areas of intelligence are presented in Table 4.1, along with examples of each as it applies to nursing practice.

I have incorporated this theoretical framework into my teaching to be more effective, especially with regard to minority students. For example, in the African American culture, music is a large part of our being and plays an important role in our understanding of the world. It is through music that we find comfort and utilize a large degree of our creativity. Visual stimulation, which taps into spatial intelligence, is another potentially effective strategy in educating minorities.

Prior to nursing school, as far back as grade school, my mother made me audiotape myself and play back items that I needed to hear repeatedly to learn, for example, spelling words. In nursing school, I remember my classmates teased me about my colored pencils. Every semester I would purchase a box of colored pencils. During class I would write my notes and then underline all of the important topics with different colors. I would also underline categories and main headings. When it was time to study, the words would "jump out" at me because the color-coding made sense to me and was visually pleasing. I would also draw body parts or create visuals to understand concepts. A friend of mine from the Philippines found a greater understanding of nursing concepts by creating mnemonics to help her memorize information. I have learned over the years that people learn in so many different ways and that we have many senses that can be stimulated into learning. Nursing naturally taps into multiple intelligences, at least in the clinical settings, as evidenced by Table 4.1.

Table 4.1

MULTIPLE INTELLIGENCES AND NURSING PRACTICE

TYPE OF INTELLIGENCE	APPLICATION TO NURSING
Verbal—Linguistic ("word smart")	■ Documentation—how we express in writing our patient care and giving report (hand off communication) ■ Choosing words and verbal communication style to promote comfort and healing
Logical—Mathematical Intelligence ("number/ reasoning smart")	■ Calculating dosages, managing time ■ Understanding graphic and numerical indicators of community health
Spatial Intelligence ("picture smart")	■ Assessing—abnormal vs. normal ■ Assessing the body language of patients, families, and colleagues ■ Assessing the community by looking at patterns of movement/activity
Bodily—Kinesthetic Intelligence ("body smart")	■ Performing nursing care ■ Functioning as a professional nurse
Musical Intelligence ("music smart")	■ Attending to clinical alarms, codes ■ Using music for healing ■ Creating an environment free of auditory distractions
Interpersonal Intelligence ("people smart")	■ Team building ■ Delegating ■ Interviewing and listening for understanding ■ Developing therapeutic relationships with patients and families
Intrapersonal Intelligence ("self smart")	■ Understanding how one fits in the role of a nurse ■ Understanding self ■ Developing a reflective practice
Naturalistic Intelligence ("nature smart")	■ Increasing awareness/consciousness of your role and those around you ■ Attending to environmental conditions that heal ■ Engaging natural forces and sources of strength to aid in healing

I incorporate the theory of multiple intelligences in every class I teach—theory or clinical. I make every attempt to "turn students' brains on" to what is being taught and to assist them in full comprehension. Each area of intelligence is paired with a specific nursing task, thereby ensuring that a variety of intelligences are incorporated into the teaching/learning process.

To illustrate, one clinical day a Code Blue for cardiac arrest was called on the oncology unit. I asked the students to stop and listen (musical intelligence); for me it was second nature to hear the operator "call a code"; however, they were confused. I repeated what the operator stated (verbal—linguistic intelligence); then I took two students to the location of the code to see the emergency response (spatial intelligence). After the code concluded, we debriefed, and I explained the role of the primary nurse (interpersonal intelligence) and other staff nurses (interpersonal intelligence, bodily/kinesthetic intelligence). We talked about the large doses of medications given during a code (logical—mathematical intelligence), how the charge nurse managed the environment (spatial and interpersonal intelligences), and the difference between dying at home and in the hospital (naturalistic intelligence). We reflected on what the students felt (intrapersonal intelligence). This is one example of how to utilize the theory of multiple intelligences in educating nurses.

Every class should incorporate at least three of these interactive techniques in order to be effective. In so doing, nurse educators have more opportunities to reach the learner, by "turning on one of the computers." The first step in teaching is to do an assessment of how students learn; this is critical. My assessment is always discreet. When meeting my students, I ask them their name, why they chose nursing, and what their hobbies are. The hobbies are my clue. People take pleasure in their hobbies; hobbies are also a key to how people learn. Another assessment tool is to ask students what teaching/learning strategies they find effective or what has given them the best results.

Some students can identify with these intelligences and recognize what helps them learn. The tape recording of myself studying and playing it back multiple times is a demonstration of musical intelligence; hearing myself on the tape helped to ingrain the information in my mind. The example of utilizing colored pencils while taking notes to have concepts "stand out" is an example of visual intelligence. Learning is fluid; it is not the same for everyone, so we must be creative.

THE IMPORTANCE OF CLINICAL SUCCESS

Students spend less quality time in clinical practice today than they did in the days of diploma graduates. I often tell the story of my mother, a diploma graduate, who worked every day on the clinical unit and learned to suture, autoclave, and manage four to five patients upon graduation. Today, many student nurses graduate without managing more than one or two patients, few learn suturing, and some even graduate without ever giving an intramuscular injection. Clinical time must be maximized to create a workforce of nurses that are confident, secure, and competent.

RECOMMENDATIONS FOR SUCCESS!

In addition to incorporating the theory of multiple intelligences into nursing education, nurse educators need to make expectations for the clinical setting transparent to create a supportive environment for all students. I have created recommendations for all participants in the clinical setting (Hill-Cill, 2005)—the clinical instructor, the staff nurse, the nurse manager, and the student nurse—to ensure that students from all cultural backgrounds have a robust and successful clinical experience. Many of my students are minorities, and these tips have helped them to be successful and have also helped to create a supportive clinical environment. My recommendations for success are as follows:

Recommendations for Clinical Instructors

- Arrange a preclinical visit to the hospital to tour the assigned unit, to examine paperwork and protocols, and to introduce yourself and allow staff to ask questions.
- Educate staff on what the students can/cannot do on the day of clinical.
- Create and post an assignment sheet, post students' duties during clinical shift, and communicate this information to staff nurses.
- Create a communication report sheet. Students should use this sheet as a written report of what they do.

Recommendations for Staff Nurses

- Mentor students—staff are experts of their units; they are essential in the learning process.
- Encourage students—seek out students to observe procedures.
- Communicate appropriately—contact clinical instructor about any procedure the staff would like the student to perform.
- Students and staff nurses should be clear on what duties the student can perform.

Recommendations for Nurse Managers

- Announce the dates students will be on the unit and describe student activities.
- At staff meetings, encourage staff to participate in students' learning.
- Nurture relationships—encourage your staff to participate in student activities and reward staff when they partake in student learning.
- Create opportunities—enroll your unit in internship and externship programs.
- Help maintain a student-friendly environment—let the students know you want and need them there.

Recommendations for Student Nurses

- Be resourceful—ask yourself the question first and see if you can answer it or get the answer yourself.
- Communicate with the nurse—write down and report important information for the nurse.
- Be thorough—complete all tasks.
- Be aware of nurses' time.
- Remember: Nurses are your resource, not your crutch.

QUESTIONS FOR DIALOGUE

1. What ideas or concepts did you find most meaningful in this chapter? Identify your insights and questions to bring to a dialogue with your colleagues.
2. How could faculty help students develop strategies to deal with racism in the clinical encounter? Give specific examples

of incidents in which education, kindness, and/or confrontation were or would have been effective responses.

3. How can faculty balance the need to hold students accountable with the need to be sensitive to the complexities of their lives?
4. What procedures are in place in your institution for a student such as Keri to appeal a clinical faculty's performance evaluation? Could Keri have successfully challenged her evaluation at your institution? Why or why not?
5. Often minority nurses use their personal knowledge and experiences of overcoming discrimination to develop approaches to eliminate or minimize similar experiences for other students. Dialogue with colleagues about how Hill-Cill was able to accomplish this with her students and give them the strength and courage to persevere. Give additional examples from your own experience.
6. In what ways could nursing curricula expand upon Hill-Cill's application of the theory of multiple intelligences to nursing education?

REFERENCES

Covey, S. (1998). *Seven habits of highly effective people.* New York: Free Press.

Gardner, H. (1993). *Frames of mind: The theory of multiple intelligences.* New York: Basic Books.

Gladwell, M. (2005). *Blink: The power of thinking without thinking.* New York: Time Warner.

Hill-Cill, D. (2005, Aug 29). The path to proficiency. *Nursing Spectrum,* 17A, 18.

Maxwell, J. (2007). *Failing forward: Turning mistakes into stepping stones for success.* Nashville, TN: Thomas Nelson.

McNally, D. (1990). *Even eagles need a push: Learning to soar in a changing world.* New York: Dell.

PART II

Pedagogical Innovations in Nursing Education

5 Coming Home to Nursing Education for a Hmong Student, Hmong Nurse, and Hmong Nurse Educator

AVONNE YANG

As an ethnic minority Hmong refugee in the United States, I grew up with a racial consciousness of the Hmong as a historically oppressed people who yearn for freedom to live their lives unbothered by others. Throughout our history, from the time of the Hans (206 B.C.–A.D. 220) in China (Yang, 1993) until now, we have experienced discrimination at the hands of the Chinese, French, lowland Lao, Vietnamese, and others in the countries to which we fled after the U.S. invasion in Southeast Asia (P. Vang, personal communication, June 1, 1984). Since the Hmong first arrived in the United States in the 1970s, many of my family members and myself, Hmong friends, and other members of the Hmong community have experienced unequal treatment and/or culturally insensitive health care that we feel would not have occurred were there more Hmong health care providers, such as Hmong nurses. Thus, I am acutely aware of the implications posed not only by a nursing shortage but also by the lack of diversity in the nursing profession.

As a Hmong woman who has been a nursing student, nurse, nurse researcher, and nurse educator in the United States, the scars from unequal treatment and/or culturally insensitive care remain long after the transgressions. Sometimes, a new incident of unequal treatment or cultural insensitivity will trigger old memories and bring back floods of anger, sadness, despair, and hopelessness that I thought time had healed. When these trigger moments happen, I am heavily burdened with the knowledge that while I can forgive, I cannot forget the harm that was done to me, to my loved ones, and to others in the Hmong community. In this chapter, I share my story and insights so that nurse educators and administrators can gain insights into how to create a more culturally inclusive environment in which minority students can learn and succeed.

EXPERIENCE OF BEING A HMONG NURSING STUDENT

My first experience of blatant cultural insensitivity in nursing occurred in a maternal–child clinical rotation when I was a nursing student. One of the White nurses made a derogatory statement about the squatting position Hmong women have traditionally used for labor, and she laughed in mockery. I do not know if she even cared that I was Hmong. None of the other nurses in the group challenged her inappropriate remark. In fact, they joined in the mockery with laughter. I was initially offended, but this quickly gave way to fear and mistrust. Because of this experience, I no longer trusted these nurses to provide respectful, kind, and maybe even safe care for me and for the many Hmong women who came there to deliver their babies. The thought entered my mind, "How sad that we Hmong patients have to continue to come here as dictated by our health insurance policy." At that time, this facility was a major community hospital that served a large Hmong population. As a neophyte, I was eagerly soaking in what seasoned nurses were teaching me and expected them to socialize me into becoming a caring nurse. This incident of cultural denigration was perpetrated by seasoned mentors. It shook my faith in the image of the nurse as someone who is caring and tolerant of patients' cultural differences.

At this time, there was no professional circle of support in which I could process this experience. My classmates were White. My instructor was White. The nurses involved in the incident were White. The nursing faculty was predominantly White. In a previous incident outside of class, a nursing classmate had made a negative comment about Hmong people, so I did not feel safe with my classmates. In this sea of Whiteness, I did not feel safe to seek support.

Other more subtle experiences of cultural insensitivity that Hmong patients have experienced include not being provided with linguistically appropriate services or same-sex health care providers. As a student, I knew that all patients who did not speak English were entitled to interpreters. Yet, I regularly witnessed nurses not requesting interpreter services for Hmong patients who did not speak English. These Hmong patients were so glad to see me. For Hmong women, who consider modesty to be of the utmost importance, it was unsettling to have male physicians on the maternity ward walk in to provide care without anyone explaining to the patient why a same-sex provider was not available. Provision of linguistically appropriate services in the first place might have allowed the women to express their preference for female providers. Cultural competency on the organization's part would prevent such situations of culturally incongruent care. Due to limited resources, it is understandable that same-sex providers may not always be available. However, at least an attempt should be made to explain to the patient that this is the case. I saw no such attempt. I felt psychic pain from these experiences because they were reminders of the historical oppression experienced by Hmong people.

Inevitably, when different cultures meet, there will be instances of cultural conflict, but when those conflicts occur, minority students need a safe space to process their experiences of cultural insensitivity without fear that their experiences will be invalidated or be used to define them negatively. Prior to becoming a nursing student, my experiences of racial discrimination had been invalidated by White individuals whom I trusted. Too often I found that Whites with whom I shared my experiences quickly became defensive or said that my perceptions were incorrect. They responded that I have an unfounded bias against Whites or that not all Whites are racist, or they came up with explanations that invalidated my experiences. One trusted White high school instructor even asked me, "Are you sure you don't have a chip on your shoulder?" This expression implied that my hurt feelings were not real and neither was the incident of racial discrimination. This pattern of White behavior over time built up a pattern of fear in me that my experiences of racial discrimination and cultural insensitivity would be invalidated by Whites. Because there was not a sure way of telling which White individuals I could trust, it was safer to simply not share my experiences with Whites at all. I did not want to feel isolated or singled out or to have my experiences invalidated anymore.

What I was seeking in sharing my stories was acknowledgment of my experiences. To acknowledge is to listen nonjudgmentally, to hear the story and the feelings behind it, and to respond with compassion to the storyteller. In order to experience timely healing, I needed to hear another human being, especially a White person because it was White individuals who had hurt me, acknowledge my experiences. Acknowledgment does not mean that the listener agrees with my version of the story or is being asked to see all Whites as racist or as having done me or other minorities wrong. Acknowledgment shows caring and respect for my feelings and respect for my willingness to reveal my human vulnerability by sharing the experience. Contrary to being acknowledged, there was no meaningful dialogue to find out what had happened that made me feel the way I did or to find out how I could be supported. This worsened the original pain. Because of these experiences, I decided not to share my stories in clinical postconference.

Clinical postconferences typically meet right after clinical is over. Fatigue and time are critical factors because students and faculty are tired by the end of clinical and ready to go home. In the postclinical conferences I experienced as a nursing student, students and faculty discussed lessons learned from the clinical experience. While every student was encouraged and expected to participate, no explicit rules for sharing or role modeling were provided to assure participants that the dialogue would be respectful and nonjudgmental. No guarantee was made that every student would be given time to speak. This type of postclinical conference did not make me feel safe nor assured that I would be heard without being invalidated. Since that time, I have thought about how postclinical conferences could be handled differently.

TRANSFORMING THE POSTCLINICAL CONFERENCE

Postclinical conferences can be made more meaningful in several ways, one of which is by using a talking circle on a nonclinical day, which would neutralize the fatigue and time constraint typical of postclinical conferences and increase the potential for every student to participate and be heard. The talking circle, which is derived from American Indian culture, has been used as a tool for American Indians to discuss how racial oppression in North America is related to their lived experiences (Struthers et al., 2003). American Indian racial consciousness and awareness that life experiences have emotional ties to past racial oppression is similar to that of the Hmong. Similar to the American Indian talking circle, when Hmong families gather together for important discussions, everyone takes a turn talking in a circular fashion starting with the eldest. Thus, the talking circle holds great potential as a tool for Hmong students to share experiences of cultural insensitivity. Even among Hmong students who have no racial consciousness of oppression or no experiences of discrimination, the talking circle still serves a useful purpose because it allows them a chance to share their experiences like everyone else. The following faculty–student exemplar is presented as an alternative to the typical postclinical conference.

The instructor explains the concept of the talking circle to the students. The instructor explains that a rock will be passed around. The person holding the rock gets to speak while others listen. When the person has finished speaking, he or she passes the rock to the next person. The instructor explains that each person is to be respected and listened to without judgment. Before talking begins, the instructor passes out copies of the American Nurses Association (ANA, 2005) Code of Ethics for Nurses with Interpretive Statements *and the International Council of Nurses (ICN, 2006)* Code of Ethics for Nurses. *The instructor reviews the codes and asks everyone to share stories about their clinical day and relate it to the codes. She starts off the talking circle by sharing a story of her own first.*

Because of past experiences with being invalidated, I am afraid to share my story. When it is my turn to talk, I share something totally unrelated to my hidden story. At the close of the conference, the instructor says that any concerns, questions, or thoughts, no matter what they are, are important because of the insights they can provide to all. The instructor then asks each student to write down any concerns, questions, or thoughts that were not shared but that are important to the student. This is to be turned in to the instructor and will be discussed in privately arranged one-to-one conferences. She emphasizes that students are welcome to speak to her about any concerns or issues throughout the semester.

I am still fearful of having my story be invalidated, but I work up enough nerve to share my story during the one-to-one end-of-semester conference. The instructor asks me how the experiences made me feel and asks for my suggestions on how I need to be supported in dealing with them. I am relieved just to have a nonjudgmental person hear me out. At the close of our dialogue, I feel that nothing can be done immediately that would change the situations that have already passed. I suggest to my instructor that perhaps after I have received my nursing degree, I might come back to give an inservice on cultural competency to the organizations involved. The instructor asks if it is okay if she shares my stories with the nurse managers of the organizations and nursing units involved. I tell her not to do this because I am still a vulnerable neophyte and am fearful of repercussions for my future economic opportunities. She honors my request. I come away from the experience feeling supported and experience decreased psychic pain.

This exemplar holds many lessons. By sharing her own story, the instructor role models that it is safe to share one's experiences and vulnerability. By assuming the role of the supportive listener, the instructor facilitates healing, growth, and professional development for the minority student who is experiencing discrimination. By asking how the student feels, listening nonjudgmentally, and being supportive without jumping in to offer interventions or solutions, the instructor allows for the expression of painful emotions that would otherwise remain bottled up inside. Timely release of painful emotions clears the student's mind to focus energy on finding creative solutions to the problem. By asking the student how she would like to be supported, the instructor is not forcing her own agenda upon the student but empowers the student to reach for her own solutions.

Another lesson from the exemplar is that the use of the codes of ethics for nurses can help students identify the boundaries of ethical professional behavior. The codes of ethics require respect for persons (ANA, 2005; ICN, 2006). Had my clinical instructor used the codes of ethics for nurses as a framework for discussions, as a vulnerable neophyte, I would have felt greater reassurance that the nursing profession did not condone the behaviors I observed. This would have made me more willing to share my experiences in the postclinical conference setting because I would have felt that greater emotional safety existed when the moral authority of the codes of ethics was openly espoused by a mentor, the instructor. In addition, for students of color, including immigrant students, the sense of emotional safety may be greater when the mentor or instructor is a person of color, too.

ROLE OF MINORITY FACULTY FOR STUDENTS OF COLOR

In my experience as a learning lab instructor, students of color consistently sought me out. White students rarely did this. Most revealing is what the White students did not say and what the minority students said. White students did not mention racial, ethnic, or cultural issues negatively impacting their education. Minority students did. Students of color, including immigrant students, discussed feelings of cultural isolation and difficulties with immigration authorities and revealed great stress related to these issues. The stress was interfering with their education, and they appreciated the extra time and attention I gave them. They did not feel that their White classmates and the White faculty understood them as well as I did. They were appreciative that I listened to their concerns and provided the extended personal attention and time they needed in order to focus on mastering their skills.

Students detailed the disparities they faced. Black students in particular revealed stories of White patients and faculty perceiving them as less qualified than White individuals simply because of the color of their skin. Black students stated they felt it was critical that they master skills so as to appear fully competent. They were appreciative that, as a person of color, I understood their situation. Hmong students shared their difficulty trying to juggle the individual responsibilities of being a student and taking care of the collective needs of their family, such as helping to take care of children and in-laws. The Eastern philosophy of duty to one's family was at times difficult to fulfill while trying to complete numerous nursing assignments in addition to attending clinicals. They appreciated my willingness to give them the attention and time needed to practice procedures repeatedly so they could master skills. I understood their needs because I had once been in their position.

Students of color benefit from seeing successful role models at school and work and from hearing encouragement from them. For many of them, residential segregation has resulted in a lack of role models to inspire their career aspirations. According to Wilson (1987, as cited in Williams & Collins, 2002), residential segregation limits economic opportunities for Blacks by limiting their access to social networks and role models who have stable employment and could serve as leads to potential jobs. The social isolation that results from residential segregation can also promote cultural responses that decrease commitment to a set of norms and values essential for economic success (Williams & Collins, 2002). Shihadeh and Flynn's (1996) work indicates that chronic exposure to concentrated poverty and its associated conditions can discourage a strong work ethic and belief in the value of academic success while removing negative stigmas associated with imprisonment, academic failure, and economic failure. Although minorities may experience enhanced mental health when living together in concentrated communities (Williams & Collins, 2002), the downside is fewer role models to influence academic and career aspirations (King & Multon, 1996). While not every community of color experiences the problems described in the literature and not every minority student comes from segregated or poor communities, the mere fact that there are generally so few minority role models does suggest that the literature has indeed not overstated the importance of role models for the academic and career success of minorities.

In nursing, the presence of minority role models promotes self-confidence in minority nursing students that they, too, can succeed. Self-confidence strengthens students' beliefs that they can become a nurse like the role model, leading to a self-fulfilling prophecy, referred to in the literature as the Pygmalion Effect, which posits that a person lives up or down to the expectations that others have of him or her (Von Bergen, Soper, & Foster, 2002). According to DeAngelis (1995, as cited in Von Bergen et al.), if women believe their employment and promotion are based on gender and not ability, they tend to devalue their own abilities, choose less taxing responsibilities, and devalue female colleagues. The implication is that if these women had *self-confidence* in their abilities and therefore *belief* in their abilities, their performance would improve. In the case of Hmong and other minority nursing students, the presence of role models promotes *confidence* and the *belief* that they can succeed, too, which can help students to succeed in areas in which they have difficulty, for example, on written examinations. In sum, minority students live *up* to the expectations of their role models.

My lived experience provides evidence for me of the need for more nurses of color to serve as role models and mentors for future minority nurses. Being surrounded by a sea of Whiteness is in itself for nursing students of color an intimidating environment but especially for talking about issues of race, culture, and ethnicity. Environments that reflect diversity and a tolerance for diversity lay the groundwork for an atmosphere of nurturance and support for minority students. The presence of minority nursing faculty is an essential aspect of creating this supportive, nurturing educational environment.

ADDRESSING DISPARITIES IN THE RECRUITMENT AND RETENTION OF MINORITY FACULTY

Like minority students, minority nurses yearn to talk with other nurses who look like them and come from their culture or who at least understand the pressure of being in a White nursing environment. The shortage of nurses of color has its roots in culturally insensitive nursing education environments. To address the shortage, nursing faculty of color and nursing education administrators must take the lead. I believe nursing education can be transformed so that it is part of the solution, not part of the problem. Each time a nursing school has a Hmong student, it holds in its grasp a future Hmong nurse and the promise of increased culturally sensitive care. It has the opportunity to guide and nurture Hmong nursing students toward success and the larger goal of transformative practice. The same holds true for other minority groups. As my lived experience has shown, minority nurse educators are a vital source of guidance and nurturance for minority nursing students; they are needed as role models.

Nursing education administrators are in a position to actively recruit more minority nurse educators. They can advocate for competitive salaries for nurse educators in order to attract more minority nurse educators. Minority nurses may not be attracted to nursing education if the economic rewards are not commensurate with what they could get in higher-paying positions. While this is also true for majority nurses as well, it is especially critical for minority nurses; because there are so few of them, they are in relatively higher demand. If they come from a racial consciousness of oppression as I do, they are likely to be highly gifted overachievers who will "go with the highest bidder," so to speak. In other words, compared to a White candidate, they may paradoxically be in a position of having greater freedom to "write their own ticket," meaning they have greater freedom to choose from among many prestigious and high-paying positions. In this scenario, the educational institution that does not offer a competitive salary will lose out on a valuable chance to "catch" these nurse educators.

In addition, minority nurses are more likely to have greater family and community financial commitments than their White counterparts. Furthermore, White nurses are more likely to have inherited wealth from previous generations, including wealth generated by the work of people of color, as well as disproportionate access to property—sources of White privilege that are not often acknowledged. Most of the minority students I have encountered come from minority residential communities with high concentrations of poverty and have the pressure of being the *first* or among the *few* in their communities to pursue nursing education. They have the pressure of being role models in their communities. They also have the moral duty of someone who is more fortunate to take care of the less fortunate members of their communities, including family members. In addition, immigrant nurses may have entire extended families in their home country to support. A competitive salary is essential. If nursing education administrators fail to recognize the additional financial responsibilities of minority nurses, they may fail to attract or retain them as nurse educators.

To increase the visibility of nursing education as a viable career path for minority nurses, nursing education administrators could work in partnership with minority nurse educators, minority nurses in the community, White colleagues, and professional nursing organizations to do outreach work that builds mentor–mentee relationships for aspiring minority nursing students. Such relationships would certainly enhance the visibility of minority nurses and minority nurse educators as role models, as well as increase the visibility of the nursing profession, which might spark more interest in the nursing profession and in nursing education. If there are few or no nurse educators of color and/or nurses of color in the institution and in the community, this is all the more reason to build partnerships to *create* more nurses of color and more nurse educators of color.

Nursing education administrators need to be mindful of not overloading minority nurse educators, who in addition to reaching out to recruit minority students take on added responsibilities of mentoring minority students who seek their support and guidance. A reduction in teaching load may be needed in order for minority nurse educators to be able to fulfill all these responsibilities. The same would hold true for other nurse educators who participate in this valuable effort.

Smedley, Stith, and Nelson's (2002) report underscores the need for actively recruiting minority nurse educators. They found that racial and ethnic differences do not fully account for all the racial and ethnic health disparities in the United States, and they point out that minority health care providers are more likely to practice in minority and underserved communities. As a result, Smedley et al. recommend an increase in minority health care professionals to help reduce disparities in health care. This brings us full circle to my point that nursing education must be a part of the solution to the shortage of minority nurses, including Hmong nurses.

Nursing education administrators should partner with administrators in other disciplines to publicly acknowledge that inclusivity is a nonnegotiable part of the college or university's culture and that a supportive infrastructure needs to be in place. A diversity council made up of culturally diverse individuals should be established to address diversity concerns expressed by all students. Members of the diversity council should come from the institution and the community. In addition, nursing education administrators should establish formal assessment mechanisms that allow all students to identify what instructional practices and institutional practices have promoted their learning and their professional and personal growth, to identify which have been an impediment and why, and to recommend changes. Such an initiative would require using a variety of assessment formats, not just the traditional questionnaire where students are asked to fill in boxes. Nursing education administrators and nursing faculty need to analyze the assessment findings in relation to the performance of minority students as well as the performance of nonminority students, identify what changes need to be implemented, make the changes, and evaluate the outcome. This process strives for the recognition and participation of all students, and it uncovers educational and assessment practices that operate from a position of cultural bias.

MULTIPLE-CHOICE NURSING EXAMS: A MAJOR IMPEDIMENT TO SUCCESS

The shortage of minority nurses creates a critical need to invest in exploring the factors that impede or enhance the success of nursing candidates. In my experience, students of color who were not making passing grades on multiple-choice examinations had no trouble in clinical rotations. They said they were not "stupid" and could not understand why they did poorly on multiple-choice exams. I emphasized that test questions are only just that, test questions, and, as such, they do not define one's intelligence or clinical competence, as evidenced by the students' acknowledgment that they had no problem in clinical. In our dialogue, we talked through patient scenarios and came to realize that there may be several equally excellent answers. This led me to question the conventional belief that students who do poorly on multiple-choice tests have weak critical thinking skills.

If the students truly had weak critical thinking skills, they would not have been able to identify many equally good solutions and would have come up with only one solution or no solution at all. I began to suspect that the students had not yet been socialized to become excellent multiple-choice test takers. Indeed, studies have found that nursing students actually experience a decline in their critical thinking skills after completion of a specific educational program (Nokes, Nickitas, Keida, & Neville, 2005) or a whole nursing program (Staib, 2003). It occurred to me that perhaps the emphasis on *one* correct answer in a nonclinical context, such as on a multiple-choice test, was stifling the students' creativity, inquisitiveness, and ability to think critically.

The premise of current nursing education is that written examinations, particularly multiple-choice examinations, provide proof of students' *critical* thinking ability and, thus, of their *clinical* thinking ability. This belief presupposes that students who perform well on multiple-choice tests will be safe clinical practitioners. There is no proof of this in the literature (Tanner, 2005). I trusted rather in the dialogic process to help the students and me uncover what they needed to work on.

Because poor performance on written multiple-choice examinations was one of the main reasons why students came to see me, I also taught them test-taking strategies. Quite revealing was the admission by all, after improving test-taking skills, that their worst enemy was not a lack of "test" intelligence but rather a lack of self-confidence. This lived experience left me pondering whether the present state of nursing education, which promotes memorization of only one right way to do things (such as "select the best answer" on multiple-choice exams), needs to be supplemented with other ways of assessing learning so that students who fail multiple-choice tests do not end up questioning their own intelligence and self-worth. It was only through my developing a relationship of trust with the students that their confidence in themselves flourished.

NURSING THEORY INVITES ME BACK HOME

In hindsight, I realize that when I entered into dialogue with students about their lives, what they found to be meaningful, and how they might solve clinical problems, I was not playing the "God" role of determining all the right answers. Students participated in the discussion and asked questions, and together we cocreated what would be appropriate choices and discussed why *one* particular choice might be chosen in the context of a written multiple-choice test versus what might actually happen in real life. This partnership process embodied Margaret Newman's (1994) theory of health as expanding consciousness (HEC) and also involved using narrative pedagogy (Diekelmann, 2001; Ironside, 2003) because of its congruence with HEC. I had stumbled upon HEC and narrative pedagogy by chance. But, as I began to teach nursing guided by HEC and narrative pedagogy, I began to truly see the relevance and importance of theory-guided education for nurses and the need to explicate the linkage between nursing theory and clinical practice early on in each nurse's education. In sharing my lived experience of how I came to this conclusion, I offer another voice to the discussion on nursing education, a voice of one lone Hmong nurse. There is a dearth of literature on nursing education from the perspective of Hmong educators and nurse educators of color in general. My hope is that my minority voice adds another colorful thread to the discourse on nursing education transformation.

HEC HELPS FRAME THE EXPERIENCE

What does HEC have to offer that is relevant to my experiences of unequal treatment and culturally insensitive care as a person from the Hmong culture, to Hmong nursing students, and to nurse educators? Health as expanding consciousness defines health in terms of a person's seen or explicate pattern and unseen or implicate pattern of the whole. The visible pattern includes what we typically label disease, which is a disorganized state that presents opportunity for the individual to search for meaning (Newman, 1994). Once this meaning is uncovered by the individual, she or he knows what actions need to be taken and thus experiences expansion of consciousness, which Newman defines as "a process of becoming more of oneself, of finding greater meaning in life, and of reaching new heights of connectedness with other people and the world" (Newman, 2008, p. 6). When one experiences expansion of consciousness, one experiences deeper love (Newman, 1994). The nurse's role in this experience is not to intervene or provide the solution but to create a caring environment that promotes the expansion of the patient's consciousness.

In hindsight, I can now see that I was embodying this HEC philosophical perspective in my relationships with students. Rather than holding rigidly onto the conventional idea that they were not thinking critically and that was the reason for their failure, I searched along with them for the reason behind their academic struggle, and together we found an answer that was meaningful. The Hmong and Black students came to realize that there was nothing "wrong" with them and that they needed to trust their ability to succeed. I came to realize that relying solely on conventional pedagogy, with its heavy emphasis on lecture and passive memorization by students, was not serving all students. I lived out the HEC perspective when my relationships with Hmong and Black students who were having difficulty with multiple-choice exams left me pondering if there was more to education than outcome-based questions that always had only one right answer.

Health as expanding consciousness values the creation of a caring environment that is meaningful to individuals and their cultural communities.

For example, if we Hmong women find that the squatting position facilitates labor, then we can expect to be supported by nurses when we employ this culturally congruent practice even though it is different from the norm of the larger culture. Nurses who practice with the HEC perspective will not disrespect and deride us as the nurse in my maternal–child clinical rotation did.

The HEC perspective provides a unitary-transformative view of the human being as an irreducible open system that is interconnected with all other human beings and the universe, such that the parts contain their own patterns while their patterns are also simultaneously contained in the larger pattern of the whole (Gunther, 2006; Monti & Tingen, 2006; Newman, 1994). Reflecting its unitary-transformative paradigm, HEC defines the concept of pattern as information organized into centers of consciousness to form individuals, families, communities, and the overall center of consciousness called the larger pattern of the whole (Brown, 2006; Newman, 1994). In HEC, the human being is a pattern of consciousness interacting within the pattern of the family, which in turn is a pattern of consciousness interacting within the pattern of community, and so on (Newman, 1994). This interconnectedness means that consciousness is present throughout the universe (Brown, 2006; Newman, 1994).

In HEC, movement is considered to be a manifestation of consciousness (Newman, 1994). Movement in space, as a conscious manifestation of the implicate order, is interconnected, containing all movements through space of all points in time (Newman, 1994). Time is holographic, in that each movement in space contains all other movements at all points in time (Newman, 1994). Movement makes time and space become real (Newman, 1994). Humanity is constantly moving and changing both internally at the cellular level and externally via bodily movements and environmental action (Brown, 2006). Such motion through space and time provides each individual with a unique experience of reality (Brown, 2006). Motion is the vehicle for the individual to experience reality and to change (Newman, 1994).

Hmong Cosmology and HEC

The nurse who practices from the HEC perspective is operating from a holistic perspective, which is congruent with Hmong cosmology. In Hmong cosmology, space and time are defined by nature, not by humanity. Traditionally, Hmong depend on the cock's crow in the morning, the light of the rising sun, the dusk of the setting sun, and other natural changes in the environment to determine time. Hmong life ways are patterned around nature's laws. For example, people wake up at sunrise when the cock crows and work until dusk, when the sun sets. Breakfast, lunch, and dinner are prepared according to this schedule provided by nature, and they are served when everyone has arrived, not when a certain "clock" time has been reached. The human being must coexist in harmony with nature because every thing, living and nonliving, has a spirit that must not be disrespected. In this coexistence, all spirits must strive for love in all interactions with each other in order to earn the privilege of returning home to their original source of creation, the universal consciousness. Hmong cosmology embodies the unitary-transformative paradigm, which sees the human being as a pattern interacting with the larger pattern of the whole. The Hmong concept of a universal consciousness is equivalent to HEC's concept of the larger pattern of the whole, which is the overall center of consciousness.

A transgression against a spirit, whether it be the spirit of a living or inanimate object, will result in retribution if corrective action is not taken. A person may suspect that he or she has committed a transgression when "bad" things occur. The bad things could be anything the person perceives to be negative, but typically, they are such things as illness, disease, injury, or death. The person may seek confirmation of the suspicion from a shaman or other religious person, such as a Buddhist monk, who will find out from the spirit world what needs to be done to appease the offended spirit. If the offended spirit is not appeased, retribution could occur in this lifetime or the next or the next and so on. Death in this lifetime does not buy freedom from retribution. Time and space do not wipe out the transgression or release the wrong-doer from retribution. It is as if now is yesterday, and yesterday is today as well. One's karma or fate today is the result of actions taken in the past. One's actions today determine one's future karma. Good actions are those that create love. The more good actions one takes, the more love one experiences for oneself and others, and the closer to enlightenment one gets. Enlightenment is when a person has achieved unconditional love for the self and others. An enlightened person is free of retribution because he or she has learned to do only good. According to Hmong cosmology, all actions through space and time are interconnected, and each reveals the influence of one on the other; time is holographic, and space-movement-time is a manifestation of consciousness, just as Newman asserts in the HEC perspective (Newman, 1994).

Newman (1994) also bases HEC on the concept that there is order even in disorder. Disorder is when a person experiences illness or disease, and order is achieved once a person has uncovered meaning in the illness or disease. One is complementary to the other, and there is not a good–bad dichotomy (Newman, 1994). The Hmong cosmic view that a person has a choice to change his or her karma through corrective action illustrates an embodiment of the concept of order within disorder. Randomness or disorder lies in the fact that the person does not know what his or her future karma will be. It all depends on the choice the person makes today. Order lies in the fact that once a person makes a choice, there is indeed a specific karma associated with it.

Hmong cosmology views spirits as timeless, formless consciousness that do not die, even though their "shells" (i.e., the human body) die. Traditionally, Hmong believe in reincarnation. Reincarnation is when the spirit is reborn in the flesh. The spirit keeps being reborn until it has achieved enlightenment. When a spirit has achieved enlightenment, it returns to the universal consciousness from which all spirits come. This "home coming" signifies that it is free from further reincarnation. The universal consciousness is love, just as Newman has characterized expansion of consciousness in HEC as love (Newman, 1994).

Hmong cosmology has a fluid concept of time. This fluidity is evident in the more flexible time that Hmong families allow for guests to arrive for meals during social events, such as New Year's celebrations. In this instance, for example, although a family may invite guests to eat dinner at say, 5:00 P.M., the actual time when the meal is served may be later than this, varying by as much as one to several hours later. This allows extended family members time to finish their life tasks and to gradually stream in. This fluidity reflects the cosmic view previously described about human beings organizing their life tasks around the laws of nature rather than imposing human "clock" time on nature. This may be frustrating for outsiders. At times, it is also frustrating for Hmong who have acculturated to Western ways, who may mean exactly 5:00 P.M. when they say dinner is at 5:00 P.M. They may become frustrated like Westerners do if dinner is delayed, but if they still retain some of the traditional Hmong thinking, they will not fret about it as much as Westerners do. Understanding about the Hmong cosmic view can help Western health care professionals provide more culturally congruent care to Hmong clients. For example, health care clinics that allow walk-ins instead of just appointments are more congruent with the fluid concept of time in the Hmong cosmic view.

More serious cultural clashes between Western health care and the Hmong cosmic view include incidences in which Hmong families refused Western health care treatment because of their belief that it was the patient's karma to have the "medical" condition that the Western health care providers insisted must be "cured" or "treated" with drugs or surgery. For example, a traditional Hmong family may view an epileptic child as being in disharmony with the spiritual world. For the sake of discussion, let us say that the family had committed a transgression by fleeing from the war in Laos without providing proper burial for an elder. The elder's restless spirit lets the family know its displeasure by causing the child to have seizures. In the beginning, the cause for the seizures is unknown. Later, a shaman is consulted. The shaman tells the family that the reason for the seizures is the lack of a proper burial of the elder. The shaman tells the family that appeasement can be brought about through burnt offerings of paper money. (There is a specialty paper used for this purpose, not literally real money.) This intervention is carried out. It may take several shamans and several interventions before the seizures stop, or the seizures may never stop because the appeasement was not enough. From the traditional Hmong perspective, the Hmong family is taking excellent care of the child; their actions make perfect sense according to the Hmong cosmic view. However, to Western health care providers, the family's response is not "rational," and the family is stubborn, backward, and medically negligent and is not providing good care for the child.

From the HEC perspective, the child's seizures serve as an opportunity for the family to find meaning. When the family finds that the meaning of the illness is retribution for wrongdoing, they acknowledge their improper act and fulfill their moral duty to the deceased elder. The nurse who practices from the HEC perspective creates a caring environment for the family. Through dialogue, culturally congruent care can be realized and increased health becomes a greater possibility.

Lest the reader is left with only negative examples of Hmong cosmology, I would like to present a positive example. Women and girls stitch intricate hand-sewn embroidery called *pan dao*. The Hmong did not have a formal alphabet until the 1950s, and many Hmong elders are illiterate, so *pan daos* are an effective visual means to tell a story. Over the last three decades, since the end of the war in Laos in 1975, the Hmong *pan dao* has undergone a revolution to include scenes of the war in Laos, scenes of Hmong fleeing the war, and scenes of current life in Western countries. The current *pan daos*, which portray the life experiences of the Hmong in the past and in the present, will become history in the future. Yet, while they are "history" in the future, they will continue to tell the Hmong where they came from and why and how they got to the point they did. In this way, the *pan dao* unfolds the past for the Hmong while also enfolding the present. This means that as Hmong women and Hmong girls carry out the act of stitching the *pan daos,* they are manifesting the concept of space-movement-time described by Newman (1994).

In the current state of disorganization, in which the Hmong do not have a "Hmong" country and are scattered all over the world, the *pan dao* can serve as a tool to help the Hmong recount their life experiences, find meaning in their lives, and discern potential actions to take to adapt to life in foreign lands. In this capacity, the *pan dao* may be especially appropriate for elderly Hmong women because they are the group most likely to be illiterate. I gained this insight while doing HEC research with Hmong women with type 2 diabetes (Yang, Xiong, Pharris, & Vang, 2006). Because *pan daos* require considerable skill and time to create, I used pictorial scrolls to help the Hmong women with diabetes reflect on the patterns in their lives. The Hmong women found the pictorial scrolls useful and were able to discern meaningful ways to move forward with their lives.

While Hmong cosmology can serve as a tool for understanding Hmong culture, one must remember that cultures evolve and change. For example, if one encounters a Hmong family who believes that epilepsy has a biological cause and wants anticonvulsant drugs, one should not get confused why this family does not embody Hmong cosmology. The beauty of practicing nursing guided by the HEC perspective is that the nurse operates from a partnership stance, where the nurse is engaged in a dialogue with the patient to find out what an illness or disease means for him or her. With the focus on the patient's meaning, there is very little danger that the HEC nurse will prescribe meaning to the illness or disease for the patient. So, too, with Hmong nursing students, educators will find a wide variety of views related to traditional and Western health practices. Therefore, the most important lesson I want the reader to come away with is that it is critical to dialogue with the Hmong patient, Hmong student, Hmong nurse, and Hmong nurse educator about what is meaningful to them and not make assumptions beforehand. Knowing about Hmong cosmology enhances cultural understanding if in the dialogue it is uncovered that the Hmong person subscribes to Hmong cosmology, but even Hmong cosmology evolves and changes over time.

A partnership engaged in dialogue is not only critical to prevent incorrect assumptions; it is also an important aspect of creating a culturally inclusive nursing education environment.

HEC AS PRAXIS: CREATING A CULTURALLY INCLUSIVE ENVIRONMENT IN NURSING EDUCATION

Nurse educators whose practice is guided by the HEC perspective will engage students in a dialogue through which meaningful events can be recounted, and the educator can find out what is not working or helping students learn. This approach holds the potential for identifying corrective actions to take. I do not suggest that HEC-guided education will be perfect, but I do believe that such a program will be more likely to point out institutional barriers that need to be corrected. Instead of focusing solely on the deficits of students, it uncovers the deficits in the educational system itself. This is a best practice that would benefit all students, not just ethnic minority students like the Hmong.

Health as expanding consciousness also has relevance for a specific area of concern—that of communicative style, which is often raised by nurse educators when students' communication styles differ from their own. My supervisors, who were all White women, and other nursing instructors pointed out to me and other Hmong nursing students that we were too shy, too quiet, and too unassertive. From the Hmong perspective, being "shy" or "quiet," in particular "shy" and female, does not carry with it the negative connotation that it does in the dominant culture. Nor does it indicate that such a person is not assertive. If a nursing supervisor or instructor feels shyness, quietness, or unassertiveness is negatively affecting the Hmong nurse's job performance or is hampering a Hmong student's learning, the supervisor or instructor should first have a respectful dialogue with the Hmong person to find out what it means to be "shy," "quiet," or "unassertive" in Hmong culture. The supervisor or instructor should find out how the Hmong person views herself or himself and take this into consideration.

Too often, I have seen supervisors or instructors automatically label a Hmong nurse or student "shy" or "unassertive" and attach the negative connotation that this is an undesirable trait. The message is clearly that the Hmong person needs to change to conform to the dominant culture's standards of being open, authoritative, and "assertive." Too often there is no meaningful dialogue, and no allowance is given for how the

Hmong person views herself or himself, as opposed to the supervisor's or instructor's view. I know that I am a shy person, but I do not attach a connotation that this is an undesirable trait. Furthermore, I do not regard my quietness as "unassertive." Quite frankly, in all my experiences with Hmong patients, they have been receptive and seemed reassured in response to my quiet and sometimes even shy approach, especially the frail and elderly.

Interestingly, when my White supervisors first told me that I needed to be more assertive, even though I did not agree, I tried to change and become "assertive." To my surprise, my Hmong mother chastised me for having become too "aggressive," even though she had no knowledge of what had transpired between my supervisor and me. I had to quickly tone down my assertive behavior that was so highly prized by my supervisor. This experience has taught me that behaviors have to be taken in context in order for their meaning to be fully understood. Nursing education guided by HEC would encourage us to engage in caring partnerships to discover the meaning behind our patterns of behavior and not simply jump to intervene by telling Hmong students they need to change when, in fact, sometimes no intervention may be necessary. In other words, without dialoguing with a Hmong nurse or student, one cannot simply jump to the conclusion that she or he needs to change because she or he is too shy or not assertive enough for the profession or for the job at hand.

It is important for Hmong nurses to be aware that the dominant culture may judge their behaviors in the same negative way that my White supervisors judged me. In accord with HEC, a nurse educator who notices a "shy" or "quiet" Hmong student may best help the student by first dialoguing with him or her. Through the dialogue, if the educator still thinks the student has a problem, but the student disagrees, then the educator could point out the possibility of being judged negatively by future employers, as I also was, and by patients of the dominant culture. This at least forewarns the student of the reality of the pressure from the dominant culture to change. The educator should emphasize that the cultural differences do not mean that Hmong culture is inferior. The instructor could also plant the idea that perhaps between "now and graduation," the student could reflect on what was discussed in the dialogue and investigate several resources on cultural diversity and communication style, which the educator could even provide. The purpose of the instructor's dialogue with the student should be to help the student self-strategize in a nonthreatening way without imposing behavioral changes upon the student.

The HEC emphasis on exploring meaning with students also opens the door for alternative pedagogies. Rather than having students just focus on tasks to be memorized, especially when those tasks may no longer be meaningful or helpful in the care of patients (Ironside, 2003), instructional technology can be put in place to help teach the content that students need to learn in order to pass the national licensure examination, thereby freeing nurse educators to spend more time creating relationships with students, as I have done, and helping students explore what is most meaningful to them and their patients (Pharris & Endo, 2007). One such alternative pedagogy is narrative pedagogy.

NARRATIVE PEDAGOGY

Narrative pedagogy goes hand in hand with HEC-guided education. Narrative pedagogy emphasizes a safe, fair, respectful, and site-specific learning community in which students and educators work in partnership to come up with what is meaningful to the person being cared for (Ironside, 2003). Narrative pedagogy (Ironside, 2003) shares with HEC (Newman, 1994) the importance of dialogue focused on discovering meaning for the individual.

Picard and Henneman (2007) invite nurses facing complex situations to consistently ask the questions "What is happening here?" and "What are we doing here?" (p. 41). Their viewpoint resonates with me as I think about what is going on in nursing education. Study after study has not been able to document increased *critical* thinking skills in nursing students following completion of a whole nursing program (Staib, 2003). Yet, we continue to dole out multiple-choice tests as if the scores on these tests measure students' critical thinking. There is a paucity of research linking *critical* thinking to *clinical* thinking or clinical competency (Tanner, 2005). There is article after article on the *definition* of *critical* thinking, yet we have no effective tool to measure it (Tanner, 2005). What are we doing here? The world's population of people of color is growing; yet, there is a worldwide shortage of nursing students of color, nurses of color, and nurse educators of color. What is going on here? What is happening to nursing students of color? What is happening to nurse educators of color?

THEORY-GUIDED PRACTICE: THE KEY TO COMING HOME

Carol Picard and Elizabeth Henneman (2007) call for nursing education and practice to be theory-guided so that nurses live out the values and philosophy that underpin nursing theories. They assert that many nursing faculty have not had the experience of doing this, thereby contributing to the current state of nursing education in which theoretical courses are taught separately from other nursing courses and strong linkages to clinical practice are not made. When nurses studying the meaning of experiences for students, patients, and their families do not make reference to applicable nursing theories, the nursing knowledge generated is weakened, which ultimately leads to disciplinary incoherence.

I am a nurse who thought I had abandoned theory-based practice many years ago only to realize that all the time I was grounding my practice in values and philosophy that coincide with HEC. This realization led me to theory-guided practice based upon HEC. My lived experience pointed the way to a narrative pedagogy. I have found the combination of HEC and narrative pedagogy useful in my work with Hmong students and with Hmong patients. Hmong cosmology and HEC both share the ultimate goal of love. All of humanity yearns to be loved. No wonder when I embraced HEC, it was like embracing a family member—and coming home.

I value very highly my lived experience because it has taught me to focus on the meaning of experiences for Hmong students, Hmong patients, and their families. It has pointed the way back to theory for me when I was lost. As Carper (1978) pointed out in her seminal article on "Fundamental Patterns of Knowing in Nursing," voices like mine, based upon lived experiences, even if not based upon formal empirical research, provide worthy evidence to be taken into account in transforming nursing education.

RECOMMENDATIONS FOR NURSE EDUCATORS

Based on my lived experiences, I make the following recommendations for nurse educators and nursing education administrators to create a more culturally inclusive environment in nursing education:

1. Design your office to be welcoming to culturally diverse students.
2. Clearly and consistently post your schedule of availability and also verbally emphasize to students that you are willing to see them outside of these times if necessary.
3. Emphasize before and after postclinical conferences that *any* concerns students have are important to you, too.
4. Tell students to write down concerns, thoughts, and ideas they want to talk to you about but feel uncomfortable sharing in groups.
5. Learn about a variety of pedagogies.
6. Learn about nursing theories, and use them as guides to reflect upon one's pedagogy.
7. Get some teaching experiences in other countries and communities, if possible, where your minority student populations come from.
8. Utilize the talking circle format to discuss clinical as well as academic issues.
9. Bring copies of the code(s) of ethics for nurses to postclinical conferences and use the code(s) in discussions.
10. Participate in cultural diversity activities in your community and in your institution.
11. Talk to students of color and ask them how things are going from the beginning in order to build a relationship early on.
12. Share your own stories of vulnerability as a student or novice.
13. Explicitly state the rules of respect for persons and of being nonjudgmental during postclinical conferences and in any discussion.

RECOMMENDATIONS FOR NURSING EDUCATION ADMINISTRATORS

1. Actively recruit nurse educators of color.
2. Do research to find out why nursing students and nurse educators of color leave your institution.
3. Take action to address the reasons why nursing students and nurse educators of color leave your institution.
4. Use research findings to back up your recruitment efforts of nurse educators of color.

5. Do surveys and/or talk to your nurse educators of color to find out what challenges they are facing and what students of color are saying about their experiences in your institution.
6. Advocate for competitive salaries for nurse educators.
7. Establish a formal assessment mechanism to find out from students which instructional practices and institutional practices have promoted their learning and professional and personal growth, which have been an impediment and why, and what changes they recommend.
8. Use a variety of assessment formats, not just the traditional questionnaire, which require students just to fill in boxes.
9. Identify, in conjunction with nurse educators, how assessment findings are related to the performance of minority students as well as the performance of nonminority students; identify what changes need to be implemented, make the changes, and evaluate the outcome.
10. Collaborate with other disciplines to establish an institutional policy of inclusivity and publicly acknowledge inclusivity as a part of the institution's culture.
11. Form community partnerships to build mentor–mentee relationships with communities of color.

QUESTIONS FOR DIALOGUE

1. What ideas or concepts did you find most meaningful in this chapter? Identify your insights and questions to bring to a dialogue with your colleagues.
2. Do the postclinical conferences in your nursing program provide an environment in which students feel comfortable sharing incidents of racist and/or culturally insensitive encounters in the clinical setting? Why or why not? What suggestions do you have for creating a safer environment for these kinds of dialogues?
3. Using the talking circle process discussed by Yang, dialogue as a faculty or student group about incidents of racism and/or cultural insensitivity in your nursing program and strategize how to create a more culturally inclusive and welcoming environment.
4. Discuss the additional responsibilities that minority faculty are expected to shoulder in historically White schools of nursing.

To what extent are minority faculty justly compensated for the many committees, diversity initiatives, and panels they participate in and the mentoring of minority students they take on? To what extent do minority students and faculty from different ethnic minority backgrounds support each other, both formally and informally, in your program?

5. Has your institution made a public declaration that "inclusivity is a nonnegotiable part of the college or university's culture"? To what extent is there a supportive infrastructure in place? To what extent does the racial and ethnic makeup of your nursing faculty reflect your student body and the community you serve? If not, in what ways is your program seeking to increase faculty diversity?
6. What formal assessment mechanisms are in place to evaluate the extent to which your program has promoted the learning and professional and personal growth of all of its students? Does your program use a variety of assessment formats? If not, what suggestions do you have?

REFERENCES

American Nurses Association (ANA). (2005). *Code of ethics for nurses with interpretive statements.* Washington, DC: Author.

Brown, J. W. (2006). Margaret A. Newman: Health as expanding consciousness. In A. M. Tomey & M. R. Alligood (Eds.), *Nursing theorists and their work* (6th ed., pp. 497–521). St. Louis: Mosby Elsevier.

Carper, B. A. (1978). Fundamental patterns of knowing in nursing. *Advances in Nursing Science, 1*(1), 13–23.

Diekelmann, N. (2001). Narrative pedagogy: Heideggerian hermeneutical analyses of lived experiences of students, teachers, and clinicians. *Advances in Nursing Science, 23*(3), 53–71.

Gunther, M. E. (2006). Martha E. Rogers: Unitary human beings. In A. M. Tomey & M. R. Alligood (Eds.), *Nursing theorists and their work* (6th ed., pp. 244–266). St. Louis: Mosby Elsevier.

International Council of Nurses (ICN). (2006). *The ICN code of ethics for nurses.* Geneva: Author.

Ironside, P. M. (2003). New pedagogies for teaching thinking: The lived experiences of students and teachers enacting narrative pedagogy. *Journal of Nursing Education, 42*(11), 509–516.

King, M., & Multon, K. (1996). The effects of television role models on the career aspirations of African American junior high school students. *Journal of Career Development, 23*(2), 111–125.

Monti, E. J., & Tingen, M. S. (2006). Multiple paradigms of nursing science. In W. K. Cody (Ed.), *Philosophical and theoretical perspectives for advanced nursing practice* (4th ed., pp. 27–41). Boston: Jones and Bartlett.

Newman, M. A. (1994). *Health as expanding consciousness* (2nd ed.). Sudbury, MA: Jones and Bartlett (NLN Press).

Newman, M. A. (2008). *Transforming presence: The difference nursing makes.* Philadelphia: F. A. Davis.

Nokes, K. M., Nickitas, D. M., Keida, R., & Neville, S. (2005). Does service-learning increase cultural competency, critical thinking, and civic engagement? *Journal of Nursing Education, 44*(2), 65–70.

Pharris, M. D., & Endo, E. (2007). Flying free: The evolving nature of nursing practice guided by the theory of health as expanding consciousness. *Nursing Science Quarterly, 20,* 136–140.

Picard, C., & Henneman, E. A. (2007). Theory-guided evidence-based reflective practice: An orientation to education for quality care. *Nursing Science Quarterly, 20,* 39–42.

Shihadeh, E. S., & Flynn, N. (1996). Segregation and crime: The effect of Black social isolation on the rates of Black urban violence. *Social Forces, 74,* 1325–1352.

Smedley, B. D., Stith, A. Y., & Nelson, A. (Eds.). (2002). *Unequal treatment: Confronting racial and ethnic disparities in health care.* Washington, DC: The National Academies Press.

Staib, S. (2003). Teaching and measuring critical thinking. *Journal of Nursing Education, 42*(11), 498–508.

Struthers, R., Kaas, M., Hill, D. L., Hodge, F., DeCora, L., & Geishirt-Cantrell, B. (2003). Providing culturally appropriate education on type 2 diabetes to rural American Indians: Emotions and racial consciousness. *Journal of Rural Community Psychology, E6*(1), 1–12.

Tanner, C. A. (2005). What have we learned about critical thinking in nursing? *Journal of Nursing Education, 44*(2), 47–48.

Von Bergen, C. W., Soper, B., & Foster, T. (2002). Unintended negative effects of diversity management. *Public Personnel Management, 31*(2), 239–251. Retrieved from EBSCO database.

Williams, D. R., & Collins, C. (2002). Racial residential segregation: A fundamental cause of racial disparities in health. In T. A. LaVeist (Ed.), *Race, ethnicity, and health* (pp. 369–390). San Francisco: Jossey-Bass.

Yang, A., Xiong, D., Pharris, M. D., & Vang, E. (2006, April). *The experience of Hmong women living with diabetes.* Presentation at Midwest Nursing Research Society 30th Annual Research Conference, Milwaukee, WI.

Yang, D. (1993). *Hmong at the turning point.* Minneapolis, MN: WorldBridge Association.

6 Journeying Beyond Traditional Lecture: Using Stories to Create Context for Critical Thinking

SUSAN GROSS FORNERIS AND SUSAN ELLEN CAMPBELL

Well, here it is, my first clinical day ever . . . I'm not sure I'm ready for this . . . I just have to walk through the door . . . I am entering the room to have a conversation, provide support. I love listening to people; I actually find it fascinating. It is a way to understand people, to learn about them, hear their story . . . understand who they are. Those are the words I told myself as I recalled my first patient. The information I had about my patient only filled half a sheet of paper. I knew about her medical diagnosis, her medications . . . I didn't know anything about the person she was . . . I knew I would learn something new because she was elderly and from a culture different than mine. I started to feel anxious . . . doubt my abilities. As we began, our communication was a bit on the reserved side . . . I was kind of focused on my communication skills and had to remind myself to relax and just listen to the words of my patient. I found she started to relax while telling me about what brought her to the hospital . . . In the past, I have visited with elderly people many times, and I have learned that they have many stories. Even though they might speak more slowly, they can still be very aware of what is happening. With my first patient, I saw the importance of good communication and developing a therapeutic relationship. I felt a real sense of accomplishment by just having spent time with my patient listening to her because it really made all the difference in understanding her needs, beginning to understand her culture . . . her story.

John Dewey, an American pragmatist, believed that education should prepare individuals to understand the nature of the world in which they live by developing their capacity to think, see problems, relate facts, and enjoy ideas but, most importantly, to think critically (Alexander, 1987; Dewey, 1933, 1958). Students do not learn from just textbooks and lectures but from their ability to discuss and apply their own experiences and ideas, like the nursing student above. Information is best taught relative to its relationship to nature—encouraging student observation, inquiry, testing, and reflection. Many of the teaching and learning processes in nursing education, while seemingly effective at enhancing students' critical thinking abilities in structured learning situations, do not prepare them to manage the uncertainties that actually exist in practice. Teaching and learning processes need to move students from knowing what to knowing how and knowing why so that students can determine what is meaningful and relevant within the context of practice. Engaging students to move along this continuum of knowing is the challenge for professional nursing education, for knowing is not always easily articulated. The growing number of culturally diverse nursing students along with diverse learning styles creates an impetus for nurse educators to move along this continuum of knowing.

The purpose of this chapter is to discuss the design and implementation of a contextual reflective case-based teaching process to help students with diverse learning styles and cultures make meaningful connections in their learning. Contextual learning is a process of teaching that involves the examination of the context of practice and incorporates the use of dialogue combined with the use of narratives or stories. Storytelling is one of the oldest means of communication and exists in every culture. The use of storytelling as a teaching technique helps students embrace important aspects of their culture as they begin to blend and adapt to new ways of coming to know (Koenig & Zorn, 2002). The American Academy of Nursing Expert Panel on Cultural Diversity (1992) discusses the need for more educational models that address the cultural diversity of student nurses. Newer conceptual models in nursing education have emerged that emphasize the use of context and personal experiences in the teaching and learning process (Rew, 1996). These models provide insight into how nurse educators can embrace the diversity of experiences among students, creating a process of learning that becomes an empowering experience that may be more consistent with their culture's ways of knowing than traditional didactic models of learning. This chapter describes the contextual case-based teaching process in detail. The authors begin with a brief exploration of the philosophical and theoretical underpinnings of this approach, followed by a discussion of the instructional methodology that was used in implementing the approach in an introductory professional nursing assessment course. Lessons learned from this initiative are discussed in light of possible revisions.

BACKGROUND: PERSPECTIVES ON THINKING

Without a doubt, learners need ways to connect their classroom knowledge with their everyday lived experience and to recognize the role culture and experience play in refining values and beliefs. Learning connections are generally made at the individual level as learners think about their unique experiences and make connections in meaningful and practical ways. Teaching and learning processes in the discipline of nursing need to take into account these unique experiences and the cultural influences that guide student thinking. As nurse educators contemplate ways to create meaningful learning across diverse learners, they can draw on these words by philosopher Milton Mayeroff (1971): "I grow by becoming more self-determining, by choosing my own values and ideals grounded in my own experience instead of either simply conforming to the prevailing values or compulsively rejecting them" (p. 13). Mayeroff suggests that there is a relationship between growth and self-determination. He also engages us to appreciate the relationship between values, beliefs, and human experiences. Learners come to us with values and beliefs grounded in unique experiences. Recognizing and celebrating this uniqueness assists learners in their process of becoming more self-determined. Like Dewey (1933), Mayeroff's words embrace the notion that teaching and learning are processes of engaging these unique experiences to appreciate the values and beliefs that ultimately guide thinking. Engaging learners to reflect on their experiences so they come to know their values and beliefs not only helps them to understand the nature of the world around them but also engages them in a process of thinking critically.

Critical thinking in nursing is described as purposeful, outcome-oriented thinking that is driven by patient needs (Alfaro-LeFevre, 1999). Critical thinking described in this way is based on the principles of the nursing process and scientific method and is viewed by some in the discipline of nursing as synonymous with scientific method. As such, critical thinking is equated with the process of identifying a problem, collecting data, outlining a solution, testing hypotheses, and evaluating findings in an evidence-based manner. In the discipline of nursing, this format of thinking is described as the nursing process of assessment, diagnosis, planning, implementing, and evaluation.

Regardless of how effective the nursing process may be in helping nurses to think systematically, other scholars in nursing believe that critical thinking involves more than the nursing process (Benner, 1984; Diekelmann, 1993, 1995, 2001; Peden-McAlpine, 2000; Tanner, 2000). As the discipline of nursing continues to define and expand its body of knowledge, it has become clear that the complexity of practice requires more than a sequential approach to thinking. It requires critical thinking that is imaginative, creative, dynamic, and reflective and an approach to practice that involves the *examination of context* to improve not only the practice itself but, more importantly, the outcomes for our patients (Argyris, 1982; Brookfield, 1990; Forneris, 2004; Freire, 1970; Mezirow, 2000; Ruth-Sahd, 2003; Schon, 1987; Tennyson & Breuer, 1997). Through this process of critical thinking, we learn by being involved in the world and with others. We compare and share information that focuses on the nature of the world around us, taking into account different cultures, values, and beliefs—*context*. Context is the nature of the world in a given moment and includes the culture, underlying assumptions, facts, rules, beliefs, and principles (Forneris, 2004). By creating a greater awareness of the relevant issues within the given context of a situation, we can critically discriminate between facts and ideas and differentiate how knowledge may change given context. Meaning emerges as we critically discriminate differences and make sense of the world around us. Through our experience of being and interacting in context, we come to understand. Engaging context within the teaching process creates an opportunity to acknowledge each learner's uniqueness, influencing the way he or she creates meaning and builds a knowledge base.

Thinking as Narrative: Nursing Education Research

Within the nursing education literature, several recent studies have been instrumental in developing a process of teaching that involves the examination of the context of practice. These studies use dialogue combined with the use of narratives or stories (e.g., narrative pedagogy) to study nursing students' reflective thinking (Andrews et al., 2001; Diekelmann, 2001; Ironside, 2003). Narrative pedagogy involves dialogue through the sharing and interpretation of stories. Through public conversations, students and teachers share and discuss their reflections on their practice experiences in the context of nursing education. Diekelmann's (2001) 12-year study used narrative pedagogy and a phenomenological approach to study the common experiences and shared meanings of over 200 nursing students, teachers, and clinicians. She concluded that as participants discussed and reflected on their stories, they were able to communicate in a manner that (a) moved beyond issues of power, (b) embraced questioning that went beyond critique, and (c) remained open to future possibilities.

Building on the work of Diekelmann (2001), Andrews et al. (2001) also used narrative pedagogy to explore reflective thinking with nursing faculty and students, who gathered to share their teaching and learning experiences. The findings suggested that students learned to dialogue about what really matters and were able to identify the lens through which they examined their experiences, making visible the nature of their thinking within the context of practice. The researchers also noted that through dialogue about stories, faculty was able to highlight the relevancy of a clinical situation given its context.

Also building on the work of Diekelmann (2001), Ironside (2003) used narrative pedagogy to study reflective thinking with 15 teachers and 18 students from all levels and types of nursing schools in the midwestern United States. Two themes emerged: (a) thinking as questioning and (b) practicing thinking. These themes suggest that reflective thinking in practice moves beyond answering questions to questioning everything known and unknown in nursing practice in an effort to interpret situations accurately.

The significance of these three studies was the use of stories as a teaching process to operationalize students' reflective thinking. The studies illustrated that this teaching process provides opportunities for students to attend to the practice of thinking. Reflective thinking combined with dialogue results in students' increased open-mindedness, increased ability to understand the viewpoints of others and to challenge the practice of others, and, most importantly, greater awareness of relevant issues and an overall emergence of the client as the center of care. Narrative pedagogy in particular facilitates a critical dialogue (i.e., encouraging students to challenge perceptions, asking questions beyond expository or declarative knowledge) and makes visible the nature of thinking to broaden perspectives and reframe thoughts and insights.

The use of critical dialogue as a model to assist students and faculty in understanding and creating an empowering learning experience for culturally diverse students has also been explored in the nursing education literature. One such theoretical model, Pathways (Rew, 1996), promotes relational interaction between faculty and students. The Pathways Model uses the analogy of travel as a metaphor to create this relational learning experience. The model emphasizes three major concepts: (a) *recognizing the diversity of roads* traveled by students, (b) creating a *learning landscape* that embraces diversity in the educational process, and (c) building unique *pathways* that lead the student into professional nursing practice. The model emphasizes the important interaction between context and human development. Faculty engage students in dialogue to recognize unique experiences and their impact on the learning process. This model was introduced among a small core of faculty in a school of nursing (Rew, 1996) and applied with a diverse population of students. The model facilitated an increased comfort level in the learning process between diverse students and faculty. The model provides insight into how students come to know through the use of their own personal stories as context blended with the context of their learning environment.

Thinking as Narrative: Case-Based Teaching

Drawing from the nursing education literature on narrative pedagogy and critical dialogue, faculty involved in teaching an introductory professional nursing assessment course integrated stories into their teaching approach in an effort to begin developing a foundation for students to *think within the context of nursing practice.* Students involved in the course had few clinical experiences both prior to and within the first two months of the course. This lack of context limited the students' abilities to share and reflect on their own stories as a process of learning. Therefore, faculty improvised by creating stories and a context for practice and sharing them through a case-based teaching approach, moving to the use of personal narratives later in the course.

The contextual, case-based teaching approach used is derived from the philosophical and theoretical notions of narrative or story. The use of stories or storytelling has been a part of many cultures as an oral tradition and primary means of passing on information or knowledge intergenerationally (Koenig & Zorn, 2002). As such, storytelling is one of the oldest and most effective approaches to teaching and learning. Stories provide an opportunity for diverse students to share what is important from their cultural upbringing that may impact the way in which they are thinking about their learning and how they engage and embrace new educational concepts (Bartol & Richardson, 1998; Diekelmann, 1995; Sandelowski, 1991).

Stories (as narrative) capture temporal aspects of the human experience as it changes over time. Peden-McAlpine (2000) and Pieper (Eberhart & Pieper, 1994) discussed the use of narrative (stories) as a way to organize human experiences into actions and events. They contend that we are better able to understand experiences and actions when we actively read and reflect on stories. Through reflection, we focus on the context of the story through which the implicit meanings can be understood. Therefore, narrative understanding is the form through which life experiences are organized and meaning can be interpreted. Stories provide the mechanism for understanding as they can be reflected on, reanalyzed, and reinterpreted.

Instructional theorist Roger Schank uses stories in his instructional methodology of case-based teaching (Riesbeck & Schank, 1989; Schank, Berman, & Macperson, 1999). Schank et al. (1999) assert that stories are easily remembered because they are stored in memory via the sights, sounds, and smells of our experiences and are then retrieved by the cues in the environment. Therefore, learning that occurs within the context of a story has a greater chance of being recalled and transferred to other learning situations (Schank et al., 1999). Schank et al. also assert that teaching through stories: (a) the *process of thinking* or the *how to* of learning as opposed to the factual knowledge or the *what* of learning, (b) achieving goals that are relevant and important to the learner given the context of an experience, and (c) learning within context, rather than decontextualized learning.

Case-based teaching as a reflective pedagogy engages the learner in a process of critical reflection, *unveiling the reality* in a story through reflection. The learner is provided with a foundation of stories to begin to structure their knowledge and understanding. As the learner progresses to the use of their own real-life experiences, they begin to create their own stories. The learner reflects on these stories to understand their meaning within the context of real life experiences. Understanding new educational experiences as stories helps the learner to problem solve. In the discipline of nursing, as experts encounter problems in practice, they compare the current problem to past practice experiences. Experts in practice apply past experiences or stories from memory to inform new situations (Peden-McAlpine, 2000). Case-based teaching provides the stories as context for beginning nursing students to inform new situations.

TRANSFORMING THE LECTURE: A JOURNEY OF CASE-BASED TEACHING

The case-based teaching approach used in this introductory nursing assessment course encompasses two main components: case-based scenarios and guided reflection. The course was a 15-week nursing assessment course that encompassed a variety of practical clinical experiences (e.g., preschool screening, school-age assessment, and health education), culminating in a 3-day sub-acute care clinical experience.

Case-Based Scenarios

The purpose of using case-based scenarios is to provide a nursing practice context to assist the nursing students in their thinking and learning about professional nursing assessment. Stories capture and accentuate context. Through the use of nursing stories as an educational strategy, the context of practice situations is revealed through reflection of the how and why of specific actions in specific context. Adapted from Schank's instructional methodology (Riesbeck & Schank, 1989; Schank et al., 1999), the goals for each class discussion on assessment focus on (a) the students' understanding of the components of a comprehensive professional nursing assessment (e.g., physical assessment, professional communication, and establishing therapeutic relationships) and (b) the nurse educator demonstrating professional nursing assessment through role-play in the classroom setting. Topics are introduced to the student in the form of case-based scenarios that include patients' stories.

Students are guided through the assessment process through case-based scenarios that focus on developing an understanding of assessing the whole person without assumption or bias. For example, students are asked to read the scenario for Lucas Hernandez (see Appendix A) and complete the following tasks: (1) answer questions regarding the patient's history and physical assessment; (2) apply principles of therapeutic communication in the interview process; and (3) identify assumptions, values, and beliefs related to race, ethnicity, and sexual orientation that may influence the student's thinking about the patient.

Students prepare their course reflections prior to attending class. During the classroom discussion, students meet in small groups to share their reflections. Specific instructional time is allocated to dialogue and reflect on the narrative stories. The nurse educator then guides a large group discussion and has students share their reflections and insights from their small groups. The reflections and discussions form the basis of the students' notes on the topic. This teaching process moves the nurse educator's role from lecturer to guide in facilitating students' thinking. Using the stories, the nurse educator guides the students' thinking about the main ideas of each course topic, helping students to make connections between topics. Similar to the Pathways Model and travel analogy outlined by Rew (1996), the students and faculty interact to guide safe passage through the learning landscape. As the course progresses, the nurse educator engages the students to reflect on past and present learning experiences to help them make sense of new learning situations. Through a contextual case-based approach to teaching, the students and educators embrace new ways of coming to know by working together to create an awareness of social and cultural values and beliefs, which enhances our understanding of and communication with our clients.

Guided Reflection

Guided reflection questions are used in conjunction with the case-based scenarios as outlined previously. As the students begin to engage in their own clinical experiences (e.g., 3-day clinical component), guided reflection becomes a more personal reflective learning activity. The student's 3-day clinical experience occurs over the course of three weeks with each clinical day lasting approximately 5 hours. The main learning objectives for the clinical component include: (a) performing a history and physical assessment, (b) integrating communication skills to establish a therapeutic relationship, and (c) completing a plan of care. Students prepare a reflective journal by documenting their clinical experiences in the form of a story. Using guided questions (e.g., what factors influenced your thinking, what assumptions did you have, what sources of knowledge influenced your thinking, etc.), they reflect on their written story and describe how they will integrate this learning into their future practice.

At the end of the clinical experience, students meet individually with a nurse educator to discuss their nursing care plans and reflective journals. The nurse educator then guides each student in a reflective dialogue to illuminate the connections the student is making. For example, students often share stories that highlight their insecurities around practice experiences. The following is an exemplar of a story shared by a European American student:

I began my clinical day feeling lost and nervous to a moderate extent, but as soon as I met my patient those feelings began to dissipate as he was very talkative and friendly. Just being able to have a conversation with him and smile gave me the feeling that I was accomplishing something . . . At the end of the morning, my patient's family and his primary nurse came into the room to have a nurse–client teaching session. I noticed that my patient's family spoke to him as though he didn't really understand what they were saying. They spoke to him like one would speak to a child. As I observed this, I began to wonder why . . . he cannot articulate his words very well due to dysarthria . . . his family might assume he has a lag in comprehending as well. Then I started thinking, "If I hadn't spent so much time . . . listening to him, I probably would have assumed that he couldn't comprehend things very well either" . . . What influenced my thinking was the knowledge that communication is key, and knowing some of the pathophysiology of Parkinsons—in that dysarthria is a speech deficit not a thinking or comprehending deficit . . . being patient and listening is key.

Using their own stories, students are coached in their reflection to consider assumptions and beliefs and their impact on the learning process. For example, using this exemplar, the student was coached during her conference with the faculty member to talk about assumptions surrounding her knowledge and beginning clinical skills. To facilitate critical thinking and questioning, the nurse educator helped the student to identify important aspects of conversation with her patient that were missing from the story. These discussions opened the door to how this new learning might impact future clinical experiences.

For all students, but particularly those from highly relational cultural backgrounds, guided reflection provides an opportunity to reflect on past personal experiences and how cultural context can blend with a new learning context to create valuable learning connections. In the following exemplar, a Hmong American student uses her experiences with her grandmother to blend contexts that ultimately guided her learning connections around working with a European American elderly patient:

I could feel myself shiver. It wasn't the cold-shiver, but instead it was the nervous-shiver. After the introduction with the nurse, we were told to go to our patient . . . Standing in the hallway—unsure of what to do—I walked down and peeked into the patient's room. . . . I stood on the side of the door, reading thru my quick notes of the assessment, trying to remember everything. Then I realized I have to enter the room. I was not getting anywhere by standing there for so many minutes now. I entered and introduced myself to the patient. From this point on, I realized I have been so nervous

> *for nothing. . . . I felt so proud of my interaction with her. I didn't just go into the room to do an assessment, but also, to listen to her concerns and thoughts . . . Prior to going to clinical, I knew my patient had came close to death, and I made sure to be sensitive to this topic. I was not going to bring this up until she was comfortable bringing up the topic of why she was there. I wanted to let her talk when she was comfortable . . . My own experience with my grandmother had made me realize life wasn't about the quantity, but rather the quality. I went in the room with an open mind and listened to what my patient had to express . . . It wasn't about collecting just the data, but also, to have the caring component in the relationship–trust . . . During the conversation she did explain what had happened and why she chose what she had chosen for the code status. I made sure I was present throughout the entire assessment, but especially, when she brought this up.*

Using the student's story, the nurse educator and student dialogued about being present for the patient, and the connection between the student's past experiences with her grandmother blended with the new learning experience of the patient's near-death encounter. Dialogue focused on how cultural values and beliefs played a role in the student's interactions with the patient and how the blending of her cultural context and the new clinical context connected personal knowledge of elderly developmental tasks with theoretical knowledge. Guided reflection on stories provides an opportunity for students to assess their thinking, develop their knowledge base, and sharpen their critical thinking skills.

ASSESSING STUDENT THINKING THROUGH STORIES

While the course continued to use some traditional methods to assess thinking and learning (e.g., multiple-choice exams), stories were incorporated to provide a qualitative approach to assess how students might organize their thinking and begin to make important learning connections. The following discussion will focus on the use of stories to assess students' thinking and their knowledge and performance on nursing assessment and communication.

The use of case-based scenarios and guided reflection created an opportunity for reflective, self-directed learning. Preparation for small group discussion and sharing of insights was required prior to each course meeting. Each student was required to provide evidence of having completed the self-directed learning materials prior to the beginning of each class discussion with this activity weighted at 30% of the total course points. Student compliance with self-directed learning was outstanding at 99%–100%. More importantly, the reflection on stories and the sharing of insights created a classroom discussion that was rich and engaging. The guided reflection questions gave students an opportunity to structure their learning individually and then share and discuss their thinking with their classmates.

Case-based scenarios were also used to creatively assess students' therapeutic communication skills. In one example (see Appendix B), students read a scenario about Ellen James, an African American female. Students wrote out questions they would ask in response to statements made by the patient. They also reflected on how their own culture, values, beliefs, and assumptions might impact the way they established the relationship. Such guided reflection questions can provoke meaningful dialogue between faculty and students about hidden assumptions and biases about patients based on their race and ethnicity that may block a therapeutic relationship and quality care.

Building communication skills within a racialized context also provides students with an opportunity to reflect on how their own personal experiences impact their communication. It provides students from various cultural backgrounds an opportunity to share their cultural perspective and how this cultural perspective influences their thinking around communication. The following is an example of a Chinese American student's reflection on communication concerning the scenario provided in Appendix B:

> *When considering a culture, it is important to consider my own and Mrs. James's culture because actions can convey different meaning to Mrs. James and me. In my culture, touching is a way to show understanding and communication. On the other hand, Mrs. James's culture could misinterpret touching as a sign of aggression and/or she might not accept touches from other people than her family members . . . If I was in the room with Mrs. James and she was telling me about her concerns with the midcycle vaginal bleeding she had for the last two months and I suddenly touch her as a way of showing empathy, she could withdraw from me and feel betrayed because in her culture this is something that they don't accept from other people than family members and/or it could convey to her that it was a sign of aggression, therefore, this event [could] jeopardize the therapeutic relationship I am trying to build with Mrs. James.*

Building on communication skills in this way provided an opportunity for students to reflect on important principles of communication and blend new knowledge with their personal perspectives and life experiences, creating more of an awareness of how knowledge changes given the context. It also provides an opportunity for dialogue with students about stereotypes and the need to critically examine stereotypes about other cultures in deciding how to approach patients as individuals. For example, the student's perception that Mrs. James might not want to be touched could be a subject for dialogue and research. Indeed, not being touched might be perceived by Mrs. James as a sign of racism or lack of caring. Students can reflect on, research, and discuss the role of touch in patient care and contexts in which it may or may not be therapeutic, as well as whether broad cultural knowledge can be applied to individuals. The students can also role-play therapeutic touch and ways to gauge patients' comfort with touch.

Finally, students' use of their own personal stories and guided reflection at the end of the course provided an opportunity for nurse educators to assess important learning connections the students were making with nursing assessment across the course. The following is an exemplar of a story shared by a European American nursing student in her final clinical reflection:

> *This week's clinical was spectacular, I went in to this week not allowing myself to get nervous. I did a fair amount of preparation for this week and looked over [many times] all the information I needed to get . . . which helped me a lot . . . One aspect of my clinical experience that left me with feelings of accomplishment was that at the end of my time with the patient, she thanked me and said I will be a wonderful nurse . . . encouraging her to continue her PT at home, increase her activity, and having her explain to me how she was going to manage her medical cares as well as emotional outlets while at home left me feeling like I helped this patient more when she was able to leave the hospital . . . [I was thinking] what can I do now that will last when she is at home . . . The sources of knowledge that influenced my thinking was mainly I tried to think of what was taught in class on patient education and interventions that would help her current status and help her in the future. Some of my teaching she was not able to grasp or refused to admit were true (due to too much internet surfing on her part . . .) but all in all I hope I left her with some helpful information . . . past clinical experiences that helped me this last week . . . I learned how to ask questions and get information in the way of a conversation and also to tell just enough about myself to gain their trust. I truly think this clinical experience has made a positive impact on me . . . I will keep in mind what I have learned for future practice.*

The guided reflection gave students an opportunity to focus on their overall learning experiences and the thinking that guided their nursing actions. Stories, such as the previous one, help nurse educators gain insight into their students' thinking, what they were thinking about during their experiences, what guided their thinking, and what their personal learning accomplishments are.

Guided reflection and stories also provide a window into how culture and diversity impact overall learning. The use of the story and reflection questions creates more awareness for nurse educators of how diversity and culture impact meaningful learning. The following is an exemplar shared by an African American student:

> *Week 3 of clinicals was my best week . . . First of all, I had a female patient who I felt very comfortable with. She talked a lot and was very cooperative. She told me a lot about herself, and this made it easier for me to ask her the history questions. I took her vitals and did a head-to-toe assessment on her. She was eager to have her shower that morning . . . When I found out that my patient was female, I was relieved. I have had positive experiences working with elderly females at the elderly home where I work. I approached this situation with the assumption that my patient would be comfortable with me since we were of the same gender. I had at least one thing in common with her. With my previous patients, I believed that I had nothing in common with them since I was Black and female and they were both Caucasian and male. Those differences made me hold back a little bit and hindered my interaction with them. I was hesitant because I was not sure of how my patients viewed me or how they felt about me providing care for them . . . Thinking back on all of my interactions with my patients, I have learned that there will always be circumstances where I might not necessarily have anything in common with the people that I provide care for. This should not get in the way of my interactions with them. The two men that I [previously] cared for turned out to be really cooperative and appreciative of me regardless of our differences. In the future, I will approach such situations with less apprehension. I walked out of the [facility] feeling relieved and satisfied with the job I had done.*

The use of stories gave all students an opportunity to reflect and share how their unique perspectives challenged their learning. The student recognized how her assumptions and her previous experiences impacted the way in which she approached this care situation. This story also provided an opportunity for the nurse educator to discuss with the student her prior experiences, concerns, and fears about racism, which can impact learning. Students have an opportunity to talk through what they would have done had things gone differently.

Personal stories also create recognition of the importance of meeting the diverse needs of learners and understanding how culture impacts meaningful learning. In the following exemplar, a Mexican American student shares how the influence of her culture helped her to make important learning connections in the assessment of her patient:

> *At about 7:30* A.M. *after the group meeting I had the chance to meet my nurse. She was very nice and gave me a report on my patient. I felt nervous when I was following the nurse around, because I wasn't sure on what I was supposed to do. I watched the nurse take the patients vital signs. I didn't get to talk to my patient since she was using her asthma device and couldn't talk through it. But I introduced myself and asked if it was ok that I am here. She nodded her head up and down indicating yes . . . As I started getting information about my patient's history and get to know her better I felt a sense of satisfaction that I was accomplishing my tasks and having fun doing them. . . . What influenced my thinking was . . . I used my beliefs that is respect the elders. I believe older people have a lot of wisdom and knowledge to offer; therefore I used my full attention towards my patient and listened to her. I had a great time listening to what my patient had to say and I loved to hear the stories that she told about how St. Paul has changed since she was a child. The sources of knowledge that influenced my thinking were knowledge I learned growing up with my family. My family taught me to respect others. I also used the knowledge that I learned in lab. For instance I used some of the questions in the book to see if my patient's perception was intact. Such as "what is the date today?" My clinical experience taught me that nurses do important work for people. We can make a difference in a person's day and life. I noticed that by me listening and being interested in my patient it made her feel good about herself. I learned that head-to-toe assessment is an important aspect of a nurse's job and nurses need to do them right away to find out if there is anything wrong with the patient. The earlier the assessment the better care we can give. That lesson I will take with me throughout my career.*

Stories provide an opportunity for students to experience a sense of acceptance and support. In the previous story and reflection, the student was empowered by the meaningful connection she had made between her own beliefs and knowledge and the new knowledge she was using and, in the process, retaining a sense of her own cultural identity and family values. Nursing is brought to life through the use of stories engaging students and nurse educators as partners in learning. While formal evaluation tools are necessary to assess learning (e.g., written care plans and exams), the use of students' stories provides an additional perspective on their thinking and learning. Stories help students discern what aspects of their culture and which personal and family values they will weave into who they become as a nurse and to reflect on how that serves their patients.

RECOMMENDATIONS FROM THE JOURNEY OF CASE-BASED TEACHING: ROAD MAP CORRECTIONS

After faculty reflected on the teaching experience of using stories to enhance context, a number of key factors were noted that could be refined to enhance this teaching approach. First, course evaluations reflected a *redundancy* with guided reflection questions. While it was important that the questions focus on helping students to structure a foundation for learning, the questions should also be more intentional about the nature of the learning connections students should be making. In this way, students could be presented with different questions that build on previous questions each week, helping to eliminate the redundancy and enhance the small group discussions and guided discussion with the nurse educators. In addition, nurse educators noted that while using stories and guided reflection was a useful approach to help them transition from *lecturer* to *guide,* it was difficult to avoid slipping into the lecture mode when it appeared that students were not making important learning connections. There is a fine balance between assuring that foundational learning is taking place and that students are creating that foundation in their own meaningful way.

Second, guided reflection takes time! Nurse educators were overwhelmed with the amount of time guided reflective dialogue would take in order to make learning meaningful. The nurse educators worked individually with approximately 24 students each. The current course structure allowed little seminar time for small group interactions. As a result, instead of being able to engage students in a meaningful reflective dialogue, small group time was often limited to giving feedback to the students on the development of the nursing care plan and discussing issues that arose during the course of their clinical experiences. While students also created a journal encompassing their stories, the lack of seminar time and individual time impacted meaningful feedback. Nurse educators briefly reviewed the students' journal entries and had limited discussions during final conferences, but they acknowledged being unable to engage many students in a reflective dialogue. Therefore, the quality of faculty feedback was impacted given these time constraints and may have limited the faculty's ability to capture gaps and important connections with learning through the students' stories. The sheer volume of journal entries required of students over the course of three weeks became a factor in the *nature of the students' reflection.* Some of the students' stories were not actual stories but an evaluation of their clinical experience with limited discussion about the nature of their thinking about the story. Perhaps reducing the number of required journal entries by having students journal specifically in preparation for a small group seminar would make the journaling more meaningful and help the nurse educators prepare to guide a more reflective dialogue.

Third, nurse educators involved in the course need to enhance their dialogue skills with students. Dialogue should be a critical conversation with students that guides students' thinking. Critical conversations help students to integrate their prior learning and practical experiences. Students move from *telling what they know* to *why they know.* The use of stories gives students an opportunity to share their knowledge in unique ways. Educators can capitalize on these stories by guiding conversations that help students interpret their knowledge and achieve understanding of their actions. Dialogue in this regard also opens the door for students to integrate multiple perspectives into their thinking. Providing nurse educators with a series of reflective prompts or guided questions would help to enhance their dialogue and approach to conversations with students. This would also enhance the consistency with teaching and learning across the multiple nurse educators involved with students in one course.

Finally, Rew (1996) talks about the importance of faculty development in the process of teaching and learning across diverse student backgrounds. Providing more opportunities for nurse educators to share their own stories of engaging in this case-based approach to teaching enhances faculty awareness and sensitivity around diversity. Sharing their students' stories creates an opportunity to enhance their own knowledge about varying cultures and individual variation within cultural groups. In addition, sharing stories about individual teaching experiences creates opportunities for faculty to reflect on new learning strategies that engage diverse student learners. These discussions and faculty reflections lead to the implementation of new teaching and learning strategies, which in turn have the potential to engage all learners.

CONCLUSION

This chapter described a contextual reflective case-based teaching process that facilitated students to make meaningful connections in their learning. Students came to the course with limited clinical experiences but learned to build a repertoire of experiences through the sharing of stories and a beginning appreciation of how culture, values, and feelings guided their thinking through this repertoire of experiences.

The use of stories in a contextual learning approach helps us to envision new possibilities for nursing curriculum that creates an environment where students begin to operationalize a process of thinking that is derived not only from classroom learning but also from their own practice experiences and what they were thinking about when they cared for their patients. In keeping with the spirit of education from Dewey's (1933, 1958) perspective, students do not learn from just textbooks and lectures but also from their ability to discuss and apply their own experiences, values, cultural beliefs, and ideas. The goal of instruction becomes creating an opportunity for learning that integrates content knowledge with knowledge of the context. Nurse educators need to continue to explore the ways that new pedagogies, such as case-based teaching and the use of stories and reflection, inform self-determination and extend students' thinking, both within the classroom and within the practical clinical situation.

QUESTIONS FOR DIALOGUE

1. What ideas or concepts did you find most meaningful in this chapter? Identify your insights and questions to bring to a dialogue with your colleagues.
2. To what extent does your program incorporate case-based teaching to help students "think within the context of nursing practice" and develop critical thinking skills?
3. Given Yang's experiences as a student in the clinical setting (see chapter 5), how might this approach have provided a catalyst for deeper discussion and professional growth in the postclinical conference?
4. Dialogue with colleagues about ways in which guided reflection questions could help students process and learn from incidents involving discrimination.

5. To what extent do courses in your program incorporate case-based scenarios in the assessment of students, and what portion of final grades do they constitute? What are the advantages and disadvantages of this kind of assessment for students and faculty?
6. Reread the exemplar of the Black student taking care of a White female patient. Create guided reflection questions for your conference with this student. Share your questions with a colleague whose race is different from yours. Discuss how and why your questions are similar and/or different.

APPENDIX A

CASE-BASED SCENARIO: ASSESSING THE WHOLE PERSON

Directions: Please read the following "Story of Mr. Lucas Hernandez." Respond to each question following the story. *Your answers should show depth of thought and reflection.*

STORY OF MR. LUCAS HERNANDEZ

Lucas Hernandez, a 21-year-old college junior, arrives for his annual checkup. He has no specific health complaints, but he is concerned about juggling school and work responsibilities and the impact this might have on his health. Lucas states he is studying to become a teacher and also moonlights as a bartender four nights a week, from 7 P.M. to 3 A.M. He states he usually sleeps from 6 A.M. to noon on workdays, but he is about to start student teaching and must be at school from 7 A.M. to 4 P.M. He says he plans to sleep in two shifts.

The medical record reveals that Lucas's past health history, family history, and review of systems have been negative. His psychosocial profile reveals that he is gay and has been living with a partner for 2 years. Lucas states that he drinks only occasionally and is a vegetarian who includes eggs and milk in his diet. His physical assessment findings note that Lucas is well-groomed, speech clear, and in no acute distress. Vital signs are: Temperature 98° F; pulse 88 BPM and regular; respirations 20/mn; BP 130/80; pulse oximetry 98% room air; lungs clear. The records indicate that his immunizations are current, but he has not been immunized against hepatitis B. He declines HIV testing, stating that he is in a monogamous relationship.

Your *role as the nurse* is to perform both a *history* and *physical* assessment on Lucas Hernandez so that you can better address his concerns. After you have read and reviewed the chapters focused on nursing assessment, health history, and physical assessment, answer the following questions to help you review and understand the components of a nursing assessment relative to Lucas Hernandez.

Part 1: Answer the following questions focused on *history.*

1. Review the case study information on Lucas Hernandez. Define each of the following terms and identify examples from the case study for each term:

   Primary data source:

   (Definition):
   (Example from case study):

   Secondary data source:

   (Definition):
   (Example from case study):

   Subjective data:

   (Definition):
   (Example from case study):

   Objective data:

   (Definition):
   (Example from case study):

2. Using the principles of communication identified in your reading, write out one question that you would ask Lucas about each of the following:

   a. Current health status.

      Provide a brief rationale for why you are asking the question.

   b. Past health history.

      Provide a brief rationale for why you are asking the question.

   c. Family history

      Provide a brief rationale for why you are asking the question.

- **d.** Review of systems

  Provide a brief rationale for why you are asking the question.
- **e.** Psychosocial profile

  Provide a brief rationale for why you are asking the question.

Part 2: Answer the following questions focused on *physical assessment.*

1. Examine the case information of Lucas Hernandez. What were you thinking about as you read about Lucas? (Think about the questions that ran through your mind; think about the assumptions you might be having regarding the information Lucas shared. How do your values and beliefs influence your thinking?)
2. Based on Lucas's concerns, would you perform a complete health history or a focused health history? Describe the four techniques of physical assessment and how they would be used in your physical assessment of Lucas.

Adapted with permission from *Nursing Health Assessment: A Critical Thinking, Case Studies Approach,* by P. Dillon, 2003, Philadelphia: F. A. Davis.

APPENDIX B

CASE-BASED SCENARIO: COMMUNICATING THERAPEUTICALLY

Directions: Please read the following "Story of Mrs. Ellen James." Respond to each question following the story. *Your answers should show depth of thought and reflection.*

STORY OF MRS. ELLEN JAMES

Mrs. Ellen James is 29 years old, married, and the mother of one 4-year-old child. She complains of scant midcycle vaginal bleeding for the last two months. She has taken oral contraceptives since the birth of her child 4 years ago. She takes no other medications except occasional aspirin. She has no history of sexually transmitted infections (STIs). Family history is remarkable, including mother with breast cancer age 54, osteo-

porosis, and a fractured hip at age 63. Father has hypertension and had a myocardial infarction (MI) at age 68. Both parents are alive and well as are two healthy female siblings, ages 33 and 35. There is no family history of gynecological carcinomas (cancer). Mrs. James reports no serious problems relative to review of systems. She attended 1 year of college after high school and is currently a homemaker. Her husband is a stockbroker for an investment banking company. Review of systems is negative and general survey is unremarkable. Mrs. James appears to be a reliable source whose affect is very pleasant. Psychosocial profile includes a daughter who goes to daycare 2 days a week during which Mrs. James volunteers at an indigent health care facility. Her exercise/leisure activities include gardening, reading, and outside activities with her family. She was walking on a daily basis but has stopped this in the last year due to lack of time. She reports that she eats a balanced diet and has had an unexplained 10-lb. weight gain in the last year. She has never smoked, drinks a glass of wine with dinner 2–3 times per week, and denies using illicit drugs. Family attends church most Sundays. Describes loving relationship with spouse and states they intend to have three more children. Enjoys being a homemaker. States she has good relationship with siblings and parents. She uses prayer, friendships, and family support to deal with stress. Mrs. James has come for her annual wellness examination. As part of this examination, your role as the RN is to assess and promote wellness.

Question 1

An important component in your role as a professional nurse is the type of therapeutic relationship you establish with your clients. As you begin to establish a therapeutic relationship with Mrs. James, why is it important to consider how your own culture, past experiences, values, beliefs, and assumptions impact the way you establish this relationship? In addition to your response, *please give an example* (the example does not need to be a personal example; the example should help to illustrate the point(s) you are making).

Question 2

Review the information contained in Mrs. James's story.

Recall the characteristics of wellness discussed in theory class and also in your reading. Based on Mrs. James's story, identify three questions that you would ask about her wellness and provide your rationale for each.

Question 3

Use Erikson's developmental theory to identify the Developmental Stage for Mrs. James and two Developmental Tasks.

Question 4

During your visit with Mrs. James, you discuss her concerns surrounding her scant midcycle bleeding. Mrs. James makes the following statements. How would you respond? Provide your rationale for your response.

(a) "I'm afraid that I might have to have surgery." Your response might be:

(b) "Nurse, could this bleeding mean cancer?" Your response might be:

Question 5

During Mrs. James's visit to the clinic, you overhear another nurse talking with her. You identify pitfalls in this nurse's communication with Mrs. James. Read each of the following statements. After you have read the statement, identify the communication problem or pitfall. Provide a more therapeutic response.

(a) "Experiencing a bit of a weight gain at your age is really quite normal. Even if you haven't changed your routine much, I'm sure you have nothing to worry about." (Response to Mrs. James' concerns about her unexplained 10 lb wt. gain.)

(b) "If you want my advice, with your history of breast cancer, I would consider discontinuing taking your oral contraceptives."

(c) "You're not a victim of domestic abuse, are you?"

Adapted with permission from *Nursing Health Assessment: A Critical Thinking, Case Studies Approach,* by P. Dillon, 2003, Philadelphia: F. A. Davis.

REFERENCES

Alexander, T. M. (1987). *John Dewey's theory of art, experience, and nature: The horizons of feeling.* Albany: State University of New York Press.

Alfaro-LeFevre, R. (1999). *Critical thinking in nursing: A practical approach* (2nd ed.). Philadelphia: Saunders.

American Academy of Nursing Expert Panel. (1992). American Academy of Nursing Expert Panel Report: Culturally competent health care. *Nursing Outlook, 40,* 277–283.

Andrews, C. A., Ironside, P., Nosek, C., Sims, S. L., Swenson, M. M., & Yeomans, C. (2001). Enacting narrative pedagogy: The lived experiences of students and teachers. *Nursing and Health Care Perspectives, 22,* 252–259.

Argyris, C. (1982). *Reasoning, learning and action: Individual and organizational.* San Francisco: Jossey-Bass.

Bartol, G. M., & Richardson, L. (1998). Using literature to create cultural competence. *Image, 30,* 75–79.

Benner, P. (1984). *From novice to expert.* Menlo Park, CA: Addison-Wesley.

Brookfield, S. (1990). Using critical incidents to explore learners' assumptions. In J. M. Associates (Ed.), *Fostering critical reflection in adulthood: A guide to transformative and emancipatory learning* (pp. 177–193). San Francisco: Jossey-Bass.

Dewey, J. (1933). *How we think: A restatement of the relation of reflective thinking to the educative process* (2nd ed.). New York: Heath.

Dewey, J. (1958). *Philosophy of education.* Ames, IA: Littlefield, Adams.

Diekelmann, N. L. (1993). Transforming RN education: New approaches to innovation. In N. L. Diekelmann & M. L. Rather (Eds.), *Transforming RN education* (pp. 42–58). New York: National League for Nursing.

Diekelmann, N. (1995). Reawakening thinking: Is traditional pedagogy nearing completion? *Journal of Nursing Education, 34*(5), 195–196.

Diekelmann, N. (2001). Narrative pedagogy: Heideggerian hermeneutical analyses of lived experiences of students, teachers, and clinicians. *Advances in Nursing Science, 23*(3), 53–71.

Dillon, P. (2003). *Nursing health assessment: A critical thinking, case studies approach.* Philadelphia: F. A. Davis.

Eberhart, C. P., & Pieper, B. B. (1994). Understanding human action through narrative expression and hermeneutic inquiry. In P. L. Chinn (Ed.), *Advances in methods of inquiry for nursing* (pp. 41–58). Gaithersburg, MA: Aspen.

Forneris, S. G. (2004). Exploring the attributes of critical thinking: A conceptual basis. *International Journal of Nursing Education Scholarship, 1,* 1–18.

Freire, P. (1970). *Pedagogy of the oppressed.* New York: The Continuum International Publishing Group.

Ironside, P. M. (2003). Implementing and evaluating narrative pedagogy using a multimethod approach. *Nursing Education Perspectives, 24*(3), 122–128.

Koenig, J. M., & Zorn, C. R. (2002). Using storytelling as an approach to teaching and learning with diverse students. *Journal of Nursing Education, 4*(9), 393–399.

Mayeroff, M. (1971) *On caring.* New York: Harper.

Mezirow, J. (2000). *Learning as transformation: Critical perspectives on a theory in progress.* San Francisco: Jossey-Bass.

Peden-McAlpine, C. (2000). Early recognition of patient problems: A hermeneutic journey into understanding expert thinking in nursing. *Scholarly Inquiry for Nursing Practice: An International Journal, 14*(3), 191–222.

Rew, L. (1996). Affirming cultural diversity: A pathways model of nursing faculty. *Journal of Nursing Education, 35*(7), 310–314.

Riesbeck, C. K., & Schank, R. C. (1989). *Inside case-based reasoning.* Hillsdale, NJ: Lawrence Erlbaum.

Ruth-Sahd, L. A. (2003). Reflective practice: A critical analysis of data-based studies and implications for nursing education. *Journal of Nursing Education, 42*(11), 488–497.

Sandelowski, M. (1991). Tell stories: Narrative approaches in qualitative research. *Image, 23,* 161–166.

Schank, R. C., Berman, T. R., & Macperson, K. A. (1999). Learning by doing. In C. M. Reigeluth (Ed.), *Instructional design: Theories and models* (Vol. 2, pp. 161–183). Mahwah, NJ: Lawrence Erlbaum.

Schon, D. (1987). *Educating the reflective practitioner.* San Francisco: Jossey-Bass.

Tanner, C. (2000). Critical thinking: Beyond nursing process. *Journal of Nursing Education, 39,* 338–339.

Tennyson, R. D., & Breuer, K. (1997). Psychological foundations for instructional design theory. In R. D. Tennyson, F. Schott, N. Seel, & D. Sanne (Eds.), *Instructional design: International perspectives* (Vol. 1, pp. 113–135). Mahwah, NJ: Lawrence Erlbaum.

7 INDE Project: Developing a Cultural Curriculum Within Social and Environmental Contexts

VICKI P. HINES-MARTIN AND ALONA H. PACK

An undergraduate nursing student in her junior year develops a care plan for an African American, low-income, expectant teen to whom she has been assigned as part of her clinical experience. Her care plan is approved by her clinical faculty. It includes a list of needed baby items that include a crib, a changing table, children's toys, and a rocking chair. She discusses with the teen the places she can go with her mom to purchase these items . . .

An undergraduate nursing student is providing health information to a group of inner-city seniors at a center located in a public housing community. He discusses several areas for health maintenance related to aging. At the end of the presentation, he says to the audience—"Thanks for attending. You can find the information that I discussed at www . . . (Web site address)" as the final statement in this educational presentation . . .

Two African American undergraduate nursing students stop by the office of an African American nursing faculty member and begin to talk about their worries about nursing school, "College is not like high school . . . I always did well in math and science . . . I didn't know it would be like this. I study more, but I am still having problems." They also identify their frustration with many clinical experiences, "Why can't I go to the clinic or community setting in my neighborhood? I would like experiences like those, too!"

Each of these vignettes presents common situations that nursing faculty and nursing students have experienced as part of the educational process. These exemplars reflect one or more areas in which faculty and students lack cultural awareness, knowledge, and the ability to formulate meaningful nursing interventions relative to the diverse needs of others—their culture, their social and economic context, and their literacy. How schools of nursing can best address these needs is complex, challenging, dynamic, and uncertain. What *is* certain is that understanding and addressing diversity is an essential task that all of nursing education must address.

INTRODUCTION

Velde, Wittman, and Bamberg (2003) found that the population of the United States represents over 100 ethnically and racially diverse groups and may be more diverse than any other nation in the world. According to the 2004 U.S. Census Bureau report, approximately 31% of U.S. residents are members of racial or ethnic minority groups. Sixty-nine percent are Caucasian, but by 2050, that figure will drop to 50% (U.S. Census Bureau, 2004a). Wealthier nations throughout the world are experiencing similar demographic shifts. These changing demographics have had a significant impact on a multitude of human service agencies, such as law enforcement, schools, and health services, leading them to adapt to a myriad of language and communication differences (Smith, 1998). Due to changing demographics, there has been an ever-increasing awareness of the need for cultural competency for health care providers (Ndiwane et al., 2004). Dreher and MacNaughton (2002) contend that "cultural competency is really nursing competency" (p. 181) and should receive as much investment as any other standard of professional practice. Cultural competency, as the preferred approach to address changing demographics, has infiltrated into all health care environments as a result of governmental and accrediting agency mandates and professional standards of practice including contemporary nursing practice. Dreher and MacNaughton (2002) refer to two major categories in which clinicians need to be culturally competent. First, during the health care encounter, the communication process should reflect the ability of the health care provider to meet the needs of each client; and second, providers should be knowledgeable about the various cultures they encounter with respect to lifestyles and culturally determined health beliefs and behaviors.

CULTURAL DIVERSITY IN HEALTH CARE

Although there is much agreement on the need for cultural competence and culturally appropriate care, how that can be accomplished and supported in nursing education and nursing practice continues to evolve. One approach that has been supported in the literature is the increase of culturally diverse health care providers. The Sullivan Commission on Diversity in Healthcare Workforce (2004) identifies that in the United States the enrollment of diverse populations in nursing and other health professions has stagnated despite growing diversity in the general population:

> While African Americans, Hispanic Americans, and American Indians, as a group, constitute nearly 25% of the U.S. population, these three groups account for less than 5% of dentists, 6% of physicians, and 9% of nurses. Examining the education and training environment in which health professionals learn and develop is critical to efforts to increase the number of health care providers who can, and will, address health care needs. The absence of a diverse health care workforce may be an even greater cause of disparities in health access and outcomes than the lack of health insurance for tens of millions of Americans. (The Sullivan Commission, 2004, p. 1)

The literature demonstrates that minority health professionals are more likely to work with underserved and/or minority populations (Cooper & Roler, 2003; Komaromy et al., 1996), and minority persons are more likely to accept health care with the availability of minority health care providers and the culturally competent care they provide (The Sullivan Commission, 2004). In summary, there is a clear mandate to educate and graduate more minority nurses. The intent of this chapter is to outline a project designed to increase the graduation rate of African American nurses and improve the cultural competence and sensitivity of nursing faculty and students toward diverse clients and their families.

UNIVERSITY OF LOUISVILLE SCHOOL OF NURSING: THE SETTING OF THE PROJECT

Schools of nursing with limited numbers of minority students and graduates have sought new and unique approaches to address the national challenge to increase cultural diversity in their student populations and support cultural competence in nursing education. The University of Louisville School of Nursing (ULSON) in Louisville, Kentucky, is one of those schools, and its growth toward those goals has resulted in critical assessment, planned change, increased awareness, and some unintended outcomes.

The University of Louisville (U of L) is a public metropolitan university located in Louisville, Kentucky, which is one of the largest metropolitan areas in a primarily rural state. Louisville has a combined city–county government and a population of 687,235 citizens (U.S. Census Bureau, 2004b). The African American population in Louisville is 136,143 (19.8% of the population, compared to 7.3% of the state population). African Americans comprise 30% of the Louisville public school's elementary and secondary students and only 5.78% of the active registered nurses. African American per capita income in this metropolitan setting is approximately $18,335, compared to $36,071 for Whites. The largest segment of Louisville's African American population resides in the western portion of the city. This community experiences the highest rate of poverty, the lowest level of education, and limited social and economic resources (U.S. Census Bureau, 2000).

The same health disparities currently experienced by African Americans nationally are reflected in the health of African Americans in the Commonwealth of Kentucky. The *Health Status Assessment Report* (Office of Policy, Planning & Evaluation [OPPE], 2004) states that in Kentucky the death rate is the 10th highest in the nation, but the rate for African Americans exceeds the rate for Whites by 38%. The African American infant mortality rate is more than two times the rate among Whites, and low birth weight is highest among African American mothers, almost twice that of Whites. African Americans have higher mortality rates from heart disease, lung cancer, stroke, and accidental deaths than Whites. The diabetes death rate for African Americans is 74% higher than the rate for Whites (OPPE, 2004). The ULSON is part of a community that has significant health disparities. There continues to be an urgent need to address those disparities through culturally appropriate health care provided by an increasingly diverse workforce reflective of the community.

The ULSON nursing faculty reflects the demographics reported by the American Association of Colleges of Nursing (AACN). The AACN (2002) survey found that the overwhelming majority of nursing faculties are White women. Only 9.2% of faculty members come from racial/ethnic minority groups, and 3.7% are male. The ULSON has approximately 40 full- and part-time faculty members. Of that number, there has been an average of three African American female faculty members and two White male faculty members since 2000.

The ULSON has BSN, MSN, and PhD educational programs and a student population of almost 400, of which 10% are minority students (across all programs), the majority of whom are African American. At the U of L, BSN students are officially admitted into the upper division after completing their first 2 years of required preprofessional course work. Upper division includes the junior and senior level clinical instruction component of the curriculum and requires application and admission by committee. It is a competitive admission process, and admission is based on academic achievement. Although ULSON has more African American BSN students than other programs in Kentucky, it is still a relatively small number given the numbers needed to reflect demographics in the population. In the fall semester of 2001, African American students comprised 15% (23 of 153 enrolled in upper division nursing courses) and in fall 2002, 14.4% (20 of 139 enrolled). Additionally, the Kentucky Council on Postsecondary Education (the state's regulatory body over the colleges and universities), the University of Louisville, and the ULSON had identified as a priority the need to increase African American admission, retention, and graduation for all higher education including nursing.

DESCRIPTION OF THE INITIATIVE FOR NURSING DIVERSITY EXCELLENCE (INDE) PROJECT

In July 2003, the ULSON Initiative for Nursing Diversity Excellence (INDE) project was funded through June 30, 2006, by the U.S. Health Resources and Services Administration (HRSA)/Division of Nursing/Nursing Workforce Diversity program. The development of the INDE project was based on the conceptual definitions of culture and cultural competency developed by Cross, Bazron, Dennis, and Isaacs (1989), which identified these concepts as follows:

> *Culture* is the integrated pattern of human behavior that includes thoughts, communications, actions, customs, beliefs, values, and institutions of racial, ethnic, religious or social groups. *Competence* is the capacity to function effectively using a set of congruent behaviors, attitudes, and policies that come together in a system, agency, or among professionals and enable that system, agency, or those professionals to work effectively in cross-cultural situations. A culturally competent system of

> care acknowledges and incorporates—at all levels—the importance of culture, the assessment of cross-cultural relations, vigilance towards the dynamics that result from cultural differences, the expansion of cultural differences, the expansion of cultural knowledge, and the adaptation of services to meet culturally unique needs. (p. iv)

The purpose of the project was to increase the number of African Americans in the nursing profession and to increase activities to improve the cultural sensitivity and competence of faculty and students at the School of Nursing toward minority clients. The primary outcome of the project included increased enrollment of African American students admitted into upper division nursing with successful completion of the U of L BSN program. Barriers for African American students to upper-division admission, retention, progression, and graduation were identified as: disparities in academic preparation, financial constraints, and lack of peer and professional mentoring support during the educational process. These barriers had been previously identified through educational data, meetings with African American students, and faculty feedback.

As with other schools of nursing, ULSON had sought to increase its overall enrollment to address the nursing shortage. However, African American students are at additional risk for underrepresentation in the ULSON BSN program not only because of the educational, financial, and social disparities they have experienced, but also because of the rapidly rising numbers of applicants to nursing schools and limited class size, which have created an increasingly competitive environment. The INDE project focused on addressing all these barriers to African American representation.

The INDE project was a 3-year project composed of a set of complimentary programs that focused on activities aimed at increasing recruitment, retention, and graduation of African American students in the nursing profession (see Table 7.1 for description of all INDE components). INDE's programs were *voluntary,* and those that targeted the enrolled lower-division students provided academic and peer-mentoring support and stipends to those who qualified financially. The Tutoring Program was conducted in the following manner. First-semester freshmen students were assigned tutors in math/algebra, chemistry for health professionals, introduction to biology, and history/world civilization, as these courses were previously identified as the most challenging for the students. Lower-division students were scheduled for tutoring

Table 7.1

INDE PROGRAM COMPONENTS

COMPONENT	ACTIVITY/ FOCUS
Summer Enrichment Program	Invite incoming freshmen students to a 5-week session to provide a "jump start" in academic enrichment in the key freshmen lower-division courses. This activity also provides insight into the nursing profession as presented by guest speakers.
Tutoring	Provide academic support in math/algebra, chemistry for health professionals, introduction to biology, history/world civilization, psychology, microbiology, and anatomy and physiology.
Nursing Enrichment Program	Promote ongoing peer relationships and peer support. Provide information on previous student success and the nursing profession and specialties with presentations by former students and members of KYANNA Black Nurses Association, and seek student mentors.
Parents Day	Invite Future Nurses Club members' parents and parents of incoming freshmen to inform them of the nursing profession and the School of Nursing's undergraduate curriculum in order to promote student success and family support. Provide information from the admissions office, financial aid, and area local hospitals.
Future Nurses Clubs	Provide pre-entry academic preparation activities and information on the nursing profession to high school, middle school, and elementary school students. Also invite students to attend the school's Fall Open House.
Stipends and Scholarships	Stipends: Maximum of $1,500 per semester distributed monthly based on demonstrated financial need. Scholarships: Upper-division nursing students only. Maximum of $5,000 per year distributed at the beginning of the semester based on demonstrated financial need.

1 hour a week per course for 14 weeks. The tutors, who were referred to as Student Academic Managers (SAMS), also functioned as monitors and provided the SON academic advisor/project director with biweekly progress reports on tutored students indicating attendance, targeted grades, and strengths and weaknesses. Students who progressed in the lower-division curriculum were also provided with tutoring in microbiology, anatomy and physiology, and psychology. In addition, the university has an academic resource center, which students could utilize in the event an INDE project tutor was not available.

Lower-division students who demonstrated financial need were also awarded monthly stipends with a maximum award of $1,500 per semester. Students who received the stipends were required to attend relevant tutoring sessions unless they demonstrated they did not have academic need. Lower-division students receiving stipends were also required to attend Nursing Enrichment Program meetings, which are further described later.

The INDE program also included the Nursing Enrichment Program, which focused on both lower- and upper-division nursing students. This component included peer mentoring, professional support, and community outreach initiatives. The Nursing Enrichment component later evolved into the Black Student Nurses Association (BSNA), which continues to be an officially recognized university student organization that currently includes both lower- and upper-division students. It is an active organization that continues to provide mutual support, professional minority nurses as speakers and mentors, and student-led community health outreach.

Upper-division students who were progressing in their coursework and demonstrated financial need were awarded HRSA scholarships with a maximum award of $5,000 per year. Students were not permitted to receive both stipends and scholarships concurrently. Financial assistance in combination with the other components of the INDE project were developed as mediators against the multiple barriers to educational matriculation and progression that had been identified prior to the implementation of the program. It was hoped that these mediators would assist in ensuring INDE students' successful completion of the nursing curriculum and graduation.

The INDE project also provided activities through the Future Nurses Club that focused on academic preparation and exposure to the nursing profession for students at selected middle and high schools who demonstrated an interest in the nursing profession. Parents of students who were part of the Future Nurses Club were also provided with information about the nursing profession and the ULSON.

Lastly, INDE included a component that focused on entering undergraduate freshmen students who had declared nursing as their major and their parents. The focus of this component, the Summer Enrichment Program, was to help students and their parents make the connection with the ULSON and to get a jump start on the academics of the undergraduate curriculum. INDE project staff and select faculty members met with these students and parents to provide information and answer questions.

The goals of the Future Nurses Club, Summer Enrichment Program, and activities for parents, such as Parents Day, were to promote an interest in nursing, familial support of a career in nursing, and knowledge about the ULSON, in hopes of ensuring a competitive pool of African American students for admission into the upper-division nursing program in the future.

In addition to the aforementioned activities, goals were developed to enhance cultural awareness, cultural sensitivity, and cultural competence at the ULSON with each of these goals focused on both students and faculty as they relate to client care. Furthermore, these goals were to assist nursing faculty in teaching and supporting diverse students through the educational process.

INDE and Cultural Needs Assessment

The cultural aspect of the project included assessment, intervention, and evaluation components and was developed according to the following plan. Assessment areas included cultural sensitivity, knowledge, and competency within the nursing faculty and upper-division students. Attitude and competency assessment toward culturally different patients was originally scheduled for ULSON faculty and students at data points prior to, during, and following the INDE program. The assessments included self-assessment measures and discussion sessions with faculty and students as separate groups.

Assessment instruments were identified and administered at baseline to evaluate characteristics among the faculty and upper-division students. The assessment process during year one focused on gaining an understanding of what the current state of cultural awareness was on the part of students and faculty alike. The assessment instruments selected and used at baseline were the Cultural Self Efficacy Scale (CSES)

(Bernal and Froman, 1987) and the Ethnic Attitude Scale (EAS) (Rooda, 1992).

Findings from the initial assessment measures did not provide direction for the development of the INDE interventions or program evaluation, as anticipated. With respect to the CSES, both faculty and students reported confidence and competence in providing care to the African American population, with an average score of 69%. Changes in the course of the INDE project, which will be discussed later, made reassessment at the end of the 3 1/2-year period using the CSES inappropriate to the project's goals. The results of the EAS were also problematic in that this measure was too lengthy and a significant number of faculty and students did not complete it in its entirety during the initial administration. Therefore, the extent of the changes that might have occurred during the course of the project could not be adequately determined due to missing data.

On the other hand, qualitative data collected during the course of the project were invaluable in our understanding, direction, and evaluation of the project. Qualitative data were collected from faculty members through discussions during faculty meetings. Faculty discussion centered around their experiences with students of different racial and ethnic groups as well as their own assessment of their cultural attitudes, knowledge, and competence related to helping students with diverse patients. The undergraduate nursing faculty also participated in scheduled discussions with the INDE project director during faculty meetings, which provided ongoing data about faculty responses to ethnically and racially diverse student issues and the effects of the INDE project from their perspectives.

Faculty members exhibited a mixture of responses to the initiation of the INDE project. Some, who had an interest in expanding their cultural knowledge, were active in identifying the advice and resources they needed to become more culturally competent. Others felt they were competent in meeting the needs of multicultural students and patients. Those members who felt confident in their skills were either interested in facilitating the project or felt no need for involvement. There were several faculty members who expressed concern that the INDE project was focused on only one population and that other racial ethnic populations should also be targeted as part of this program. A few faculty members indicated that African American students were getting "special treatment." Issues of student confidentiality, lines of communication regarding minority student progress, responsibilities of the faculty in the project, the effects of the project on nonminority students, and the role of the INDE project director were all part of faculty discussions. These data were incorporated into the development, modifications, and evaluation of the project.

Qualitative data were also gathered by INDE staff from students participating in the project's Nursing Enrichment Program at regularly scheduled meetings. Faculty members were not a part of the meetings at which student data were collected. Students agreed to allow unidentified comments and discussions during the meetings to be used as part of the INDE assessment and evaluation process. Student feedback at meetings provided critical information on faculty and majority (nonminority) students' expressed cultural attitudes and demonstrated competencies. INDE students also provided their perception of the cultural competence needs of these two groups and their own impressions of the INDE project, which identified what was working, what could be modified, and areas for outcome evaluation.

The African American students reported they would appreciate more opportunities for clinical experiences in their own community to provide services to their people. They also felt that majority students needed to have these experiences, as well. They also expressed concern about a few incidences in which they perceived that majority students exhibited insensitivity through comments regarding other racial/ethnic groups, such as: "We take good care of our migrant workers" and "Why can't we have better patients?" when referring to minority patients. A comment from a majority student asking for the input of an African American student on how to care for an African American patient was perceived negatively by the African American student as she felt she should not be utilized as the "expert" resource.

Students also discussed issues related to the tension between meeting school requirements and family responsibilities. Several students were female with children and some were single parents. Most African American students were employed while attempting to keep up with school and clinical responsibilities. Most students were the first in their family to attend college, and their expectations of college education required adjustment. In addition, African American nursing students reflected similar economic and social circumstances as other members of their community. These sessions with students also afforded the INDE staff opportunities to problem solve with students about how to handle a variety of situations involving encounters with other students, faculty, and clients in clinical situations that were less than welcoming or supportive. For example, students were given strategies on how not to become defensive but to try to express their feelings using techniques that would convey their concerns in a professional manner. Assertiveness techniques and conflict situations were discussed, role modeled, and practiced. Students were also directed to discuss incidences that were perceived as offensive or insensitive with an assigned faculty member.

INDE Interventions

Interventions were developed to increase cultural sensitivity, knowledge, and competence for both students and faculty. The INDE project sponsored annual cultural diversity workshops for faculty and students. Speakers were identified at the local, national, and regional levels, in that order, to present at the ULSON. Additionally, the committee responsible for curriculum oversight at the ULSON was identified as the body to evaluate the content in each junior- and senior-level course for cultural components in their annual review of the undergraduate program and ensure that any recommendations for change were implemented. By the end of year one, interventions had occurred ahead of the timeline.

Implementation of interventions were undertaken in the following areas: (a) resources for the faculty on culturally appropriate teaching methodologies, models, and evaluation tools; (b) work with undergraduate faculty on teaching strategies; and (c) development of two seminars for junior- and senior-year students focused on culture care. These interventions were implemented during the first 2 years of the project. In year three of the project, the ULSON sponsored a faculty-wide program on culturally appropriate teaching strategies. This faculty-wide program was a nationally presented teleconference on multicultural teaching strategies.

Although Cross's model of cultural competence was the conceptual underpinning of the project, Cross's definition could not be used operationally within a nursing education setting. How to translate that into specific nursing approaches proved challenging. Therefore, in the development of the INDE project, a comparative cultural model, which was congruent with Cross's constructs, was identified. Giger and Davidhizar's (1999) Transcultural Assessment Model was initially viewed as advantageous because both students and faculty could gain needed information about, and appreciation for, people belonging to diverse groups. In addition, the model provided a systematic approach to cultural assessment.

Phase One of the interventions was to focus on increasing cultural knowledge in the faculty about specific cultures. This phase began with an assessment of faculty knowledge and perceptions about diversity and culture care, as previously discussed, and information about the INDE project. Secondly, a presentation of general concepts about diversity in educational settings was given to the faculty and staff. Eight months into the project, a nationally known speaker on diversity teaching presented a day of faculty development, which was attended by all full-time faculty members. In conjunction with that activity, a process was undertaken by a team of two faculty members and the INDE project director to identify key components in building a comprehensive cultural curriculum. As these processes were co-occurring, ongoing feedback was received regarding the faculty development effort, and faculty input was sought to develop the curricular components and teaching strategies. Feedback from students, as previously discussed, was also integral to the development of the cultural curriculum. What emerged from feedback from faculty *and* students was an increasing understanding that the chosen approach of a comparative cultural model was not adequate as a comprehensive foundation for developing cultural competence in the specific setting of ULSON.

These messages from faculty *and* students clearly identified the following three critical issues that were *not* adequately addressed by any comparative cultural model: first, *differences that were reflected in client and student populations, such as sexual orientation and disability, were not included in the definition of cultural diversity;* second, *concern about potential stereotyping of populations based on their race or value system;* and third and most important, *the impact of the socioenvironmental context on the lives and health of diverse students and patients.*

In addition to the messages we were receiving from our faculty and students, there is a growing body of literature on health disparities that identifies the impact of social and environmental influences (or context) on health decisions and health status. The literature on social determinants of health increasingly highlights the impact of community resources, urban versus rural settings (geographic location), social status, history, language, and economic power on health (Gustafson, 2005; Pincus, Esther, Dewalt, & Callahan, 1998; Syme, 2004; Wilkinson & Marmot, 2003). The Institute of Medicine report *Unequal Treatment: Confronting Racial and Ethnic Disparities in Health Care* reviews hundreds of health disparities research studies and concludes that unequal treatment is a major factor underlying disparities (Cooper & Roler, 2003;

Smedley, Stith, & Nelson, 2003). The broader definition of diversity, influential social factors, and racial discrimination in the health care setting are not addressed within the comparative culture model.

The INDE project director identified the need for a broader understanding of the influences on human health behavior, and as a result, the INDE project's concept of cultural diversity expanded beyond the values, beliefs, practices, and customs of different cultural groups, as identified at the onset of the project. Our initial strategy for faculty development provided *facts and perspectives* that were not perceived as fully encompassing the experiences of faculty and students in our evolving community and lacked the historical, social, and environmental context of our setting that would assist faculty members in implementing the curriculum to the benefit of our students.

So, a shift was made from the initially chosen approach for both students and faculty, and a cultural curriculum was developed based on a newly identified definition of diversity, modified to reflect the following:

> Variations in culture, behavior, values, characteristics, biologies, customs and histories are all considered important aspects of human experience and diversity that are included in the developing curriculum. Factors such as gender, sexual orientation, disability, language, race, religion, ethnicity, geography, social/economic status, and health disparity reflect the complexity of human expression and need. These complex expressions of diversity require competence in nursing care and are the focus for cultural competence at the ULSON.

This definition of diversity continued to be compatible with Cross's conceptual definition and included the critical elements of the comparative model but also reflected the importance of social and discriminatory contexts that affect health and health care. Most importantly, this definition reflected the experiences of faculty and students within our environmental context, and as a result, our definition of diversity became more closely aligned with the sociological concept of the *Social Determinants of Health* (Wilkinson & Marmot, 2003), which has been identified as a key component in addressing health disparities in a variety of settings.

The exemplars provided at the beginning of this chapter reflect this expanded definition of diversity. They illustrate the obvious as well as hidden variations among humans that can function as barriers to understanding clients and providing care. They illustrate assumptions and disparities related to economic resources, familial relationships, technology and health, history and social expectations, and community and race. These exemplars also served as important data on which change and new directions in the ULSON nursing curriculum were built.

Based upon that shift in perspective, the INDE project focused on developing the following programmatic elements within the curriculum for faculty and students: (a) identification of the skills that students would possess as they entered the workforce (student educational outcomes), (b) broadly defined diversity concepts that would be integral to the educational process, (c) curricular placement of essential content and educational and outcome measurement strategies across the upper division of nursing courses, (d) educational resources for use in the classroom, and (e) areas for faculty development that support minority student retention and facilitate culturally competent educational outcomes for all students.

The developed curriculum demonstrates the importance of diversity as newly identified across the curriculum and fosters cultural awareness, knowledge, and competence within a specific socioenvironmental context. The curriculum also includes avenues for discussion of disparities in health care delivery. Factors such as gender, sexual orientation, disability, language, race, religion, ethnicity, geography, social/economic status, and health disparities are integrated throughout the upper-division curriculum. In addition, topic areas and resources to assist faculty members to incorporate these diversity factors into the curriculum are identified. The curriculum with all five programmatic elements is illustrated in Table 7.2.

OUTCOMES OF THE INDE PROJECT

At the project's end, the outcomes of the project fell within several areas. Student-related outcomes were to increase the number of African American students who were admitted to the upper division of nursing over the course of the project and to retain and graduate these students. Thus, one major project goal was to increase the total number of upper-division admissions to 32 over the 3-year project period. Prior to the implementation of the INDE Project, 14 African American students were admitted in 2001, 4 in 2002, and 8 in 2003. Six graduated in 2001, 8 in 2002, and 8 in 2003, for a total of 22 graduates during this timeframe. From summer 2004 through summer 2005, the first full year of the grant, 31 African American students were admitted into the

Table 7.2

CULTURE IN THE CURRICULUM (UNDERGRADUATE)

STUDENT EDUCATIONAL OUTCOMES	KEY CONCEPTS	CURRICULAR PLACEMENT EDUCATION STRATEGIES AND OUTCOME MEASUREMENT STRATEGIES (OMS)	EDUCATIONAL RESOURCES FOR USE IN THE CLASSROOM	FACULTY DEVELOPMENT 5 AREAS
1. Self Awareness; Biological Variations	Cultural Theories Ethnocentrism Cultural Self-Assessment & Knowledge Ethnicity Cultural Diversity Race Health Disparities	*First Semester—Junior Year* Theoretical Frameworks Communication & CLAS Standards Self-Awareness Assessment Physiologic Variations in Health Assessment **OMS:** Paper and clinical group assignment	Kentucky Health Report Louisville-Metro Health Status Report Clinical Focus Sheets Self-Assessment—Instruments/Activities CLAS Standards Select Cultural Theories Physical Assessment Components	*Online Resources* Kaiser AHRQ Commonwealth xculture.org omhrc.org Institutes of Medicine World Health Organization
2. Sociocultural Variations & Influences	Transculturalism Multiculturalism Cultural Knowledge & Awareness Health Disparities Research	*Second Semester—Junior Year* Theoretical Frameworks Cultural Variations & Implications for a Variety of Health Settings Evidence-Based Practice and Health Disparities Research **OMS:** Individual clinical assignment	Select Cultural Theories Select Research in Culture & Health Focus Sheets on Diversity Select Web sites Economic data Community data Gender data	*Cultural Modules of Care/Health* Campinha-Bacote Leininger Giger-Davidhizar Purnell Social Determinants of Health

3. Culturally Appropriate Health Resources	Cultural Sensitivity and Health Policy Health Literacy and CLAS standards Cultural Congruence	*First Semester—Senior Year* Cross-Cultural Communication Cultural Exposure: – Language – Religion – Lifestyle Culturally Compatible Community Resources **OMS:** Group assignment to peers	Health Disparities Reports —IOM, AHRQ, Kaiser, etc. Community Settings—Experiential Activities Select Web sites Regarding Health Education for Diverse Groups http://louisville.edu/nursing/healthcarediverse.htm	*Self-Awareness* Activities—Use & Evaluation *Policy* Regulatory & Guidelines Related to Multiculturalism and Cultural Competence Sullivan Commission Report
4. Culture Accommodation	Cultural Competence	*Second Semester—Senior Year* **OMS:** Concept paper on organizational cultural competence Client focused synthesis paper with diverse population	Guidelines for Evaluation of Cultural Competence in Health Service Organizations Peer Evaluation	*Health Disparities Research* Interdisciplinary Nursing Specialty

upper division of nursing, almost four times the average number of African American students admitted in the three previous years. They constituted 12.4% of all students admitted in the program. Of this group, 18, or 58%, participated in the INDE project. From fall 2005 through spring 2007, 31 African American students graduated, of whom 19, or 61%, participated in the INDE project. Although the numbers are from overlapping cohorts, there was a 100% retention and graduation rate of African American upper-division nursing students as compared to a graduation rate of 88.4% for majority students during the same period.

In addition to the increased admission, retention, and graduation of upper-division African American nursing students, those lower-division students who participated in the INDE project received and benefited from microbiology and anatomy and physiology tutoring and financial and mentoring support services prior to entering the upper-division nursing program. African American students who chose not to be a part of the INDE program were involved in the student seminars on cultural diversity and were recipients of the implemented culture curriculum during their educational experience at ULSON.

Furthermore, student and faculty perceptions about their cultural competence increased. At the end of the project period, the project director compiled qualitative data from faculty and students. Quotes from these data identified that INDE project activities increased their awareness of the need to be culturally sensitive and competent as health care providers and health care team members. Faculty members expressed sentiment about the value of African American students in the program and the importance of their success. They also reported experiences with majority students who were able to identify their own cultural knowledge deficits and the opportunities that faculty took to assist these students. Finally, the project resulted in the development of a definition of cultural diversity that met the needs of our setting. With that definition, the ULSON was better equipped to identify the essential elements needed for faculty and students to develop cultural awareness, sensitivity, knowledge, and competence within a specific socioenvironmental context. The revised curriculum continues to function after the completion of the INDE project funding.

LESSONS LEARNED FROM INDE

An outgrowth of the INDE project was the awareness that many of the desired components of the project must address the cultural, social, *and* environmental needs of our students, faculty, and community. As a result, there was a critical change in what we were trying to accomplish. Culture was now viewed as a constellation of complex factors that are at play when considering the health of minority clients *and* the needs of minority nursing students. Having faculty teach about and clinically address these factors using an evidence-based approach was essential to improving nursing and addressing health concerns of diverse populations.

With this fundamental paradigm shift from perceiving culture as simply variations in beliefs, values, and cultural practices to examining those (and other) variations within the social, historical, and economic contexts, our perspective of what is the domain of nursing and nursing education changed. We identified ongoing ways in which faculty could develop cultural competence as educators and mentors to nursing students. Online resources that support culturally sensitive approaches for clinical practice and teaching were identified and evaluated for application and appropriate leveling within our curriculum. Opportunities to apply critical thinking became fundamental to the development of cultural competence. Problem-based and case study experiential activities were more closely evaluated for how they reflected our view of diversity. And finally, all faculty members were expected to become contributors in maintaining the relevancy of the cultural content in the classroom. They were held responsible for transforming principles of diversity into clinical practice experiences related to their nursing specialty in support of student educational outcomes. Community settings that reflected our definition of diversity were identified and increasingly incorporated into the ULSON nursing program. The outcomes of these efforts not only addressed the health care needs of our community but also reflected the values and experiences of our diverse student population. As a school, we have broadened the domain of diversity and, as a result, increased the need for faculty support to meet the goals resulting from that change. What became increasingly essential was identification of faculty resources and ongoing faculty development to support these processes.

Faculty members who were integrally involved in the development of the INDE project were primarily African American. The effort required to undertake such a project was significant. As the project grew, so did the challenges to implementing change. One major challenge was the potential over-reliance on minority faculty as the repositories of all project knowledge. Other challenges included responsibility for developing resources without processes to maintain those resources without grant funding. Maintaining those resources was identified as assuring currency of, access to, and ongoing development of new resources as they become needed and available. In addition, at various points, faculty involved in the project perceived lack of recognition of the degree of effort involved in project development (in terms of workload and assignments). The HRSA grant funded only one faculty position (that of the director) and staff to support INDE activities. The SON had no established faculty position for diversity education or faculty workload allotment for ongoing development of diversity curriculum. The cultural curriculum was developed under the auspices of a 10% workload allotment for each of three faculty members to complete the ad hoc curriculum project over the course of one semester. The dissonance between the expression of support for diversity and the acquisition of resources to accomplish this was an ongoing source of frustration for those faculty involved in student mentoring, select INDE program components, and curriculum development.

Beyond the INDE Project

As the project unfolded, what we have learned through planned and unintended outcomes has increased and broadened our understanding of what is essential to developing and sustaining a culturally relevant curriculum and supporting diversity in nursing in a manner appropriate for a complex, evolving, and diverse health care environment. The ULSON began a process that was new and challenging. Since the completion of the project, there have been significant changes at the ULSON. A Web page that is part of the ULSON has been developed that functions as a clearinghouse for links to national sites that provide health information to diverse populations and links that support cultural competence in health care providers. Cultural competence workshops have been provided by nursing faculty for students and health science educators. Clinical settings are now routinely located in a variety of African American and other minority communities. The culture curriculum was reviewed, updated, and verified for inclusion across the ULSON upper-division curriculum by a team of nonminority ULSON faculty during the summer semester of 2007. One ULSON African American faculty member was awarded the University of Louisville President's Award for Excellence in Multicultural Teaching partially based on her work with the development of the culture curriculum and development of Web-based resources to support cultural competence. The former INDE director currently is assigned as the advisor to African American and minority students as part of her workload. Community partnership initiatives in a predominately African American community are now underway as part of a U of L multidisciplinary faculty collaboration, which includes some faculty members from the ULSON.

There are still barriers to overcome. Resources that support cultural diversity at the ULSON continue to be limited. Diversity initiatives are undertaken primarily by those faculty members who are already committed to that effort, and participation in diversity activities is not a routine part of faculty workload or an expectation in faculty performance.

RECOMMENDATIONS FOR NURSE EDUCATORS AND ADMINISTRATORS

The experiences of those faculty members who were involved in the INDE project have led to the following recommendations:

1. Although diversity education may be focused on addressing the needs of one population, all factors that have an impact on that population must also be considered in any plan of action.
2. Cultural diversity education must include the needs of the educator as well as the needs of the students.
3. Ongoing self-assessment is the key to any cultural diversity education process. Self-assessment should include the perspectives of both students and faculty to help define and operationalize what is desired from the change process.
4. Cultural diversity education in nursing *cannot* be addressed through a time- or course-limited activity but must be diffused throughout the curriculum.
5. Although faculty and students from diverse populations may identify the need for diversity education, all faculty and students must be engaged and invested in the process to institutionalize the changes.
6. Cultural diversity curriculum development and education are essential elements of professional nursing education and, as such, require faculty time, workload recognition, and resources.
7. Students follow the lead of their role models. When we as educators are explicit in our expectation of and commitment to cultural competence, students, patients, communities, and nursing benefit.

QUESTIONS FOR DIALOGUE

1. What ideas or concepts did you find most meaningful in this chapter? Identify your insights and questions to bring to a dialogue with your colleagues.
2. In your view, what are the essential aspects of cultural competence? How does your program prepare students to work in cross-cultural settings? What are the ethical implications of having inadequately prepared students work in community settings they are not familiar with?
3. Hines-Martin and Pack begin their chapter with three scenarios. Create guided reflection questions (see chapter 6) to help students identify examples of assumptions, cultural insensitivity, and potential internalized superiority and/or internalized racism (see chapter 1).
4. Dialogue with colleagues about how to balance community needs with creating opportunities for students to gain experience working cross-culturally. What are the ethical implications of not providing opportunities for minority students to serve their own community while creating opportunities for dominant culture students to work outside theirs?
5. In your program, who is involved in diversity initiatives? Are diversity initiatives equally embraced by all faculty? If not, why not?
6. To what extent is cultural content embedded in all of your courses, as illustrated in the "Culture in the Curriculum" chart?

REFERENCES

American Association of Colleges of Nursing. (2002). *American Association of Colleges of Nursing 2002: Annual state of the schools.* Retrieved January 21, 2005, from http://www.aacn.nche.edu/media/pdf/annualreport02.pdf

Bernal, H., & Froman, R. (1987). The confidence of community health nurses in caring for ethnically diverse populations. *IMAGE: Journal of Nursing Scholarship, 19*(4), 201–203.

Cooper, L. A., & Roler, D. L. (2003). Patient provider communication: The effect of race and ethnicity on process and outcomes of health care. In B. Smedley, A. Y. Stith, & A. R. Nelson (Eds.), *Unequal treatment: Confronting racial and ethnic disparities in health care* (pp. 552–593). Washington, DC: The National Academies Press.

Cross, T., Bazron, B., Dennis, K., & Isaacs, M. (1989). *Towards a culturally competent system of care* (Vol. 1). Washington, DC: CASSP Technical Assistance Center.

Dreher, M., & MacNaughton, N. (2002). Cultural competency in nursing: Foundation or fallacy? *Nursing Outlook, 50,* 181–186.

Giger, J., & Davidhizar, R. (1999). *Transcultural nursing.* St. Louis: Mosby.

Gustafson, D. L. (2005). Transcultural nursing theory from a critical cultural perspective. *Advances in Nursing Science, 28*(1), 2–16.

Komaromy, M., Grumback, K., Drake, M., Vranizan, K., Lurie, N., Keane, D., et al. (1996). The role of Black and Hispanic physicians in providing health care for underserved populations. *The New England Journal of Medicine, 334,* 1305–1310.

Ndiwane, A., Miller, K., Bonner, A., Imperio, K., Matzo, M., et al. (2004). Enhancing cultural competencies of advanced practice nurses: Health care challenges in the twenty-first century. *Journal of Cultural Diversity, 11,* 118–121.

Office of Policy, Planning & Evaluation. (2004). *Health status assessment report.* Louisville KY: Louisville Metro Health Department.

Pincus, T., Esther, R., Dewalt, D. A., & Callahan, L. F. (1998). Social conditions and self management are more powerful determinants of health than access to care. *Annals of Internal Medicine, 129*(5), 406–411.

Rooda, L. (1992). Attitudes of nurses toward culturally diverse patients: An examination of the social contact theory. *Journal of the National Black Nurses' Association, 6*(1), 48–56.

Smedley, B., Stith, A. Y., & Nelson, A. R. (Eds.). (2003). *Unequal treatment: Confronting racial and ethnic disparities in health care.* Washington, DC: The National Academies Press.

Smith, L. (1998). Cultural competence for nurses: Canonical correlation of two cultures scales. *Journal of Cultural Diversity, 5,* 120–126.

The Sullivan Commission on Diversity in Healthcare Workforce. (2004). *Missing persons: Minorities in the health professions: A report of the Sullivan Commission on Diversity in the Healthcare Workforce-Executive summary.* Retrieved August 13, 2005, from http://www.sullivancommission.org

Syme, S. L. (2004). Social determinants of health: The community as an empowered partner. *Preventing Chronic Disease* [serial online]. Retrieved May 20, 2008, from http://www.cdc.gov/pcd/issues/2004/jan/03_0001.htm

U.S. Census Bureau. (2000). *Factfinder-Louisville Kentucky demographic data.* Retrieved April 23, 2004, from http://factfinder.census.gov/

U.S. Census Bureau. (2004a). *U.S. interim projections by age, sex, race, and Hispanic origin.* Retrieved December 7, 2005, from http://www.census.gov/ipc/www/usinterimproj/

U.S. Census Bureau. (2004b). *Factfinder-Louisville Kentucky demographic data.* Retrieved December 7, 2005, from http://factfinder.census.gov/

Velde, B., Wittman, P., & Bamberg, R. (2003). Cultural competence of faculty and students in a school of allied health. *Journal of Allied Health, 32,* 189–195.

Wilkinson, R., & Marmot, M. (2003). *Social determinants of health: The solid facts* (2nd ed.). Geneva: World Health Organization.

8 Teaching the Fluid Process of Cultural Competence at the Graduate Level: A Constructionist Approach

BARBARA JONES WARREN

We were having a reception for one of our faculty who had just received an important award. A well-known White nursing research scholar entered the room and immediately came over to where I was sitting with a group of other faculty. She commented, "You all are so quiet, we should be up celebrating." Turning toward me, she said, "Barbara, you could get up and dance!"

I just looked at her, not quite believing that she had said this to me, the only African American faculty member in the room. But then I asked her, "You want me to dance*?"*

Perhaps realizing the implication of what she had said, she began to chatter nervously, "Well, I didn't mean anything cultural. Culture is not important. I am a hillbilly myself."

I just looked at her and responded, "First, you want me to dance *and now you are saying that* culture *is not important?"*

This was not the first time that this individual had made "uncomfortable" statements to or around me, but this was the height of cultural incompetence. I remember feeling simultaneously angry and hurt. I also remember wondering how a student might feel if this happened to her or him and how worried the student might be, given the power differential.

I looked at the faculty around me and they looked as shocked as I felt. I just got up and walked away because I really was afraid of what I might say and how what I would say might be used against me, as this person is an acknowledged national leader in the nursing profession who makes many decisions that affect the careers of faculty and students. Talk about a power differential! And yet, culturally and ethnically diverse students, faculty, and patients are placed in similar situations far too often (Amaro, Abriam-Yago, & Yoder, 2006; Hassouneh, 2006; Lutz & Warren, 2007; Warren & Lutz, 2007).

When I got home that evening, I picked up one of my favorite books, Shifting: The Double Lives of Black Women in America, *and these words literally leaped off the page at me: "Shifting, all the ways that Black women navigate bigotry—as well as the emotional ripples that they experience because of it . . . knowing the realities of Black women's lives can . . . help us speak up . . . and help spur us on to bring about real change" (Jones & Shorter-Gooden, 2003, pp. 278, 279).*

It seemed clear to me from this interaction with a well-known nursing scholar that there was still much to be done to educate our nursing students and colleagues about issues of culture and diversity of thought so that their future shifting and that of their patients would be grounded in the process of cultural competence and not in bias and prejudice.

This chapter began as an academic exercise, something I needed to do to move ahead in the academic world; you know, publish or perish! However, what ultimately made this exercise more enjoyable was that it focused on diversity and the education of nurses. The exercise permitted me the luxury of merging these two content areas into something that was meaningful to me and that I hope will be meaningful for the nursing students and other educators, practitioners, and administrators who choose to read this chapter. Moreover, something else happened to me along the way during this 2-year exercise. I began to remember how I had discovered the importance of culture, how I transformed my teaching, and what motivated me to make such a commitment to the process of cultural competence, beginning with the incident with the well-known nursing scholar. My passage into developing a culturally competent framework for nursing teaching, practice, and research involved qualitative learning methods, characterized by the use of introspective thinking and discussion with others, and quantitative methods, characterized by the learning of facts about other cultures. So, I am writing this "academic exercise" using techniques related to both of those methods. I am weaving story sharing and formal academic approaches together to demonstrate how the process of cultural competence can be woven into selected nursing education, practice, and research processes.

My qualitative passage toward cultural competence began with my diverse family and community experiences. That passage continues to evolve as my professional life develops. I naively began my professional life with the thought that everyone had experienced some degree of diversity, either in their family or community settings or at least had experienced diversity of thought as they grew up. But, I have discovered that this is often inaccurate and that, in some cases, diversity of experience and thought is not always embraced within nursing environments. However, over the last 10 years, the nursing discipline has expressed an increasing interest in exploring issues of culture and diversity.

So, what does the literature say about the need for acknowledging and incorporating issues of culture and diversity within nursing education, practice, and research?

BACKGROUND FOR CULTURAL COMPETENCE IN NURSING

Patients' health care beliefs and practices develop out of their cultural values and experiences (Muñoz & Luckmann, 2005; U.S. Department of Health & Human Services [USDHHS], 2002). Recommendations out of the Surgeon General's Office (USDHHS, 1999, 2001), the Institute of Medicine (IOM; 2003), and such reports as *Healthy People 2010* (USDHHS, 2002) advise that all health care providers develop clinical assessment and treatment skills related to the cultural background and heritage of their patients (IOM, 2001, 2003; Smedley, Butler, & Bristow, 2004). In addition, research findings from nursing indicate that positive health care outcomes are contingent upon nurses' abilities to successfully communicate with their patients (Andrews & Boyle, 2003; Campinha-Bacote, 2007; Peplau, 1952). Yet, miscommunication often occurs when patients and nurses experience interpersonal conflicts grounded within their differing cultural belief systems (Giger & Davidhizar, 2004; Purnell & Paulanka, 2003). It is the ethical and professional responsibility of nurses to develop and sustain the nurse–patient relationship (Peplau, 1952) through the use of culturally congruent health care knowledge regarding their patients (Leininger & McFarland, 2006; Warren, 2003, 2007a, 2007b). This ethical and professional responsibility is based on the fact that patients' cultural perspectives are an important aspect within their lives. In fact, culture creates the meaning and existence for how persons express and practice their beliefs, values, and norms on a daily basis (Warren, 2007a, 2007b, 2008).

RATIONALE FOR DEVELOPMENT OF COURSE IN CULTURAL COMPETENCE

> A generalization about a cultural group is good in the initial exploration of helpful ideas, but absolute generalizations tend to be wrong. (Muñoz, Primm, Ananth, & Ruiz, 2007, p. 211)

Over 20 years ago, the American Nurses Association Council on Cultural Diversity in Nursing Practice (1986) issued their hallmark report on the role of cultural diversity within nursing curricula. The reaction to this report has been an interesting process within nursing academic settings. Many nursing programs of higher education have developed "cultural courses" within their curricula. However, these courses often teach facts related to cultural generalities (e.g., Whites do this, Blacks do this, Asians do this, etc.) and assessment of physical symptoms and common illnesses for defined racial, cultural, ethnic, and religious groups (e.g., African American, Asian American, Latino, Jewish, Amish, etc.). In addition, often there is norming and comparisons discussed between the "majority White culture" and "other" cultures. Some academic settings merely include case studies about persons of color, and these cases always discuss the negative physical and psychological aspects of the chosen group. Unless an explicit process is in place to uncover these practices in the nursing education system, perpetuation of their use serves to teach students negative stereotypes.

Generalized approaches seem to indicate that cultural knowledge about persons is clearly defined, static, and only meaningful for specific "minority" racial and ethnic groups. The danger in this teaching approach is that it does not consider the complex, dynamic, and fluid nature of persons' cultural experiences that may and often do alter over time (Muñoz & Luckmann, 2005; Muñoz et al., 2007; Spector, 2004; Warren, 2005). In order to avoid this type of box-like thinking, nursing educators need to develop and use pedagogical approaches that stimulate nursing students to think in a more process-oriented (e.g., contextual and fluid) manner regarding issues of culture, with fluid referring to this dynamic and evolving nature of culture. Culture is a dynamic and evolving component within people's lives. In fact, every individual has layers of culture that are added over the years. Think of yourself and how your heritage or culture of origin is layered over the years by what you do, who you interface with, and what overall work and life experiences you encounter (Spector, 2004). In my experience, in a country that is socially stratified by race and class, it is the interaction of this layering with oppressive social forces that creates greater inequities for persons from racially and ethnically diverse populations. For example, if someone is from a group of color, is poor, or has less education, she or he is more apt to have little or no insurance and less access to quality health care, live in housing and environments that may be physically and mentally unhealthy, and thus ultimately be more apt to incur illnesses that are injurious to her or his mind, body, and spirit. To fully understand the intertwined forces that shape people's lives, nursing students, faculty, and administrators benefit from a dynamic, fluid model.

In teaching this course, I use the adjective *fluid* to represent the dynamic and evolving nature of culture. A process approach to teaching and learning about culture is more effective for nursing students because it stimulates critical thinking that is needed in all levels of patient care (Warren, 2003). In addition, this approach facilitates students' development and understanding of their unique cultures. A nurses need to know themselves before they can know and work with patients (Warren, 2008). So, why is a process approach specifically needed to help nursing students at the graduate level grow and develop in their clinical knowledge?

Rationale for Graduate-Level Course in Cultural Competence

Often students are so busy learning and faculty are so busy teaching facts and skills that they forget how to truly listen. And it is this listening that brings us to a higher level of awareness and understanding regarding cultural perspectives. Members of the Cherokee Nation refer to this as the "way of the right relationship . . . an experience that flows from one day to the next" (Garrett & Garrett, 1996, preface, p. x).

Nurses and nursing students are no different than their patients in that they are guided as health care professionals both by their personal and professional cultural belief systems (Warren, in press). Hence, it is essential that all nurses comprehend and develop knowledge regarding the role of culture, not only in their lives but also in the lives of their patients and health care professionals they work with. In fact, there is a growing body of literature that supports the idea that culturally competent care leads to the achievement of successful quality health care outcomes for persons from culturally and ethnically diverse populations (USDHHS, 1999, 2001, 2002). The use of cultural competence helps identify the strengths and the weaknesses within the various layers of these individuals' lives.

According to Leininger and McFarland (2006), culturally competent approaches need to be included within all levels of nursing education, practice, and research. Moreover, these scholars advise that culturally related information needs to be a taught at the graduate level of nursing in an "enhanced" way because graduate level nurses need higher levels of interaction, critical thinking, and decision-making skills in order to address the more complicated and complex needs of culturally and ethnically diverse patients. Recommendations from the American Association of Colleges of Nursing (AACN) report on *Essentials of Masters Education* state that one of the primary competencies that needs to be included within graduate nursing education is that of cultural competence (AACN, 1998). Preliminary findings from *The Registered Nurse Population: National Sample Survey of Registered Nurses* indicate more U.S. nurses are being prepared at the advanced practice level and that there is an ongoing and increasing need for professional nurses within diverse community settings (Health Resources and Services Administration, 2006; USDHHS, 2002). Current and future nurses will be working in a variety of settings and will have responsibility for a variety of culturally and ethnically diverse patients. Furthermore, nurses who are prepared at the advanced practice level and are knowledgeable regarding cultural competence may also become nurse educators or administrators within clinical and academic settings. Hence, it is critical that these nurses have a strong academic foundation in culturally competent knowledge that can facilitate not only their professional care of patients but also their ability to educate other nurses and staff about the role and importance of culture and the process of cultural competence within clinical and academic settings.

Moreover, as little information is available that details how to develop a graduate-level course on the process of cultural competence, this chapter describes how to develop such a course using a constructivism paradigm and transformative learning theory. The use of these approaches is key to helping nursing students, faculty, and researchers begin to develop and continue to grow in the process of cultural competence.

THEORETICAL PERSPECTIVES FOR THE PEDAGOGY OF CULTURAL COMPETENCE

> To transform your thinking you have to "Suspend your disbelief, appreciate your experience" so that "a new healthier culture will arise." (Brandman, 2007)

The teaching and learning strategies described in this chapter are grounded in the *transformative learning theory* described by Mezirow (2000). This theory addresses both the cultural beliefs and values of the learner as well as the strategies that are used in changing and/or transforming the learner's thinking processes (Haw, 2006). Transformative learning theory recognizes the importance and use of personal experiences and reflective discussions as critical in transforming the learner's thinking about issues.

Using transformative learning theory, nursing faculty facilitate classroom discussions in which students feel free to share their experiences, express their thoughts, and interpret meanings regarding their actual experiences of cultural issues within nursing practice. Additional components of this theory involve classroom discussions about judgments and assumptions underlying student and faculty interpretations of cultural issues.

Transformative learning theory is grounded in the *constructivism learning principle* (Mezirow, 2000). This principle promotes the idea that learners, who have a variety of previous life experiences, can work collaboratively within group environments to problem solve work/life dilemmas. This constructivism learning principle is appropriate for use with graduate-level nurse practitioner students. All of these students have previous educational experiences (i.e., a minimum of a Bachelor's degree, many with one or two Master's degrees, and some with Doctoral degrees), and many come from other career paths (e.g., biochemistry, physiology, dietetics and nutrition, teaching, etc.). In addition, many of the students have been in management-level positions in which they facilitated collaborative problem-solving within their work environments.

Definition of Cultural Competence

Cultural competence is an ongoing learning process whereby a nurse illustrates a level of proficiency in developing not only an awareness of the importance of culture for persons but also an understanding of individual and system variables that affect the quality and appropriateness of health care for persons from culturally and ethnically diverse communities.

The process of cultural competence leads students and faculty toward a transformation of their knowledge development and teaching strategies. Hence, there is no end point to culturally competent learning because the transformation in learning is always in progression, in development. I developed and continue to develop the course described in this chapter through knowledge-seeking techniques (e.g., immersion in a variety of cultural environments, attendance at culturally based workshops and seminars) and use of introspection regarding my own cultural background and that of the students, patients, faculty, and health care professionals whom I interact with on an everyday basis. This developmental process continues to alternate between use of introspective thinking and discussion with others, a qualitative approach, as well as learning facts about cultural experiences and environments, which is more of a quantitative approach. Hence, cultural competence is an ongoing developmental (i.e., unfolding, evolving) process by which a nurse develops understanding, appreciation, and knowledge regarding cultural expressions and world view concepts and then incorporates or enculturates these concepts into the care of his or her patients and during interactions and communication with students, faculty, and other health care professionals (Warren, 2002, 2003, in press; Warren & Lutz, 2007).

MOVING FROM COGNITIVISM TO CONSTRUCTIVISM

> Don't make assumptions. Find the courage to ask questions . . . communicate with others as clearly as you can to avoid misunderstandings, sadness, and drama. (Ruiz, 1997, p. 67)

As previously mentioned, many cultural courses concentrate more on learning facts and information about specifically defined cultural groups. This approach illustrates the cognitivism model for learning (Haw, 2006), in which a faculty member imparts knowledge about cultural perspectives to students in a very sequential and mechanized way. This is the "tried and true" lecture approach that is grounded primarily in the faculty person's reality, not in the student's. Moreover, there is little, if any, room for change or growth in faculty or student learning processes because the faculty member does not encourage student discussions that might focus on perspectives that are divergent from the faculty person's reality. Nursing process and concept mapping represent exemplars of a cognitivism model in which facts are collected and synthesized in a logical and ordered fashion. Of course, there are times when this approach is beneficial, and it may work better in some classes for traditional-age baccalaureate-degree students who are younger in their developmental thinking and have less contextual life experiences

(Haw, 2006). Conversely, it is not always successful with graduate-level students who have had more contextual experiences. The rationale that I hear most often from nursing faculty regarding why they do not like to use a discussion-based approach to teaching is because it slows down the faculty person's ability to "really teach" or "provide quality care" for patients in clinical environments. We, as nursing faculty, tend to want students and patients to change their lives, beliefs, and ways of living based upon what we think is best (Young-Mason, 1997). Worse yet, we ignore that students and patients often have much to offer us in our interactions with them.

In contrast to cognitivism, the constructivism approach to cultural competence is learner-focused. One way to incorporate a constructivism approach is to pose questions to students that encourage them to use their life and work experiences during discussions and in problem-solving patient situations as well as in the development of written assignments and presentations. For example, to encourage students to reflect on their life experiences and share them in class, I pose questions, such as, "What is your experience with individuals who have different beliefs than you?" and "How might your past experiences affect your interactions with other students or your clinical work with patients?" So, how have I "constructed" learning processes in this course?

DEVELOPMENT OF CULTURAL COURSE CURRICULUM

I began my work on this course over 12 years ago when I began my academic career. I had heard that students did not like the cultural course and that faculty did not like teaching it. Other faculty "thought" and expressed to me that this would be a "great course" for me to teach! I had concerns about teaching the course, but I had always felt committed to issues of culture in my practice arena and thought this commitment might be a good one for my academic career. So, I began to teach an already existing undergraduate course titled, "Transcultural Nursing." This course had been created by another faculty member of color who had retired 2 years prior to my joining the faculty. This course was created and was meant to be taught using a cognitivism paradigm, which did not "feel" right to me. Nevertheless, I began teaching it using some of the concepts of this paradigm though I did not use quizzes and tests as the primary means to measure student outcomes. I used the quiz format to ascertain whether students were reading the assignments, but the questions were based on case studies and involved more application of knowledge from the readings than memorization of facts. Furthermore, classroom dialogue, based on discussions of case studies, was the primary way in which students were evaluated.

The course as it is currently taught represents my years of reflective thinking and that of my students who have been immersed in the course. Its evolution has been interesting and challenging but has not solely been grounded in my commitment to teaching and learning about cultural issues and environments. In fact, a number of events helped me construct my thinking about the course and decide what was needed to help it grow. These events included the following:

- Development and expansion of an accelerated nurse practitioner program in the college that included the Graduate Studies Committee's alteration of the undergraduate *Transcultural Nursing* course into a graduate level course focused on cultural issues.
- Development and implementation of the AACN's (1998) *Essentials of Master's Education for Advanced Practice Nursing*.
- Development of the University Academic Plan with its emphasis on prioritization of cultural inclusion and diversity for students, staff, and faculty through the development of diversity plans across all University departments.
- Development of and my participation on the University President's Diversity Council, which helped to monitor departmental progress regarding all diversity plans.
- Development of reports out of the Surgeon General's office on issues related to mental health, race, and ethnicity.
- Development of reports from the Institute of Medicine regarding health care disparities for racially and ethnically diverse populations.

In addition, interviews with past nurse practitioner students about what they needed in their current practice settings indicated they wanted more knowledge regarding how to facilitate the cultural care of their patients, their families, and others important to them. As a result, I requested to teach the graduate-level cultural course when annual teaching assignments were being decided. So the initial reconstruction began! The next section describes course objectives, followed by teaching and learning exemplars from the current course and how those emerged from reflective thinking.

Course Objectives

The focus of the course is on development of health care concepts and techniques used by nurses and other health care professionals in providing culturally competent care of individuals, families, and communities. I was not involved in the revision of the undergraduate course into the graduate level course and would have certainly used different language to create the course focus and objectives. The content that I developed emphasizes and incorporates constructivism and transformative learning concepts. The following are course objectives that the Graduate Studies and the University Academic Affairs Committees approved:

1. Analyze health/illness-related concepts, beliefs, and values of selected ethnic and racial cultures and subcultures.
2. Assess cultural factors that influence the individual's and family's orientation to the health care system in the United States.
3. Analyze similarities and differences between traditional and Western care practices of people and the health care implications.
4. Identify areas of potential conflict between health care practices and the individual's cultural beliefs and values.
5. Explain selected cultural factors that could affect interpersonal relations between health care providers from various subcultures.
6. Use research findings and knowledge of health-related cultural and ethnic beliefs, values, and practices of different cultures and subcultures to design a plan of care for individuals and their families.

Setting the Stage for Transformative Learning

The first class meeting sets the stage for transformative learning for the course. On the first night, I talk about what I do and how I came to be so interested in cultural perspectives and issues. I also ask about the needs of the students, what cultural issues they would like to discuss, and what experiences they have had regarding cultural similarities and differences. I discuss with students the focus of the course (e.g., the process of cultural competence), emphasizing how we will all learn together over the next 10 weeks. I spend time talking about my teaching philosophy and ask students to share their expectations of me. I tell students that

I love to share my knowledge and nursing experience, my specialty of psychiatric mental health nursing, and cultural issues with students. I see it as a privilege to teach and interact with them. I tell students: "I want you to learn; I care about your experiences in the classroom. We are all part of this wonderful profession of nursing and will grow together in order to learn how to serve our clients and provide them with culturally competent care." Because the process of cultural competence is ongoing and cannot be learned via tests and quizzes, I tell students that I do not utilize these techniques in the course but rather use thoughtful discussion and critical teaching and assessment techniques. I emphasize that I welcome questions and the sharing of students' experiences in relation to the course content.

This is an important dialogue because it sets the tenor for both the students' and my learning throughout the course. I think it is also an important step in helping students improve their critical thinking techniques while finding their voices regarding cultural issues. Furthermore, this may be the first time that students have encountered this philosophical approach to teaching in their academic experiences at the college, as I think that some faculty often unintentionally correct or stifle student voices because they feel the need to teach the skills and information that nursing students need to pass NCLEX and other certification examinations. Therefore, in order to keep pace and pass courses, students begin to repress creative thinking, which can be debilitating and harmful to student growth and learning. Hence, I attempt to help students seek and find their voices within this course. And, I also talk about the fact that we all need to present comments and questions in a respectful manner, which includes listening to others, using no attacking or derogatory language, and permitting everyone the time and right to talk about their experiences and concerns as well as to express their opinions.

> [V]oice is the literal expression of one's identity, the echo of the self. (Jones & Shorter-Gooden, 2003, p. 98)

I strongly believe that students need to know themselves before they can find their voices and learn to know their patients. They need to examine their thoughts, attitudes, and feelings about their cultural heritage and origin. I dialogue with students about the fact that culture is the essence of what makes each one of us unique and that, because of this, it is very meaningful to us; culture does not just focus on what we look like or what religion we practice. Hence, our dialogues in this course focus on broadening our concept of what culture means to every person. I think this knowing of self is the initial, critical component in starting the process of cultural competence. Though not required according to our college course syllabus format, I also include the following statement in this course as well as in all the courses I teach; I think it helps to emphasize the student-centered nature of the course: "Please talk with Dr. Warren if adjustments to the course need to be done in order to meet cultural practices and needs that you want to practice or have to adhere to."

Of course, I spend time talking about the content in the course, which includes a discussion of the course assignments. Because grades need to be provided for the students, there is also discussion of the main grading components of the course, including: completion of a group presentation on a cultural issue, a final paper based on a cultural book, and weekly reaction papers regarding the weekly discussions.

TEACHING AND LEARNING EXEMPLARS FROM THE COURSE

This chapter cannot explain every aspect or all of the content of this course. However, the following exemplars of teaching and learning in the course illustrate how discussions and assignments relate to the development of the process of cultural competence for students.

A Circle Approach to Developing Reflective Cultural Approaches

> From a cultural perspective, persons from the Cherokee Nation believe that the way we grow and learn is through use of and meditation on the universal circle and the crystal vision that leads to balance, harmony and paths of peace, introspection, quiet, and spirit. (Garrett & Garrett, 1996, p. 122)

I use my expertise in the areas of therapeutic communication skills from psychiatric mental health nursing and group facilitation, as well as the technique of study circles with storytelling, to create a reflective approach for discussion and deliberation in the course. Study circles are discussions that examine a variety of diverse experiences with discussions progressing from information about a culturally based issue to personal experiences to action approaches used by others to address the issue. The purpose of study circles is to provide an environment in which "safe and open dialogue" (Ali et al., 2006, p. 4) can occur. Storytelling is an approach that can be incorporated into the study circles, and it facilitates reflective thinking for students and teachers (Koening & Zorn, 2002).

While I share my own experiences, I do not say I am the "expert" on all issues related to one culture over another. I state that I am sharing comments that are grounded in my personal and professional experiences. Moreover, I share with students my own experiences and those of my patients in order to stimulate discussions within the class so that they may also dialogue about their perspectives and experiences related to diversity issues. For example, I talk about what my experiences have been like as I have moved through my life as an African American woman and professional nurse who has a variety of other cultures within her (e.g., Native American as well as Asian, German, Scotch, etc.), as well as roles as diverse as female, sister, daughter, wife, mother, and a host of others. I always say, "I do not speak for every African American women; I speak from my own experience." I also use literature, current events, proverbs, and ethical issues in health care as a way to frame our weekly dialogues. Here is an experience that I share with students about my movement toward understanding cultural issues and culturally competent care of patients. It also presents an excellent technique to open dialogue with students about their cultural clinical experiences.

One of my earlier professional cultural nursing encounters involved my work as a nurse manager at a psychiatric mental health facility. I was working nights and had five experienced and knowledgeable staff working with me. The unit consisted of 2 floors with 30 patients on each floor. I spent most of my time on one unit because there were more ill patients on it. However, throughout the night I heard a patient on the other floor making howling sounds. My staff reassured me that they had everything under control and that the patient had calmed down. However, around 4 A.M., one of the staff from the other floor came to me and said the patient had requested medication and that she had only calmed down when she heard "the nurse was coming."

So, I proceeded to go to the floor to check her chart to see what medication had been ordered. I prepared the injection, put it in my pocket, and started to walk down the hall to the patient's room. However, I noticed that my staff was not walking very closely to me. I asked them if there was something wrong, and they said, "Of course not." However, something did not seem "right."

As I entered the patient's room, I introduced myself and asked her if I could assist her. She looked at me and said in a fearful voice, "Oh no, you are one, too."

I said, "I'm sorry, I do not understand what you mean." And I really did not; I thought she might be referring to a hallucination that she was experiencing.

She then touched her face and said, "You know, Black."

I then realized that all of us working that night were indeed Black and that the patient was White and that she was afraid of this situation. I said to her, "I'm sorry, but I am the only nurse available for you this evening. I have heard you throughout the night, and I worried about how you feel. Could you tell me about what you are feeling and seeing at this time?"

The patient proceeded to tell me about the visual and auditory hallucinations that she was experiencing and how afraid she was. I mentioned to her that I knew how upsetting this must be and asked her if she needed some extra medication to help calm her down. I told her I had checked her chart and saw that she had been given medication before to help her relax and calm down. I offered her the medication if she was interested. She said "yes," and I gave her the medication. I told her I would stay with her until she had calmed down and that I would like to come back and talk with her tomorrow about how she was feeling. She calmed down and was able to go to sleep.

I did return the next day and talked with her about how she was doing. She thanked me for helping her the night before and also shared with me the fact that she had been repeatedly threatened and even struck by another child when she was little. This child was Black and because of this experience, she felt that all Black persons were like this child she had known. She also talked about how many Black persons she had seen on TV who had committed crimes and that this always reminded her of her childhood experiences. The patient also stated, "I thought every Black person was like that and was so afraid last night when all of you were around." I acknowledged that that situation must have been very hard for her and that I hoped she felt safe at this time. She said she did, but also noted that she never thought of herself as being "prejudiced" as she lived in a neighborhood where many Black people lived and that she worked with some Black people. I said that I understood how what she had experienced as a child was affecting her adult thoughts. During the rest of her hospitalization, we continued to talk about these issues, and I think these discussions made a difference in not only her mental health and wellness but also her thoughts about Black people.

I use this situation to talk about the need for nurses to "do no harm to patients" and provide culturally competent care to patients they encounter. The students always ask me how I could react in the way I did and not be mad at the patient. I mention that I processed this encounter with a peer who I worked with to make certain that I was handling the situation in a therapeutic manner. The most important thing to me was the care of this patient and not any thoughts about the patient's "bigotry." Talk about a reflective learning and teaching experience for me and for the students! The following quote conveys my thoughts about the need for cultural competence within the nursing discipline:

> [There] are women who have . . . made the courageous decision to try to sap society's oppression rather than live with it, to fight back rather than accommodate it, to quell and rise above the pain rather than accept and internalize it. (Jones & Shorter-Gooden, 2003, p. 92)

Guest speakers are invited to the class to share and dialogue with students and me about their cultural perspectives as well as their road toward cultural competence. Examples of the speakers include persons from Laotian, Latino, African American, and Gay, Lesbian, Bisexual, and Transgender (GLBT) cultural perspectives. There is a cultural topic of discussion for each week within the course. These topics include not only the guest speakers' perspectives but also the perspectives of cultural theorists in nursing practice and health care settings; definitions and role of culture and cultural competence for individuals, families, and communities; and cultural implications for nursing education, practice, and research. Speakers often bring friends and family along and share pictures or videos about their lives. Students are also encouraged to ask about topics of specific interest to them.

Personal Cultural Heritage History

One initial learning experience for students involves the completion of a personal cultural heritage history. Students are asked to complete a portion of the history in class at the first class meeting. The cultural history questions are those provided in *Cultural Diversity in Health and Illness*

(Spector, 2004). Examples of some of the questions in the heritage tool include the following:

- What setting did you grow up in? Urban? Rural?
- Where were your parents, grandparents, yourself born?
- Did most of your aunts, uncles, cousins live near your home?
- As an adult, do you live in a neighborhood where the neighbors are of the same religious and ethnic background as yourself?

We then dialogue about student perspectives after they have had time to think about and answer the questions. This information is for their purposes, and I do not collect their answers. However, I do collect their weekly reaction papers, not just for the purpose of grading, but also to see what issues they are reflecting on or see as important. I often then adjust my teaching approaches and use some student comments to stimulate discussion for successive class meetings. For example, one student wrote, "I was really uncomfortable when we talked about gay and lesbian issues. My religion does not permit that kind of lifestyle, and I am concerned how I will be able to handle care of those persons." Interestingly enough, the student that wrote this was comfortable enough to talk about this subject in class. In conjunction with this discussion, I asked representatives from the Office on GLBT Affairs to come and dialogue with the class on this subject matter. They used the concept of study circles to talk about misconceptions, realities, and health care needs for persons from GLBT cultural groups.

Another assignment in the course involves students' weekly completion of reflection papers reacting to the current week's discussions, guest lecture presentation if relevant, and the readings. Students are asked to write their thoughts about course topics and relate how these topics may or may not be relevant for them. The two-page reflection paper is written at the end of each class session. I review the papers and use students' comments to structure the next week's discussions. For example, one student wrote:

> I found it interesting to hear other persons' opinions on race differences. I come from a small town and only had a few friends who were of different races or from different cultural backgrounds or even thought differently than my family did or than I do. Sometimes I wonder if being politically correct hasn't made racism, bigotry and hatred worse. What about emphasizing our similarities as well as our differences?

I thought, ah excellent point! So, the next week we dialogued more about the issue of similarities across cultural groups versus only focusing on the differences. According to Dr. Leininger (Leininger & McFarland, 2006), there are often more similarities across groups than within a specific group of diverse persons. For example, culturally and ethnically diverse middle-class women often have more similarities than differences in how they think and react than do women from different socioeconomic classes within the same cultural group.

Students' comments in their reaction papers illustrate their growing awareness of the process of cultural competence:

- I never thought I had a culture until I completed my cultural history. I always thought I was just White and that culture only referred to people who are Black, Asian, or Spanish.
- I have traveled a lot in foreign environments and want to know more about how I can use this experience within my nursing education and clinical work with my patients. I thought I did not have any more to learn but see that there is more than just living in different cultural environments.
- As I reflected on my family I begin to remember some of their comments about people who looked or thought differently than we did. I am surprised to discover that some members in my family are so biased about certain persons and groups.
- Thinking about my views on culture has raised more questions about what I need to learn than provide exact answers.
- I always considered myself knowledgeable about cultural issues as I lived in Italy for a number of years. However, that experience only focused on one cultural group. I have so much more to learn.
- As we continue to have more presentations, it is astonishing for me to see all of the "myths" I had about different cultures be proven wrong. I think so many people are uninformed about other cultures that the little knowledge they do have about them usually comes from an extreme news story or a startling fact that is passed quietly from one person to another.

In keeping with transformative learning theory, students are encouraged to choose from the host of nursing cultural theorists that can be found in the course texts and other professional journals, such as *The Journal of Transcultural Nursing* and the *Transcultural Journal in Psy-*

chiatry. Examples of theorists students are exposed to include: Andrews and Boyle (2003); Campinha-Bacote (2007); Giger and Davidhizar (2004); Leininger and McFarland (2006); Muñoz and Luckmann (2005); Purnell and Paulanka (2003); Spector (2004); and Warren (in press, 2002, 2005, 2007a, 2007b). Students often use a variety of theoretical perspectives to support their discussions and develop their assignments in the course.

Teaching the Integrated Cultural Assessment of Patients

One of the concerns that students have is how to assess culture with their patients. I explain that every assessment is a cultural assessment and that questions regarding cultural perspective are reflected in what a patient says throughout the nursing assessment process and are not necessarily attained by a specific "cultural" question. Students are introduced to the LEARN assessment guide, which helps nurses collect assessment data and develop strategies that are culturally competent for patients (Campinha-Bacote, 2007). As one student commented, "I think that the use of the general questions from the LEARN assessment guide can really help me learn more about myself and my patients." Components of the LEARN assessment guide include the following:

- L = Listen to the comments that the patient expresses.
- E = Explain your interpretation of what you think the patient said and ask for clarification if that interpretation is incorrect or needs to be adjusted.
- A = Acknowledge the importance of what the patient is saying and what the cultural belief means for them.
- R = Recommend strategies and collaborate with the patient in order to develop interventions that include the cultural perspective of the patient.
- N = Negotiate and collaborate with the patient and others who are important to the patient in order to provide quality and culturally competent care.

Another insightful assessment tool was developed by Kleinman (Kleinman, Eisenberg, & Good, 1978). Questions from this tool can be easily incorporated into any biopsychosocial assessment of patients:

- What do you call the problem?
- What do you think has caused your problem?

- Why do you think it started when it did?
- What do you think your sickness does to you? How does it work?
- How severe is your sickness? Will it last a short or long time?
- What kind of treatment do you think you should receive?
- What results do you hope for from the treatment?
- What are the chief problems your sickness has caused?
- What do you fear most about your sickness?

I often use some cultural exercises to illustrate the use of assessment approaches. One involves a role-play in which students interview each other based upon assigned case studies. These studies are based on patient cases that I have had as well as cases that students want to have more information about. This type of approach permits students the freedom to try out and practice any new thoughts they may have enculturated about using cultural assessment techniques. I emphasize that that there is no right or wrong, no better or worse cultural beliefs or value systems and that any cultural perspective, even though perhaps unique or different from theirs, is to be respected, valued, and incorporated into the care, education, and research approaches with our patients.

Group Presentations as Reflection for Learning

Group projects and presentations are also used as a transformative learning assignment in the course. Three weeks into the course, students decide who they want to work with for their group project and what subject they are interested in presenting to the rest of the class. Students prepare for their presentation using assigned and other readings, conducting small research studies and developing community need studies for geographic areas they are working in outside of their clinical experiences. For example, a group of students decided to experience what it was like for persons who have physical handicaps. They borrowed a wheelchair and two of them visited several malls, grocery stores, and sporting events. They had one scenario in which one student sat in the wheelchair and went to these various areas. In another scenario, one person was in the wheelchair and another person was pushing the person along. The students were surprised to find that many people reacted with a lot of bias. Most of the time the students felt ignored and many persons refused to acknowledge their presence or give them any assistance entering doors and getting things from shelves. Other members of the group kept a record of what was happening during the research experience. Upon completion of the project, the entire group processed what had occurred and discussed reasons why persons reacted as they had.

Other students have utilized role-playing techniques for case study presentations related to cultural health care situations (e.g., patients from different religions that have different beliefs regarding blood transfusions, medications, and birth and death rituals that they might have encountered in their clinical settings). One inventive group of students designed a small card with the Kleinman questions on it and presented it to all of us. This card easily attaches to clips for identification badges that we all wear in clinical environments. Other students have provided food that is representative of certain cultural groups and have created PowerPoint presentations of the faces and voices of culturally and ethnically diverse persons talking about their cultural health care needs.

Other presentations have focused on:

- The Role of the Pediatric Nurse Practitioner With Families Whose Child Is Diagnosed With AIDS/HIV
- Teaching Health Promotion and Wellness Concepts for Persons Diagnosed With Schizophrenia
- The Role of the Nurse Practitioner in Collaborating With Women From Somali Culture to Develop Community Mammogram Screening Programs
- Immunization Programs for Children From Underserved Populations
- Advanced Nursing Advocacy for Patients Who Adhere to the Jehovah Witness Philosophy

Literature as a Cultural Experience

I use literature as a means of encouraging transformative, reflective learning. I may read poems, proverbs, and portions of books and songs or include them in PowerPoint presentations to emphasize cultural perspectives. In addition, there are two texts that I often have students read: *The Patient's Voice* by Jeanine Young-Mason (1997) and *The Spirit Catches You and You Fall Down* by Anne Fadiman (1997). The book by Young-Mason consists of a variety of patient-told stories using their voices as they describe their reactions and those of their families, friends, nurses, and physicians to various mental and physical illnesses. I use patient stories for small group exercises in the class. Each group has time to read the case study and then decide on a culturally competent plan that is appropriate for the circumstances. Students then share their ideas with the larger group. Many of them have commented that it "is hard to really figure out what a patient really needs and how can we meet their needs" and that this exercise "makes culture real in actual patient situations." Others note that "culture needs to be included as part of every assessment process."

The book by Fadiman is a compelling story of one Hmong family's experience and challenges with the U.S. health care system. Lia, their daughter, is diagnosed with epilepsy. The family views this as a wonderful thing, that the spirit has touched their daughter, which represents an honor for their daughter and for them, while Western physicians and nurses describe the source of Lia's illness as a brain dysfunction, as epilepsy. Students read the Fadiman book and then develop a paper that reflects their thinking regarding cultural issues related to their specialty areas. Students have one or two areas of nurse practitioner specialties (e.g., family, psychiatric mental health, adult, and pediatric). I provide students with comments in order to help them reflect on cultural issues for the family and the health care systems that are represented in the Fadiman text. A few such comments include the following:

- The book contains many Hmong phrases and many medical phrases, both unfamiliar to most readers. Why do you think the author included them?
- What do traditional Hmong consider to be their most important duties and obligations? What do Western doctors consider to be *their* most important duties and obligations?
- *The Spirit Catches You and You Fall Down* revolves around a small child who for much of the book is too young to speak for herself and at the end is unable to. Do you nonetheless feel you know Lia Lee? Do you believe that even though she cannot walk or talk, she is a person of value—and if so, why?
- The book has an unusual structure: Lia's story occupies the odd-numbered chapters, and background material occupies the even-numbered chapters. Why do you think Fadiman organized her narrative this way?

Students have created papers that centered on the following topics regarding "the clash of two cultures" in Fadiman's (1997) book and subsequent "divergent" cultural views and needs:

- Parental rights and custody issues in relationship to children's cultural rights and needs
- Spiritual health needs of the family in conjunction with implementation of traditional Western medicine
- Birthing and dying cultural practices for persons from Hmong cultural perspectives
- Health care misconceptions and the loss of a soul

I have consistently found that this final paper illustrates the evolution and growth in students' processes of cultural competence. Students are able to present a coherent and culturally competent approach to the care of their patients. And, at the same time they include a reflective examination of where they were regarding their process of cultural competence when the course began and where they were when it ended. They have also helped me to learn new reflections about myself and my process of cultural competence.

"When do we learn and what does it take to teach us things . . . Other people have ideas and inputs" (Giovanni, 2002, p. 2), and that is how the process of cultural competence is deepened.

RECOMMENDATIONS FOR NURSE EDUCATORS AND ADMINISTRATORS

The following are my personal and professional recommendations regarding the implementation of educational techniques that lead to the development of the process of cultural competence in students. This section is grounded in my knowledge about the process of cultural competence as well as my experiences in developing and implementing workshops, seminars, and courses on the subject.

First, the study circle technique for dialogue and discussion could be used by nurse educators and administrators within clinical settings. Case studies could form the basis of initial discussions. These case studies need to be grounded in actual case studies from the clinical settings where educators and administrators work. Real life experiences can be shared by nurses of various levels and specialties and discussed in order to solve dilemmas within clinical settings. Some of these dilemmas may involve communication challenges related to differences in cultural beliefs, values, and norms.

Second, many conflicts within clinical environments involve the unspoken and unsolved biases that staff may have about each other or about their patients. Nurse educators and administrators could use some of the cultural heritage questions that students in my course use in their self-evaluation in order to help staff evaluate their own cultural heritage. These discussions could be incorporated into brown bag sessions. In fact, nurse educators and administrators could seek continuing education credits in order to stimulate initial attendance at sessions. Moreover, some of these sessions could be based on discussions regarding the Fadiman book as it is grounded in health care situations that might be familiar to staff.

Some of these techniques I have incorporated in my work with nurse educators, administrators, and their staff. I have found that these individuals responded with the same enthusiasm and interest as the students who have taken my course. So, I strongly recommend that others use these techniques in order to develop more critical thinking and expand knowledge about cultural issues and, more importantly, move persons into development of their process of cultural competence.

SUMMARY AND REFLECTIVE CONCLUSIONS

This chapter discussed a pedagogy based on a constructivism paradigm and Mezirow's (2000) transformative learning theory that is used in a course that facilitates development of the process of cultural competence in graduate nursing practitioner students within a university setting. The course involves didactic discussions, interactive learning strategies, and study circles to promote the ongoing development of students' learning processes and movement toward the process of cultural competence. Learning situations are provided to guide the forward learning of students and facilitate successful completion of student assignments. This pedagogy is grounded in premises that encourage and facilitate the incorporation of discussions that are fluid and dynamic, safe, and open for all persons who are involved.

The use of this pedagogy has clear implications for nursing education because it creates a transformed way of thinking for the nurse practitioner students and the faculty who teach them. Such thinking is essential for use in increasingly complex health care settings. The increasing diversity and rapidly expanding health care needs must be grounded in nurses' ability to use culturally competent strategies and interactions within their academic, work, and research environments. It is important for graduate nurse practitioner students and the faculty who teach them to continue to participate in reflective cultural dialogues and discussions that reveal different approaches and meanings within clinical settings.

I will continue to think about the course and continue to listen to the cultural voices of my students and patients. In addition, many of the activities from the course also present another way in which the art of teaching and learning might be enhanced and transformed across and within other dynamic and fluid academic settings such as those in which nursing educators and administrators work. Moreover, this entire process to develop the course and this chapter caused me to reflect again upon my teaching approaches. The poem "Don't Think," written by Nikki Giovanni (2002, p. 109), helps to summarize all of this and guides my work with students:

The most important thing
I know
about teaching
is that the teacher is also learning
Don't think
you have to know it all.

So remember that none of us has to know it all. But, what we do need is to want to continue to grow and learn from each other in order to move ahead in developing new processes of culturally competent education, practice, and research. Sometimes our students and our patients are far more knowledgeable about how this may be accomplished, so continue to share ideas and learn from each other.

QUESTIONS FOR DIALOGUE

1. What ideas or concepts did you find most meaningful in this chapter? Identify your insights and questions to bring to a dialogue with your colleagues.
2. Think of the first time you realized the importance of culture in your nursing career. How has your understanding of culture evolved since then? Use the study circle technique to share your experience and reflection with colleagues.

3. Dialogue with colleagues about why it is important for students to reflect on their cultural heritage and its implications for nursing practice.
4. Develop guided reflection questions to stimulate a dialogue with colleagues on Warren's experience as the nurse manager responding to the patient in the psychiatric mental health facility.
5. Discuss the value of using literature to explore the role of culture in health and illness. What three literary works could you recommend to your colleagues as most powerful in helping to develop the "fluid process of cultural competence."
6. In your institution is there a graduate-level course in cultural competence? If not, why not? If so, does cultural competence continue to be addressed in meaningful ways in other courses? To what extent are all faculty held responsible for teaching cultural competence?

REFERENCES

Ali, R., Beesley, J., Burton, B., Gordon, J., Ingles, T., Jordan, E., et al. (2006). *Dimensions of diversity: Study circles for action and change—Illinois Central College, Summary Report.* East Peoria, IL: Blueprint Diversity Team.

Amaro, D. J., Abriam-Yago, K., & Yoder, M. (2006). Perceived barriers for ethnically diverse students in nursing programs. *Journal of Nursing Education, 45*(7), 247–254.

American Association of Colleges of Nursing (AACN). (1998). *Essentials of master's education for advanced nursing practice.* Washington, DC: Author. Retrieved February 8, 2006, from http://www.aacn.nche.edu/Publications/catalog2.htm

American Nurses Association Council on Cultural Diversity in Nursing Practice. (1986). *Cultural diversity in the nursing curriculum: A guide for implementation.* Kansas City, MO: Author.

Andrews, M. M., & Boyle, J. S. (2003). *Transcultural concepts in nursing care* (4th ed.). Philadelphia: Lippincott.

Brandman, W. (2007). *Misery or happiness: It's all about energy* [Inspirational cards]. Honolulu, HI: Valenti Print.

Campinha-Bacote, J. (2007). *The process of cultural competence in health care in the delivery of healthcare services: The journey continues.* Cincinnati, OH: Transcultural C.A.R.E. Associates.

Fadiman, A. (1997). *The spirit catches you and you fall down. A Hmong child, her American doctors, and the collision of two cultures.* New York: Farrar, Straus, and Giroux.

Garrett, J. T., & Garrett, M. (1996). *Medicine of the Cherokee: The way of the right relationship.* Santa Fe, NM: Bear & Company.

Giger, J. N., & Davidhizar, R. E. (2004). *Transcultural nursing: Assessment and intervention* (4th ed.). St. Louis: Mosby.

Giovanni, N. (2002). *Quilting the black-eyed pea: Poems and not quite poems.* New York: HarperCollins.

Hassouneh, D. (2006). Anti-racist pedagogy: Challenges faced by faculty of color in predominantly White schools of nursing. *Journal of Nursing Education, 45*(7), 255–262.

Haw, M. A. (2006). Learning theories applied to nursing curriculum development. In S. B. Keating (Ed.), *Curriculum development and evaluation in nursing* (pp. 49–60). Philadelphia: Lippincott.

Health Resources and Services Administration (HRSA). (2006). *The registered nurse population: National sample survey of registered nurses, preliminary report.* Retrieved February 8, 2006, from http://www.hrsa.gov/

Institute of Medicine (IOM). (2001). *Crossing the quality chasm: A new health system for the 21st century.* Washington, DC: National Academies Press.

Institute of Medicine (IOM). (2003). *Unequal treatment: Confronting racial and ethnic disparities in health care.* Washington, DC: National Academies Press.

Jones, C., & Shorter-Gooden, K. (2003). *Shifting: The double lives of Black women in America.* New York: HarperCollins.

Kleinman, A., Eisenberg, L., & Good, B. (1978). Culture, illness, and care: Clinical lessons from anthropologic and cross-cultural research. *Annual of Internal Medicine, 88*, 251–258.

Koening, J. M., & Zorn, C. R. (2002). Using story-telling as an approach to teaching and learning with diverse students. *Journal of Nursing Education, 41*(9), 393–399.

Leininger, M. M., & McFarland, M. R. (Eds.). (2006). *Culture care diversity and universality: A worldwide nursing theory* (2nd ed.). Sudbury, MA: Jones and Bartlett.

Lutz, W. J., & Warren, B. J. (2007). The state of nursing science—Cultural and lifespan issues Depression part II: Focus on children and adolescents. *Issues in Mental Health Nursing, 28*(7), 749–764.

Mezirow, J. (2000). *Learning as transformation: Clinical perspectives on a theory in progress.* San Francisco, CA: Jossey-Bass.

Muñoz, C. C., & Luckmann, J. (2005). *Transcultural communication in nursing* (2nd ed.). Clifton Park, NY: Thomson Delmar Learning.

Muñoz, R., Primm, A., Ananth, J., & Ruiz, P. (2007). *Life in color: Culture in American psychiatry.* Chicago, IL: Hilton.

Peplau, H. (1952). *Interpersonal relations in nursing.* New York: Putnam.

Purnell, L. D., & Paulanka, B. J. (2003). *Transcultural health care: A culturally competent approach* (2nd ed.). Philadelphia: F.A. Davis.

Ruiz, (1997). *A practical guide to personal freedom: The four agreements.* San Rafael, CA: Amber-Allen.

Smedley, B. D., Butler, A. S., & Bristow, L. R. (2004). *In the compelling interest: Ensuring diversity in the health-care workforce.* Washington, DC: National Academies Press.

Spector, R. E. (2004). *Cultural diversity in health and illness* (6th ed.). Upper Saddle River, NJ: Pearson Education.

U.S. Department of Health and Human Services (USDHHS). (1999). *Mental health: A report of the Surgeon General.* Rockville, MD: DHHS, Substance Abuse and Mental Health Services Administration, Center for Mental Health Services, National Institutes of Health, National Institutes of Mental Health.

U.S. Department of Health and Human Services (USDHHS). (2001). *Mental health: Culture, race, and ethnicity. A supplement to mental health: A report of the Surgeon General.* Rockville, MD: DHHS, Public Health Services, Office of the Surgeon General.

U.S. Department of Health & Human Services (USDHHS). (2002). *Healthy people 2010.* McLean, VA: International Medical Publications. Retrieved December 27, 2007, from http://www.healthypeople.gov/

Warren, B. J. (2002). Interlocking paradigm of cultural competence: A model for psychiatric mental-health nursing practice. *Journal of the American Psychiatric Nurses Association, 8*(6), 209–213.

Warren, B. J. (2003). Cultural and ethnic considerations. In D. Antai-Otong (Ed.), *Psychiatric nursing: Biological and behavioral concepts* (pp. 151–165). New York: Delmar.

Warren, B. J. (2005). The cultural expression of dying. *The Case Manager, 16*(1), 44–47.

Warren, B. J. (2007a). Cultural aspects of bipolar disorder. *Journal of Psychosocial Nursing, 45*(7), 32–37.

Warren, B. J. (2007b). Mood disorders: Management of moods & suicidal behavior. In M. A. Boyd (Ed.), *Psychiatric nursing: Contemporary practice* (4th ed.). Philadelphia, PA: Lippincott.

Warren, B. J. (2008). Psychosocial bases for understanding human behavior within a cultural context. In C. J. Cornwell (Ed.), *Psychiatric mental health nursing: An evidence-based approach to clinical care* (pp. 348–390). Baltimore, MD: Lippincott.

Warren, B. J., & Lutz, W. J. (2007). The state of nursing science: Cultural and lifespan issues Depression part II: Focus on adults. *Issues in Mental Health Nursing, 28*(7), 707–748.

Young-Mason, J. (1997). *The patient's voice: Experiences of illness.* Philadelphia: F. A. Davis.

9 Pathways to Leadership: Developing a Culturally Competent Leadership Curriculum for American Indian Nurses

LEE ANNE NICHOLS AND MARTHA BAKER

Over the years, we have observed many American Indian nurses adhere to traditional Indian ways when serving as nurse leaders in their tribal communities. What we quickly realized was how little information existed about American Indian nurse leadership in the literature *but* how much knowledge on leadership did exist in our oral languages, traditions, and culture. American Indian nurses, particularly nurse elders, teach each other how to be nurse leaders in indirect ways by giving back to the community, being humble, being spiritual, being an example, telling traditional stories, and being a life-long mentor. What we wanted to do was preserve this knowledge and tradition so that we could pass this unique nurse leadership perspective on to future generations of American Indian nurse leaders. And so, we as humble American Indian nurses reached into our traditional knowledge and developed Pathways to Leadership to give back to our community of American Indian nurses and to all nurses from diverse backgrounds.

BACKGROUND

American Indians (AI) are a culturally, racially, and ethnically unique population who require nursing care that is distinct and culturally sensitive to their traditional beliefs. American Indians are over-represented in health disparities with limited resources available to them to assist them in meeting their health care needs. Most AIs receive health care through the Indian Health Service (IHS) or tribal health programs. The IHS is currently decentralizing and downsizing, and many tribal entities are assuming control of their own Indian health system. These changes have created a complex health care delivery system that can be confusing even to the most seasoned nurses. Therefore, AI nurses in leadership positions have many cultural and organizational challenges to deal with in providing quality care to AI populations. Most AI nurses have minimal educational preparation to assist them in overcoming these obstacles so they can continue to provide high quality care to their patients.

PURPOSE

The purpose of this chapter is to describe the holistic experience of how an AI team of nurses developed an Indian nurse leadership curriculum titled Pathways to Leadership. The Pathways team teaches the curriculum in a way that is congruent with the Indian style of learning and traditional Indian ways. The goal of the program is to provide an educational foundation to prepare AI nurses for leadership roles in tribal health programs. In the Pathways program, AI nurses teach each other how to be leaders. American Indians share the cultural value of *being-in-becoming* mode activity. Being-in-becoming mode is contrasted with the doing-in-becoming mode of activity, in which identity is more about what one does than who one is (More, 1987). This chapter is presented in a way that reflects the being-in-becoming mode of activity. The Pathways to Leadership program was developed by AI nurses for AI nurses, and the curriculum is being continually revised and refined for future nurse leaders.

AMERICAN INDIANS

There are 4.1 million AIs in the United States, approximately 1% of the total U.S. population (U.S. Census Bureau, 2000). There are over 550 tribal entities federally recognized by the U.S. government (Bureau of Indian Affairs, 2002). Each tribe has their own unique history, language, culture, traditions, and beliefs, but commonalities across tribes exist.

Many tribes adhere to values based on harmony, spirituality, ceremony, and oral traditions (Garrett, 1999). These cultural values and Indian traditions are the cornerstone of AI community life and are the foundation of tribal resiliency and strength.

American Indians are over-represented in health disparities and experience many health conditions, including: suicide, abuse, family violence, alcoholism, diabetes, cancer, and cardiovascular disease (Parker, Haldane, Keltner, Strickland, & Tom-Orme, 2002). Factors such as historical trauma, forced assimilation, and loss of traditions have influenced many of these life-challenging situations (Struthers & Lowe, 2003). However, AIs are resilient and have survived years of forced assimilation despite the many attacks, both overt and covert, on their culture and way of life (Starnes, 2006).

Indian Health Service

The U.S. government provides many AIs with health care through the IHS (Dixon, 2001). This access to health care is based on the federal trust responsibility provided by the legal and historical relationships between the U.S. government and tribal governments. Currently, the Indian health system has evolved into a tripartite service called "I/T/U," representing the IHS, tribally operated programs, and urban Indian clinics (Dixon, 2001). The IHS has changed and become more complex because of decentralization and downsizing (Holkup, 2002; Kunitz, 1996; Parker et al., 2002). The IHS has also been turning over control of the health system to individual tribes, and many AI tribal governments have assumed the responsibility of health care for their own tribal members in tribally operated programs. A minimal amount of funding from Title 5 of the Indian Health Care Improvement Act of 1974 was used to establish Indian urban clinics in a few cities across the United States. This limited number of urban clinics was set up to provide health care to the growing number of urban AIs (Dixon, 2001).

American Indian Nurses

Many AI nurses work in tribal health programs and face many challenges in providing adequate quality care for Indian people. There are not enough AI nurses to care for the number of AIs in the United States, and this number is diminishing. There are only about 9,453 AI nurses, or

0.4% of the total nursing population, to care for the 4.1 million AIs in the United States (U.S. Department of Human & Health Services Division of Nursing, 2004). The IHS has the most severe shortage of nurses with a 14% vacancy rate and an aging population (70% over age 40). In addition, the needs of AI people are very high (Parker et al., 2002); AIs are over-represented in health disparities, and there are not enough health care resources and dollars to take care of their health needs (Holkup, 2002; Kunitz, 1996; Parker et al., 2002). American Indians require care from nurses that is congruent with their traditional beliefs and nursing care that is culturally sensitive to avoid misunderstandings and harm; AI nurses in leadership positions in particular are challenged by these circumstances (Nichols, 2004). In addition, because of all the changes occurring in the complex I/T/U system, AI nurse leaders have many difficulties to confront, such as reduced funding, restricted services, and decentralization, while maintaining quality care, staff satisfaction, and productivity (Nichols, 2004). There are a limited number of AI nurses and fewer numbers of AI nurses prepared for leadership roles in the Indian health system.

MAINSTREAM NURSE LEADERSHIP

Recently, AI nurse leaders from the National Alaska Native American Indian Nursing Association (NANAINA) and the IHS have realized the leadership style and leadership needs are different for AI nurses (Nichols, 2004). Most AI nurses are educated in nursing schools that do not educate nurses using an AI leadership cultural framework. The theories of nurse leadership presented in textbooks such as Yoder-Wise and Kowalski's (2006) *Beyond Leading and Managing: Nursing Administration for the Future* and Huber's (2005) *Leadership and Nursing Care Management* are based on the mainstream cultural value system. While that is appropriate, it leaves AI nurses (and students) struggling with a conflict of values and a need to learn to be bicultural, in other words, both AI and non-AI, in their approach to leadership.

Tannenbaum and Schmidt (1973) described three major styles of leadership that nurses are taught in the mainstream culture: authoritarian, democratic, and laissez-faire. In contrast, Indian nurse leadership style is based on a holistic framework and a cooperative shared approach. None of the three styles of nurse leadership capture the "Indian way" of nurse leadership.

Review of Literature: What We Know About Indian Leadership

The review of literature reveals a dearth of texts on American Indian *nurse* leadership; however, there is relevant information in the literature on tribal leadership that is useful in understanding Indian nurse leadership. Most of the information is anecdotal; only two research studies were identified in the literature on AI leadership. Jules (1988) and Lewis and Gingerich (1980) completed qualitative studies on general tribal leadership. *Only one* qualitative study on Indian nurse leadership conducted by Nichols (2004) was identified. These studies reveal the cultural differences between Indian leadership and mainstream leadership, which does have application for nurses working in Indian health programs.

Values and qualities related to AI leadership are distinct from mainstream leadership values. Jules (1988) proposed that AI leaders must possess wisdom by having life experiences and identified four qualities of AI leadership: leaders have to be close to the people, leaders serve rather than boss, leaders inform the people about what is going on, and leaders must have humility. Dixon (2001) described four key values related to tribal decision-making: being a good relative, inclusive sharing, contributing, and noncoercive leadership. The value of respect has been described as an important value for AI leaders to have (Hill, 1995; Sanchez & Stucky, 1999). Also, the value of native noninterference is crucial for a leader to have in order to be a successful leader in a tribal community (Good Tracks, 1973). Good Tracks (1973) stated that traditional Indian societies are organized on the principle of voluntary cooperation, which means native noninterference. American Indians refrain from using force to coerce another person; an AI leader who leads by cooperation and not by coercion respects the rights of individuals to self-determine. Elders from the tribal communities are an integral part of AI leadership. Elders provide the wisdom for successful leaders and stand beside the tribal leaders (Hill, 1995; Jules, 1988; Sanchez & Stuckey, 1999). Finally, a leader is spiritual and understands the importance of spirituality in AI communities (American Indian Research and Policy Institute [AIRPI], 1997).

The approach or style of AI leadership is different from the style of mainstream leadership. An AI leader is connected to the tribal community and the members of the tribe (AIRPI, 1997; Hill, 1995; Jules, 1988; Keltner, Kelley, & Smith, 2004). The servant leadership style is the approach many AI leaders use (Jules, 1988). Jules stated: "A leader is a person capable of directing the people without giving the impression that they are being told what to do—a facilitator" (p. 8). American Indian leaders make decisions by getting consensus from the community (AIRPI, 1997; Jules, 1988). This approach assists with protecting tribal autonomy. Finally, AI leaders are expected to consult with tribal elders about decisions related to the tribal community (AIRPI, 1997; Hill, 1995; Jules, 1988).

American Indian leaders are selected based on the person's contributions to the tribal community and are recognized and selected by the people as most suitable to lead at a particular point in time, as different types of AI leaders lead at different times (AIRPI, 1997; Lewis & Gingerich, 1980). American Indian leaders possess the highest sense of personal integrity; they are valued more for who they are and less for what they do (Lewis & Gingerich, 1980). Mainstream society may place a higher premium on the leader with academic success, whereas the traditional Indian community may value the spiritual leader, who does not have academic credentials, more. To be a leader in the tribal community, the person is expected to be wise and know the culture of the community (Jules, 1988).

Findings from two qualitative studies (Jules, 1988; Lewis & Gingerich, 1980) concluded that humility, service, personal integrity, wisdom, respect, and spirituality were the essence of a successful leader in a tribal community. Lewis and Gingerich (1980) stated that even Indian participants raised in urban settings adhered more to a traditional Indian leadership style than the mainstream leadership style. In her study, Nichols (2004) concluded that many of these same leadership qualities are essential to be an effective nurse leader in a tribal setting or health care setting servicing AI populations.

THE INDIAN WAY OF KNOWING

The Indian way of knowing is different from mainstream culture. The Indian way of knowing comes from the culture and worldview of AIs and is reflected in the traditions, ancient knowledge, indirect communication, and ways of learning of AIs. The following sections describe the Indian way of knowing in more depth.

World View and Cultural Values

American Indian cultural beliefs are based on the world view of spirituality, harmony, and wholeness (Burhansstipanov & Hollow, 2001). Each tribe has their own unique rich culture, traditions, language, ceremonies, history, and spirituality. However, commonalities in cultural values do permeate across tribes—values such as generosity, wisdom, spirituality, stewardship of the earth, humility, circularity, connectiveness, cooperation, identity, honor, holism, oneness, balance, being visionary, traditionalism, harmony, and planning for the seventh generation or future generations. Respect is a central value of the AI way of life (Ambler, 2003).

Tradition

American Indians value tradition instead of change. Some traditions are related to medicine, family, dress, ceremony, music, and language (Burhansstipanov & Hollow, 2001). For example, many AIs have Traditional Indian Medicine (TIM) available to them as a health care choice and make use of this health care alternative. In TIM, "wellness of the mind, body, spirit, and natural environment are an expression of the proper balance in the relationships of all things. If one disturbs or disrupts the natural balance of a relationship, illness may be the result, whether it is expressed in the mind, body, spirit, or natural environment" (Garrett, 1999, p. 89). Healers familiar with TIM use prayer, herbs, and ceremony to treat the illnesses of AIs (Burhansstipanov & Hollow, 2001). Each tribe has their own unique healers and TIM.

Old Knowledge

American Indian tribes also value "old knowledge" (Moss et al., 2005). Old knowledge is passed down from one generation to the next through storytelling as the mode of communication (Moss et al., 2005). Elders are considered the wisdom keepers of the tribe (Wall & Arden, 1993). They tell stories to the younger members in the community, passing the teachings related to Indian traditions and history on to the next generation.

Communication Style

Oral tradition is the most common form of communication of tribes (Moss et al., 2005). American Indians also communicate through silence, storytelling, art, color, traditions, pottery, sand painting, songs, drums, and flutes (Moss et al., 2005; Nichols, 2004). Communication is indirect and involves speaking quietly at a slower rate, use of silence and nonverbal communication, delayed response to auditory messages, and less spoken interjection (Garrett, 1999). Silence is valued in the Navajo and many other AI cultures. Bell (1994) said, "Silence is highly respected in the Navajo culture. One who hurries the conversation along may be thought rude. Long periods of silence are used to formulate thoughts so that the spoken word will have significance" (p. 233).

Traditional AI Learning Styles

Learning begins with the oral passage of knowledge. Traditional Indian learning occurs in three ways: watch, then do; listen, then do; and think, then do (More, 1987). Another learning style is through mentoring. Mentoring is usually accomplished by the elders in the tribe and occurs differently in AI communities than in mainstream culture. Lowe (2002) describes the mentoring process as becoming self-reliant. The AI is neither totally dependent nor independent but is developing by becoming responsible, disciplined, and confident. A mentor–mentee relationship becomes a life-long commitment for the AI mentor. Other ways mentoring facilitates learning is through participation in ceremony, quiet reflection, the use of silence, and through storytelling (Paterson & Hart-Wasekeesikaw, 1987). Finally, another style of AI learning is by testimony or storytelling in a talking circle. Knowledge passes from one AI person to another with energy flowing circularly between the persons to create a sense of oneness.

PATHWAYS TO LEADERSHIP

The previous literature review forms the foundation for the development of Pathways to Leadership. A discussion of the history of Pathways to Leadership, the development of the AI nurse leadership model, teaching the curriculum, the curriculum itself, and the first gathering of nurse leaders follows. However, the experiences of the Pathways team in developing and implementing the Pathways curriculum were intertwined. Although it was necessary to divide the descriptions of developing and implementing the Pathways curriculum into sections to make it easier for the reader to follow, the experience of creating the leadership program was holistic in nature for the Pathways team; therefore, there may be slight overlapping of sections.

History

American Indian nurse leaders in NANAINA, the IHS, and tribal health care programs across the United States recognized the need to develop an AI nurse leadership curriculum. In June 1997, a team of four Indian nurse leaders and one non-Indian nurse leader attended the Third Congress of Minority Nurses in Denver, Colorado. This congress was sponsored by the Health and Human Services Department Division of Nursing. Their project Pathways to Leadership focused on developing an AI nurse leadership curriculum. The original curriculum focused on traditional organizational leadership behaviors. However, the Indian team members soon identified the need to explore Indian nurse leadership further and to identify whether the dimensions of this leadership style were different from the dimensions of mainstream leadership approaches. In order to define Indian nurse leadership, NANAINA was instrumental in supporting and encouraging the development of three Indian Nurse Leadership modules that captured the concepts and constructs of Indian nurse leadership (Nichols, 2004). Later on, in response to an identified need, an Indian nurse leadership model was developed to be the guiding framework for the Pathways to Leadership curriculum.

Development of the American Indian Nurse Leadership Model

Nurse leaders from NANAINA and the IHS recognized the need to (a) partner with educators to develop educational programs suitable for AI nurses and (b) educate AI nurses (and non-AI nurses who work in tribal health programs) in alternative leadership styles that are culturally sensitive and congruent with AI culture and values (Nichols, 2004). In fall 2002, at the NANAINA Summit VIII, the Pathways team presented the first overview of the newly developed leadership curriculum to Indian and mainstream nurses. During the evaluation phase of the curriculum modules, the team members identified gaps in the curriculum and identified the need to have a guiding framework or model, not just a series of unrelated information modules.

The American Indian Nurse Leadership model was then constructed from information already gathered from focus groups conducted with AI nurse leaders at the NANAINA Summit V (Nichols, 2004). The American Indian Nurse Leadership model includes three themes: being connected as a leader, what an Indian nurse leader is, and what an Indian nurse leader does (Nichols, 2004). *Connectedness for the leader* focuses on being connected to the individual, family, and tribal community. *What a leader is* includes having a quiet presence and being spiritual, self-actualized, visionary, humble, wise, experienced, political, and recognized. *What a leader does* is mentors, role models, communicates, listens, mobilizes, inspires, and demonstrates values. The American Indian Nurse Leadership model is used as the guiding framework for the Pathways curriculum.

TEACHING THE CURRICULUM

To be truly successful the curriculum has to be taught in a manner that is congruent with AI cultural ways and the "Indian way of knowing." For example, the Indian nurse leadership modules (to be discussed) are based partly on "old knowledge" from historical Indian leaders. Communication to the group of AI nurses is delivered indirectly and taught in third person so as not to offend any participant. Cultural taboos, such as death or advance directives, are talked about in third person and with great respect and only in the presence of a respected Indian elder to guide the conversations. Elder participants are respected for their experiences and knowledge. Traditions, such as prayer and ceremony, are included as part of the teaching sessions. All of these educational strategies improve the teaching effectiveness of the content *in the Indian way.*

Curriculum

The Pathways curriculum consists of nine modules, of which six are focused primarily on traditional mainstream approaches to nurse leadership and are discussed in light of the Indian nurse leadership approach, and three of which contain primarily Indian nurse leadership content. The mainstream modules cover the following topics: (a) Knowing Self, (b) Personal and Professional Communication and Mentoring, (c) Group Process, (d) Decision Making, (e) Change Process, and (f) Being a Futurist. The Indian modules cover the following topics: (g) Being a Nurse Leader in the Indian Way, (h) Indian Nursing and Tribal Sovereignty, and (i) Indian Nursing and Indian Health Programs.

Mainstream Nurse Leadership Modules

The focus of the first six modules of the curriculum is on personal development of one's leadership skills. American Indians value personal growth and self-actualization, so emphasizing a personal perspective of leadership is compatible with Indian culture and values. The traditional mainstream leadership modules are interlaced appropriately with an AI worldview. For example, an AI nurse delegating responsibilities to health team members, which reflects the mainstream style, is considered a customary way to get patient care tasks accomplished; however, for a *young* AI nurse to delegate to an *older,* more experienced AI nurse or health care team member may not be the most culturally appropriate way to get the tasks done. A more suitable or comfortable way to delegate for a young AI nurse would be to have an older team member delegate or use cooperative and respectful techniques to delegate to team members.

The two worldviews, mainstream and AI, are compared and contrasted throughout the presentation of the mainstream modules. This provides the Indian nurse a more bicultural view of Indian and mainstream health care systems because most nurses must work within mainstream organizations as well as Indian health systems. This bicultural approach provides an understanding for the AI nurse of the values, behaviors, and skills needed in Indian and non-Indian organizations.

Originally, the textbook by Bower (2000) *Nurses Taking the Lead: Personal Qualities of Effective Leadership* was chosen as a basis for the mainstream leadership modules. This text was chosen because it focuses primarily on personal leadership development. This focus was chosen to assist the emerging AI nurse leaders with the development of bicultural leadership skills. Information was also pulled from other literature on leadership development, such as Covey's (1989) *The 7 Habits of Highly Effective People* and Porter-O'Grady and Malloch's (2007) *Quantum Leadership.* The modules introduce and review essential leadership concepts that are needed by every nurse leader. A short synopsis of the mainstream leadership concepts and modules is provided here.

Knowing Self

This is the beginning module that starts the reflection on who one is and how one's leadership style is an extension of one's personality, values, and beliefs. The similarities between the concept of self and the Indian idea of self are discussed and contrasted. The mainstream idea of self is more individualistic, while the Indian idea of self includes self, family, community, and tribe. To assist the participants in professional development, the participants are asked to write a personal mission statement based on their values and beliefs (Covey, 1989). The conceptual framework of Indian nursing (Lowe & Struthers, 2001; Struthers & Littlejohn, 1999) is introduced at this point as an example of what an Indian mission statement could look like. The participants explore the concepts and ideas of the model as they develop their own personal mission statement.

Personal and Professional Communication and Mentoring

Much of the information in this module is a review of information on communication, such as active listening, that many of the participants have been exposed to in other classes. However, in the context of this course, communication takes on a new immediacy as the participants are trying to negotiate a bicultural world with a cultural leadership style and model that does not quite fit the mainstream world. Consistent with the Indian way of learning, participants are introduced to the technique of "listening and observing." This approach encourages the leader to gather information in an indirect way and introduces the leader to the people in a quiet manner.

Group Process

The principles of groups and what makes them function are described with attention to the fact that professional and work groups are based on the values of the mainstream culture and function much differently from groups in Indian culture, and what works within AI culture may not work in the mainstream workplace. Groups in Indian culture value decisions made with the consensus of all participants rather than voting and letting the majority rule. This could be problematic in the mainstream because consensus building requires more time and a less directive leadership style.

Decision Making

A key skill needed to be a leader is decision making. The curriculum explores the process from both an AI and mainstream perspective. It is essential that the students understand how decisions are made in organizations. Additionally, they need to be aware of the real differences in how decisions are usually made in both cultures. For example, consensus is the favored method of AI decision making. However, this may not be feasible or desirable in some situations in the nursing workplace.

Change Process

Change is a fact of life. No one knows that better than American Indians as life has been constantly changing since 1492. Managing and planning that change may be a concept that needs development and exploration for the participants. The tools to be a change agent are delineated from both the mainstream perspective, using Lewin's (1947) theory of change, and the Indian way, through the use of an elder's wisdom. Methods of applying and using these tools are defined and examples given.

Being a Futurist

Looking to the future needs to be understood from the lessons of the past. Traditional ways are what ground and direct AI people when living in the present or preparing for the future. Anticipating and responding to the possibilities of the future ahead of the curve is essential to the maturation of a leader. Skills to be a futurist, while necessary, are not often addressed in nursing curriculums. Pathways attempts to introduce and explore these skills of futuristic thinking and planning in light of the traditions of the past that direct our communities and people.

Indian Nurse Leadership Modules

The team reached into the spiritual, traditional, and ceremonial Indian ways of knowing to develop the three Indian nurse leadership modules. When providing a leadership curriculum to AI nurses (and non-Indian nurses who provide care to AIs), the Pathways team felt it was necessary to engage the AI cultural worldview of the nurses and patients. This approach would encourage AI nurses to lead in a manner that was natural, instinctive, fluid, holistic, and circular, which is more in harmony with their cultural beliefs and the cultural beliefs of their patients.

Throughout all of the Indian nurse leadership modules, the importance of being a spiritual leader and being in right relationships, or in harmony with self, family, and community, is emphasized because this is a key construct that has emerged from established research and research conducted by the Pathways team. The following sections provide a brief overview of the content of each module on AI nurse leadership.

Being a Nurse Leader in the Indian Way

The initial Indian nurse leadership module introduces the models of AI nursing and AI nurse leadership. Other concepts unique to Indian nurse leadership are explored as well, including being a bicultural leader (i.e., traditional mainstream nurse leadership compared to AI nurse leadership) and issues related to tribal sovereignty and health disparities of Indian people.

First, the conceptual model of AI nursing (Lowe & Struthers, 2001; Struthers & Littlejohn, 1999) is introduced to the participants. The seven dimensions of Indian nursing—caring, traditions, respect, connection, holism, trust, and spirituality—are analyzed and explored. These dimensions are the essence of AI nursing and are connected and interwoven in AI culture and tradition. They are compared to mainstream traditional nursing concepts to introduce the participants to how nursing is defined and may be practiced differently in a tribal community.

Secondly, the facets of Indian nurse leadership and the characteristics and actions of Indian nurse leaders are discussed (Nichols, 2004). The Indian nurse leadership model is introduced to the participants. Many concepts of Indian nurse leadership, such as spirituality, humility, and self-actualization, are presented and explored in detail. The differences between mainstream traditional nurse leadership and Indian nurse leadership are analyzed. For example, being humble is expected of a nurse leader in a tribal community, rather than expressing one's accomplishments.

Finally, the idea of being spiritual in the nursing community is explored in further depth. An outline for living a balanced life, based on the work of Struthers (2000, 2001), is introduced to the participants. This information is used to encourage leaders to stay healthy in mind, body, and spirit so they can be more effective leaders.

Indian Nursing and Tribal Sovereignty

The second Indian nurse module includes the discussion of Indian political topics relevant to Indian nurse leadership. American Indian political topics, ranging from trust responsibility, tribal sovereignty, tribal politics, and self-governance, are discussed and the application of these concepts to Indian nurse leadership explored. Laws relevant to Indian health and the relevance of these laws to nursing are discussed. The participants are introduced to this key idea: *"It is important for nurses to understand that by working in the Indian health care programs, they are fulfilling the government's trust responsibility toward the Indian nations under its care"* (Parker & Nichols, 2001, p. 88). This is also a way nurses can demonstrate the cultural value of giving back to the community.

Because leadership involves working with mainstream leaders in a mainstream environment as well as with tribes, AI nurse leaders are taught how to "get political" and how to work with tribal leaders, council members, and tribal health boards. Finally, the idea of Indian community is defined and its application to AI nurse leadership investigated.

During the presentation of this module, a tribal leader from the community is invited to conduct a talking circle and discuss their perspective on being a leader and how their perspective relates to health care. For example, the former president of Navajo Nation Peterson Zah presented what he described as his three principles of leadership: "be honest to yourself," "listen to people," and "respect their culture"(Parker, Baker, & Nichols, 2003, p. 42). The participants are given the opportunity to hear orally the testimony of a tribal leader and to ask questions of the tribal leader about issues related to health care and nursing. Wisdom from an experienced leader is offered to the participants. Opportunities to share occur in a circular pattern to give and take from each other and the speaker.

Indian Nursing and Indian Health Programs

The last Indian nurse leadership module explores the history of the IHS, the Indian health system, Indian health disparities and Indian health issues, and Indian nurse ethics. Application of these topics to Indian nursing is studied, and ways to address some of the health issues are discussed with the participants.

For example, many AI nurses are uncomfortable with discussion of negative medical information (e.g., advance planning, "bad news") with AI patients (Bell, 1994; Carrese & Rhodes, 1995). This can create a potentially ethical dilemma for some AI nurses. A traditional healer and traditional ways can be used to teach nurses how to address AI ethical dilemmas. A traditional AI healer from the community can be asked to conduct a talking circle with the participants. The healer can offer Indian prayers, make offerings to the Creator, create a sacred circle, and perform a smudging ceremony to cleanse members. If participants feel comfortable, then discussion about how to approach AI clients in a culturally sensitive manner with regard to negative information may be encouraged. The participants share with the healer, and the healer teaches and heals. The nurses have the opportunity to learn from each other in a traditional setting how to address ethical situations.

Information from the traditional mainstream nurse modules and Indian nurse leadership modules are used to intertwine all nine of the modules into a complete leadership program suitable to preparing an AI nurse for a leadership position. American Indian nurse leaders (and mainstream nurse leaders) need to be knowledgeable or bicultural about both leadership styles to be effective leaders in tribal communities and improve the quality of patient care.

IMPLEMENTATION OF THE CURRICULUM: THE GATHERING OF NURSE LEADERS IN JUNE 2003

A gathering workshop for Indian nurse leaders was planned and implemented by the Pathways team and other AI nurse leaders in the Phoenix area of the IHS (Parker et al., 2003). This was the initial implementation of the Pathways to Leadership curriculum developed by the team, as described previously. The gathering lasted for one week. Seventeen nurse leaders attended the gathering. The curriculum modules were presented over the week at the rate of two per day. Consistent with tribal custom, the day began with a prayer or meditation by an Indian elder. Food and drinks were provided throughout the day, and opening circles were conducted every morning. Guest speakers were invited as exemplars of leadership, including a non-AI nurse leader, a tribal leader, and a spiritual healer. The guest speakers expressed their views of leadership in relation to the concepts discussed in the modules. An evening meal was served by one of the Pathways team members at her home during the week of the workshop, which gave the participants of the Pathways gathering the opportunity to informally network and develop relationships with their peers outside the classroom setting. Finally, following the evaluation, a giveaway, which is a tradition of the Cherokee and other tribes, was done with the participants to thank them for coming to the gathering. An ending circle was formed, and the closing ceremony was conducted by an Apache healer to send the participants on a safe journey home with encouragement to continue their leadership journey.

Evaluation was done daily, and a summative evaluation was done at the end of the gathering. The evaluation data revealed that the curriculum was well received by the participants. Almost all of the sessions were rated 4–4.25 out of 5, with 4 = above average and 5 = excellent, on a Likert-type scale. This positive evaluation was also evidenced by such comments as:

> "I am learning to be a better leader."
>
> "This workshop has been an eye opening experience."
>
> "I am glad someone recognizes not everyone is the same, our leadership is different, not bad."
>
> "This week has made a difference in my view of nursing and my struggle to lead. I am not so down about it."
>
> "I hope you do this workshop for all nurses in Indian Health Service as it would help any nurse who works with our people."

Update

Since the beginning of Pathways, many changes have taken place. The curriculum has been presented 5 times to over 80 nurses. These presentations have guided further refinement and development of the Pathways curriculum. Feedback from participants has also resulted in the addition of human resource issues and conflict management to the curriculum. The textbook has changed due to Bower's text being out-of-print. The current text is Grossman and Valiga's (2005) *The New Leadership Challenge: Creating the Future of Nursing.* This text allows Pathways to maintain the same concepts and modules of mainstream culture in the course with only minimal disruption of content. The concept of the "talking circle" as a teaching method has been expanded with great success, and according to evaluations, the AI participants have found this teaching method extremely effective in applying the concepts in the Pathways curriculum. Further research and application of Pathways will continue in the future.

In addition, participants wanted more opportunity to provide feedback in a nonobtrusive way, so, to be respectful, the Pathways team began providing the participants with a "your ticket out" form. At the end of the day, the participants wrote on the form what topics they wanted more information on, and these topics were included in the instruction for the next day. This was a continual circle of exchange and learning that occurred between the participants and the Pathways team. The Pathways to Leadership curriculum is an excellent basis to demonstrate to nurses (and students) that styles of leadership can and often do vary based on one's ethnic background and world view. This understanding of different cultures is an important step in the career development of a nurse leader or future nurse leader.

CONCLUSION: GIVING BACK

Many AIs think circular and believe life is continually evolving, so to be true to this cultural value, the Pathways curriculum continues to be refined and modified for the next generation of nurse leaders. This way "old knowledge" is retained and new knowledge is created. After each curriculum presentation, whatever the venue, the nurse participants are asked to share what they learned about leadership. Information from *past* participants is then used to refine the *present* Pathways curriculum, which is then, in turn, presented to *future* nurse leaders. After each gathering, the cycle then repeats itself. This cyclic process is the Indian way of preserving our knowledge for future AI nurse leaders. It is also a way of giving back to the community of nursing and of helping to provide high quality care to AI people.

The American Nurse Leadership model and curriculum provides an example of how different cultures approach common concepts and skills. All cultures and traditions have leaders and leadership; however, each sees the implementation of leadership in a different way. It is important to keep this perspective in mind when working with clients, students, and peers of other cultures. Perceptions may differ from group to group, but each group, when approached with respect and dignity, will be willing to share their insights with others. The American Indian Nurse Leadership model is presented to nurse educators for that purpose—in order to foster understanding of the values of one another's viewpoints.

RECOMMENDATIONS FOR NURSE EDUCATORS AND ADMINISTRATORS

Based on the experiences of the Pathways to Leadership team of nurses, the following recommendations are made for nurse educators and administrators:

1. Nurse educators and administrators should evaluate their views on leadership and recognize that differences exist within differ-

ent cultural groups. One view is not better or worse, but simply different.

2. If there are students in class who are AI, be aware of the different approach these students may bring to discussions as these students are trying to negotiate a bicultural existence.
3. While there is value in the mainstream approach and it is necessary to teach this approach, there are also concepts or lessons that can be learned and incorporated into courses on leadership from other cultural traditions. In other words, what can mainstream leaders learn from the "old knowledge" that AIs bring to the discussion? For example, is a talking circle a teaching tool that could be used in your setting?
4. Be sensitive to the fact that AI students may seem hesitant to simply jump into a leadership role. As discussed in this chapter, there may be multiple reasons for this hesitancy that have nothing to do with the student's academic qualifications.
5. Lastly, remember one of the major tenets of American Indian nurse leadership: Indian leaders are valued more for who they are and less for what they do (Lewis & Gingerich, 1980). Create opportunities for students to develop personal qualities of leadership, such as humility, service, personal integrity, wisdom, respect, and spirituality (Lewis & Gingerich, 1980). This will benefit not only AI students but all nursing students to develop such leadership qualities.

QUESTIONS FOR DIALOGUE

1. What ideas or concepts did you find most meaningful in this chapter? Identify your insights and questions to bring to a dialogue with your colleagues.
2. In your opinion, what are the essential characteristics and values of professional nurse leadership? Nichols and Baker stress that AI leaders are valued more for who they are than what they do. From this perspective, dialogue with colleagues about the role of personal character versus professional accomplishments in leadership in your institution.
3. To what extent is the being-in-becoming mode recognized and validated in your program in addition to the doing-in-becoming mode? Provide specific examples and identify needed changes.

4. In your nursing program, are group process, decision making, change process, and communication conceptualized and taught in a way that prepares students to work in AI or other indigenous communities? If not, dialogue with colleagues about changes necessary to bring about greater focus in culturally competent nurse leadership.
5. In the "World Views and Cultural Values" section, the authors list cultural values that permeate across tribes. Which of these values permeate your nursing program? Dialogue with colleagues about values and ways of being you would like to bring to the center of your program's culture and how you might do this.
6. As the authors ask, what can mainstream leaders learn from the *old knowledge* that AIs bring to leadership?

REFERENCES

Ambler, M. (2003). Indigenizing our future. *Tribal College Journal of American Indian Higher Education, 15*(1), 8–9.

American Indian Research and Policy Institute. (1997). *Traditional American Indian leadership: A comparison with U.S. governance.* Retrieved May 15, 2006, from http://www.airpi.org/research/tradlead.html

Bell, R. (1994). Prominence of women in Navajo healing beliefs and values. *Nursing & Health Care, 15*(5), 232–240.

Bower, F. L. (2000). *Nurses taking the lead: Personal qualities of effective leadership.* St. Louis, MO: W.B. Saunders.

Bureau of Indian Affairs (2002, July 12). Indian entities recognized and eligible to receive services from the United States Bureau of Indian Affairs [Notice]. *Federal Register.* Washington, DC: National Archives and Records Administration.

Burhansstipanov, L., & Hollow, W. (2001). Native American cultural aspects of oncology nursing care. *Seminars in Oncology Nursing, 17*(3), 206–219.

Carrese, J. A., & Rhodes, L. A. (1995). Western bioethics on the Navajo reservation: Benefit or harm. *JAMA, 274*(1), 826–829.

Covey, S. (1989). *The 7 habits of highly effective people.* New York: Simon & Schuster.

Dixon, M. (2001). Access to care for American Indians and Alaska Natives. In M. Dixon & Y. Robideaux (Eds.), *Promises to keep: Public health policy for American Indians & Alaska Natives for the 21st century* (pp. 253–271). Washington, DC: American Public Health Association.

Garrett, M. T. (1999). Understanding the "medicine" of Native American traditional values: An integrative review. *Counseling & Values, 43*(2), 84–99.

Good Tracks, J. G. (1973, Nov.). Native American noninterference. *Social Casework, 18,* 30–34.

Grossman, S. C., & Valiga, T. M. (2005). *The new leadership challenge: Creating the future of nursing* (2nd ed.). Philadelphia: F. A. Davis.

Hill, N. S. (1995). A community road ahead: American Indian leadership 2000. *Winds of Change, 10*(2), 22–23.

Holkup, P. A. (2002). Big changes in the Indian Health Service: Are nurses aware? *Journal of Transcultural Nursing, 13,* 47–53.

Huber, D. L. (2005). *Leadership and nursing care management* (3rd ed.). St. Louis, MO: Saunders.

Jules, F. (1988). Native Indian leadership. *Canadian Journal of Native Education, 15*(3), 3–23.

Keltner, B., Kelley, F. J., & Smith, D. (2004). Leadership to reduce health disparities: A model for nursing leadership in American Indian communities. *Nursing Administration Quarterly, 28*(3), 181–190.

Kunitz, S. J. (1996). Public health then and now: The history and politics of U.S. health care for American Indians and Alaska Natives. *American Journal of Public Health, 86*(10), 1464–1473.

Lewin, K. (1947). Frontiers in group dynamics: Concept, method, and reality in social science, social equilibria, and social change. *Human Relations, 1*(1), 5–41.

Lewis, R. G., & Gingerich, W. (1980). Leadership characteristics: Views of Indian and non-Indian students. *Social Casework, 62,* 494–497.

Lowe, J. (2002). Balance and harmony through connectedness: The intentionality of Native American nurses. *Holistic Nursing Practice, 16*(4), 1–8.

Lowe, J., & Struthers, R. (2001). Profession and society: Conceptual framework of nursing in Native American culture. *Journal of Nursing Scholarship, 33*(3), 279–283.

More, A. J. (1987). Native Indian learning styles: A review for researchers and teachers. *Journal of American Indian Education, 27*(1), 17–29.

Moss, M., Tibbets, L., Henly, S. J., Dahlen, B. J., Patchell, B., & Struthers, R. (2005). Strengthening American Indian nurse scientist training through tradition: Partnering with elders. *Journal of Cultural Diversity, 12*(2), 50–55.

Nichols, L. A. (2004). Native American nurse leadership. *Journal of Transcultural Nursing, 15*(3), 177–183.

Parker, J., Baker, M., & Nichols, L. A. (2003, Fall). Pathways to Leadership: A minority leadership development program with an exciting difference: It's culturally competent curriculum created by and for American Indian Nurses. *Minority Nurse,* 40–43.

Parker, J. G., Haldane, S. L., Keltner, B. K., Strickland, C. J., & Tom-Orme, L. (2002). National Alaska Native American Indian Nurses Association: Reducing health disparities within American Indian and Alaska Native populations. *Nursing Outlook, 50*(1), 16–23.

Parker, J., & Nichols, L. A. (2001, Summer). Tribes know best. *Minority Nurse,* 88–87.

Paterson, B., & Hart-Wasekeesikaw, F. (1987). Mentoring women in higher education: Lessons from the Elders. *College Teaching, 42*(2), 72–77.

Porter-O'Grady, T., & Malloch, K. (2007). *Quantum leadership: A textbook of new leadership.* (2nd ed.) Boston: Jones and Barlett.

Sanchez, J., & Stuckey, M. E. (1999). Communicating culture through leadership: One view from Indian country. *Communication Studies, 50*(2), 103–115.

Starnes, B. A. (2006). What we don't know can hurt them: White teachers, Indian children. *Phi Delta Kappa: The Professional Journal for Education, 87*(5), 384–392.

Struthers, R. (2000). The lived experience of Ojibwa and Cree women healers. *Journal of Holistic Nursing, 18*(3), 261–279.

Struthers, R. (2001). Conducting sacred research: An indigenous experience. *Wicazo Sa Review, 16*(1), 125–133.

Struthers, R., & Littlejohn, S. (1999). The essence of Native American nursing. *Journal of Transcultural Nursing, 10*(2), 131–135.

Struthers, R., & Lowe, J. (2003). Nursing in the Native American culture and historical trauma. *Issues in Mental Health Nursing, 24*, 257–272.

Tannenbaum, R., & Schmidt, W. (1973). How to choose a leadership pattern. *Harvard Business Review, 51*(3), 162–180.

U.S. Census Bureau. (2000). Profile of general demographic characteristics: 2000. Retrieved May 14, 2006, from http://factfinder.census.gov/servlet/QTTable?ds_name=DEC_2000_SF1_U&geo_id=01000US&qr_name=DEC_2000_SF1_U_DP1.htm

U.S. Department of Human & Health Services Division of Nursing. (2004). *Preliminary findings: 2004 national sample survey of registered nurses.* Retrieved November 11, 2007, from http://bhpr.hrsa.gov/healthworkforce/reports/rnpopulation/preliminaryfindings.htm

Wall, S., & Arden, H. (1993). *Wisdomkeepers: Meetings with Native American spiritual elders.* Hillsboro, OR: Beyond Words.

Yoder-Wise, P. S., & Kowalski, K. E. (2006). *Beyond leading and managing: Nursing administration for the future.* St. Louis, MO: Mosby.

PART III

Assessment Practices: Leveling the Playing Field

10 The Role of Intentional Caring in Ameliorating Incapacitating Test Anxiety

JOYCE VEDA ABEL

I began to explore the roots of what seemed a pervasive trauma. Trauma is the shock to the psyche that leads to dissociation; our ability to separate ourselves from parts of ourselves, to create a split within ourselves so that we can know and also not know what we know, feel and yet not feel our feelings. It is our ability . . . to hold parts of our experience not as a secret from others but as a 'foreign body' within ourselves.

—Carol Gilligan, *The Birth of Pleasure*, 2002

It was the winter semester of 2004, and I was in my first year of teaching nursing care for people with mental illness when I was approached by a diverse group of eight bright and serious nursing students. They sought my help with preparation for an exam. I knew these students well. I was supervising their clinical work with patients who had severe mental illness and serious criminal offenses. Without exception, they provided solid nursing care to volatile and potentially dangerous patients on a rapidly changing unit. Clearly, I could attest to these students' competency.

The author wishes to thank Dr. Margaret McLaughlin, Dean of Health Sciences; Dr. Alice Swan, Associate Dean of Nursing; and Dr. Thelma Obah, Director of the O'Neill Center for Academic Development at the College of St. Catherine for their support of the development, evaluation, and expansion of the STAMP/SAGE program. Additional gratitude goes to Dr. Obah for invaluable editorial assistance in the development of this manuscript.

They came to me because they knew I believed in them and knew them to be effective nursing students.

They were failing their nursing course because of their performance on multiple-choice exams. They were desperate because they could not bear to fail this class, their last class before graduation. If they failed, it would be at great financial and emotional cost to themselves and their families. The students had no idea why they were failing exams. Like the students, I had no idea what was causing them to fail. I was eager to identify the problem and find ways to "fix it." I began our first study session with questions about the content to be tested. I was surprised to discover that the students knew the material even before we began to study. Still, we studied for several hours, after which they had an even greater command of the material. Yet, they failed or barely passed the nursing exam. Not one to succumb to a poor outcome, I offered to study with them for the next exam. This one covered nursing care of people with mental illness, the subject I teach. In other words, I was preparing them for my own questions. After our study sessions, they knew the material even better than they had the previous material. Yet again, they did poorly on this exam. It was now clear that the problem was not due to a lack of hard work or to inadequate mastery of the information being tested. What was blocking these dedicated students from passing multiple-choice exams?

As I thought about their situation, I was struck by several facts. First, the students knew the material. Second, it became clear to me that these students experienced intense anxiety before and during an exam. Third, as I listened to them with what I call "free floating attention," I began to hear intimations of unspeakable traumas. As a psychotherapist with 18 years' experience, I have worked with women who have been traumatized, most often during childhood. My clients have taught me a great deal about the subtle expressions of language and behaviors that indicate overwhelming or ongoing past trauma. For example, many of my clients freeze in response to a sound or visual cue, which most people would ignore but which for them triggers the memory of a trauma experienced in childhood. For my traumatized clients the cue was, and unfortunately still is, a signal associated with imminent, often inescapable danger.

A woman I will call Riga is an example. She became nauseated and terrified when she was stuck in traffic at night but not during the day. She was feeling trapped because she had to take a night class, which meant driving in evening rush hour. For years she had avoided evening rush hour traffic, but now she had to face her fear. I asked her if she had ever been in danger and unable to move to safety while in a car at night. Riga started to say "no" when a look of disbelief came over her, and she began to cry. She said, "That's silly; it was so long ago." I said, "It isn't silly. Please tell me, what happened?" She was in Kosovo driving in a caravan when bullets hit her car and a car with her friends in it. It was dark; she was surrounded by armed soldiers and could not get to her friends, nor could she drive to safety. She was trapped and in fear for her life. After our talk she could understand why she was terrified to drive at night, but until then being in evening rush hour traffic triggered terror without any context or explanatory narrative memory. This is exactly how sensory cues associated with past danger work. One senses grave danger at times of apparent safety, which leads to feelings of confusion and self-doubt. Riga could not trust her mind to be rational and felt like she was going crazy. Now she felt normal, understood her reactions, and could find ways to cope with driving in evening rush hour.

I wondered if this was happening to my students. I began to develop a hypothesis that nursing students with very high levels of test anxiety might be re-experiencing the dread of previous trauma, triggered by cues inherent in the testing situation. I became determined to create a program that would give students with high levels of test anxiety a chance to gain control over their paralyzing response to exams. First, I had to discover if the literature supported my hypothesis and then determine how I could help. I spent the summer and fall of 2004 doing a literature search on both test anxiety and posttraumatic stress disorder (PTSD). What follows is the result of the literature search, the story of the first group of students who participated in the ever-evolving program I developed for students with severe test anxiety, and a description of the essential aspects of the program.

LITERATURE REVIEW

The Neurophysiology of Anxiety

I begin with the neurophysiology of anxiety for two reasons. Students report that, when I talk about test anxiety in terms of its neurophysiology, they feel validated, and the stigma of having an emotional problem is neutralized. Secondly, when faculty understand the neurophysiological basis for test anxiety, they report a change in attitude toward students who come to them for help with poor test performance.

Fear is a normal, healthy response to danger. Anxiety is a more global and free-floating response to danger and is therefore more difficult to address effectively. Experiences of danger activate our emergency response system, the fight or flight mechanism, which is biologically mediated and survival-based. The primary hormone of this response is cortisol, which, when released into the brain, generates a cascade of cognitive, emotional, and sensory changes. We are just beginning to understand the impact of cortisol on the capacity of the brain to function. This is possible because of our ability to do cortisol assays in the cerebrospinal fluid (CSF) and because of the ability to scan the brain while it functions by using Positron Emission Tomography (PET) and other brain scan techniques. The combination of these two techniques enables researchers to determine the correlation between brain function, anxiety, and cortisol levels (Bremmer & Charney, 2004).

Research studies have been conducted using PET scans on subjects with experimentally induced anxiety and correspondingly high cortisol levels. In these studies, subjects are scanned as they attempt to solve verbal problems without and then with experimentally induced anxiety (Bremmer & Charney, 2004). Their PET scans have identified anatomical and functional changes critical to our understanding of people with high levels of test anxiety and poor test performance. The PET scans of subjects with induced anxiety show that the regions of the brain essential for test performance are black, meaning that they are deactivated and not functioning. These areas include the prefrontal, orbitolfrontal, temporal, and parietal regions of the brain (Kent & Rauch, 2004). When these regions are inactive, it is all but impossible to think critically, solve problems, make judgments, set priorities, and, most important for test performance, recall previously mastered information. Thus, anxious students are trying to answer complex questions when the thinking part of their brains has been turned off, much like a light switch turns off a light bulb. In this case, the amygdala, the area of the brain that controls the response to danger, along with the release of cortisol, has flipped the cortex's switch to off.

The Amygdala and Test Anxiety

The amygdala plays a pivotal role in coordinating and activating our emergency response system. It is uniquely equipped to guard our survival because it receives information from several regions of the brain and determines if the alarm should be sounded. The hypothalamus sends information about the body's response to the threat, for example, a racing heart or trembling. The hippocampus relays stored memories of trauma, so the amygdala can recognize any similarities between current cues and cues of past trauma. The cerebral cortex provides an objective cognitive evaluation of the environment (Miller, 2004). It also creates a context for and narrative explanation of the experience. However, the amygdala can block the objective information from the cortex and sound the alarm based solely on the emotional response, leaving the person feeling terror without knowing why. As established by Davis (2004), even a subliminal cue associated with past trauma can trigger an anxiety state. Furthermore, Davis reports sufficient evidence concluding that activation of the subcortical amygdalar circuit occurs in the absence of awareness that a threat-related stimulus has been presented. Thus, it is possible that students such as Riga do not know why they become so anxious during an exam. As a result, they are likely to suffer grave self-doubt.

It is critical to note that the amygdala cannot distinguish danger to one's body from danger to one's psyche or psychological danger. It responds to both forms of danger in identical ways (Davis, 2004). Therefore, a student experiencing test anxiety has the same neurophysiological changes as a soldier caught in battle (Kaiman, 2003). Psychological danger is the perceived threat during testing. Psychological danger results in a wounding of one's self with feelings of shame, hopelessness, and soul pain. Soul pain is what I call the feeling of being rendered invisible and devoid of personhood. One client described feeling empty for weeks after being raped. She said, "I can't explain it because I felt nothing. No, I felt like I was nothing, but I was in the worst pain ever." Soul pain is a manifestation of the trauma response.

Posttraumatic Stress Disorder

The *Diagnostic and Statistical Manual of Mental Disorders–IV* (DSM–IV; American Psychiatric Association [APA], 1994) describes the nature of trauma and the resulting emotional, cognitive, and physical symptoms that comprise PTSD. In order to be defined as PTSD, the trauma must evoke "intense fear, helplessness, or entrapment and horror" (p. 424). The characteristic symptoms resulting from the experience of trauma include: persistent re-experiencing of the traumatic event, also known as flashbacks; persistent avoidance of stimuli associated with the trauma; psychic numbing; emotional anesthesia; and persistent symptoms of hyperarousal. The symptoms cause significant distress or impairment in social, occupational, or other important areas of functioning. In addition, the *DSM–IV* states, "This disorder may be especially severe or long lasting when the stressor is of human design (e.g., torture, rape) . . . Intense psychological distress or physiological reactivity often occurs when the person is exposed to triggering events that resemble or symbolize an aspect of the traumatic event (flashbacks)" (p. 428). Therefore, traumatized people will go to great lengths to avoid thoughts, feelings, activities, and people who trigger flashbacks.

Some of the cardinal symptoms of PTSD, which are also the most likely to negatively affect exam performance, include: impaired affect regulation, dissociative states, feelings of ineffectiveness, shame, despair, hopelessness, feelings of being permanently damaged, loss of previously sustaining beliefs, and difficulty concentrating. Herman (1992) and Ehlers, Hackman, and Michael (2004) describe the intrusive memories or flashbacks that people with PTSD experience. It is interesting to note that the physical, cognitive, and emotional experiences of flashbacks are virtually identical to the physical, cognitive, and emotional experiences that students with high levels of test anxiety experience during exams.

Immigrant populations have a higher incidence of PTSD. The authors of the *DSM–IV* (American Psychological Association, 1994) also speak about populations that may have a greater number of people with PTSD. They state: "Individuals who have recently emigrated from areas of considerable social unrest and civil conflict may have elevated rates of PTSD" (p. 426). Such individuals may be especially reluctant to divulge experiences of torture and trauma due to their vulnerable political or immigrant status. Examples of high-risk populations present among nursing students at the College of St. Catherine include Africans from countries that have been at war for many years, or that have had famines, or whose populations have been forced to relocate, such as Liberia, Nigeria, Sierra Leone, and Somalia. Other people at high risk are Bosnians, Vietnamese, Hmong, and Cambodians. However, the risk of experiencing trauma is not restricted to people born in foreign lands. People in the United States who live in poverty or in gang-controlled neighborhoods are at very high risk for experiencing trauma and developing PTSD (Purnell, 1999), as are people who have experienced family violence and sexual abuse.

A wide range of traumatic experiences can lead to PTSD. In her book *Trauma and Recovery: The Aftermath of Violence From Domestic Abuse to Political Terror*, Judith Herman (1992) identifies life experiences that leave people at high risk for developing PTSD. These include:

childhood sexual or physical abuse, especially by a trusted adult; trauma that is perceived as life-threatening; rape; witnessing violence, especially to loved ones; and loss of a child, sibling, or friend, especially if it is due to violence or living in a war zone. Personal risk factors for PTSD include: being female, a health care provider, having been coerced into silence regarding trauma, having immigrant status, and having a history of any of the following: multiple traumas, inadequate social support system, a family history of alcoholism, and a poor self-concept.

The stress of internalized racism also affects students' well-being and test performance. Cohen, Garcia, Apfel, and Master (2006) demonstrated that a chronic experience of having negative stereotypes aimed at one's group, as in racism, creates a level of psychological threat that causes decrements in academic performance. They state: "School settings can be stressful to almost all students regardless of race. However, for African American students, the academic environment involves an extra degree of threat not experienced by nonminority students, due to the negative stereotype about the intelligence of their race. This threat, on average, raises stress to levels that are debilitating to performance" (p. 1307). The experience of racism is traumatic and significantly impairs the ability of its targets to function academically.

The rate of debilitative test anxiety has increased significantly since the 1960s due to several factors (Brewer, 2002). The trends in student demographics indicate that a greater number of traumatized students are on our campuses. This is especially true for St. Catherine's where, based on our values, we strive for a diverse student population and invite women escaping from many hardships to attend. Future students are likely to report higher rates of test anxiety because more of our students will be women soldiers returning from war zones such as Iraq, foreign-born students, immigrants, and U.S. women born into poverty.

Another population that is at high risk for PTSD is students who come from families and societies that attach extreme consequences to exam performance (El-Zahhar & Benson, 1994). Students from such cultures may be severely punished for not succeeding on exams. The educational system in these cultures tends to have absolute power over students and often has the cooperation of parents who ally themselves with teachers.

Another group of students with potentially high levels of test anxiety are those raised by parents whose behavior meets the definition of narcissistic personality disorder, as described in the DSM-IV (1994). The parents have an intense need to appear perfect. Children in these families are viewed as objects to enhance the parents' image. When they do not appear perfect, they are shamed and threatened with abandonment. These parents feel threatened and exposed when their child has less than an A average. Students from such families may develop high levels of test anxiety because they have been taught that anything less than an "A" is threatening to their parents and, therefore, to themselves.

Test Anxiety Among Women

Bauer, Becker, and Bishop (1998) and Lee (1999) determined that female students have a significantly higher incidence of test anxiety than their male counterparts. Female nursing students are at an even greater risk for test anxiety than other female students. Hojat and Lyons (1998) and Brewer (2002) ascertained that nursing students scored very high on general anxiety, test anxiety, depression, and loneliness. In addition, Swanson and Howell (1989) found a significant correlation between test anxiety and passing the national licensing exam for nurses (NCLEX). Martin and Poorman (1991) and Matters and Burnett (2003) found a correlation between poor academic self-concept and performance on multiple-choice exams.

Several researchers describe the emotional and cognitive experiences of test-anxious students. Lee (1999) found that test-anxious students engaged in deprecating self-talk, sustained an internal dialogue of highly worrisome thoughts about the consequences of a poor grade, feared being evaluated, paid continuous attention to test-irrelevant cues, and felt the need to escape the testing situation. These distractions caused decrements in cognitive processing and memory. Lee observed that test-anxious students have less available working memory because a significant portion of their processing capacity is usurped by trying to cope with thoughts related to their anxiety. Tasks with time constraints, such as exams, produced the greatest decrements in memory and processing. Lee concluded that test anxiety damages performance. Lee's findings were supported by Keogh, Bond, French, Richards, and Davis (2004); McIlroy, Adamson, and Bunting (2000); Davis, Schutz, and Schwanenflugel (2002); and Wilson (1999).

Test Anxiety Among ESL Students

It is important to point out that there are groups of students who experience high levels of test anxiety who may not have experienced trauma. One such group is students who are nonnative speakers of English or who speak nonstandard varieties of English. However, it must be noted that many nonnative speakers of English are people of color who are most likely experiencing racism. They are referred to as English-as-a-Second-Language (ESL) students even though English may be their third or fourth language. In my experience, they are most often dedicated students who cannot demonstrate their command of the material on multiple-choice exams due to language barriers or poorly worded test items, not due to lack of knowledge or hard work. In addition, these students have great difficulty answering questions with emotional content because such questions are steeped in culturally determined appropriateness and make use of idioms and innuendoes. All students tend to answer questions with emotional content from their culture's perspective. This is often a great disadvantage because the authors of such questions are most often from the dominant culture and usually presume the correct answer is the one that reflects the dominant culture. Therefore, having roots in a nondominant culture or being a nonnative speaker of English can lead to a sense of futility and hopelessness resulting in high levels of test anxiety. The irony is that ESL students generally do well in clinical work with patients. Thus, they know and can apply nursing knowledge, but they cannot demonstrate their knowledge successfully on multiple-choice exams. Tragically, they begin to feel stupid, hopeless, and very anxious about failing. However, ESL nurses and those from a nondominant culture have a critical role to play in health care. They serve patients, nurses, and all other health care providers as interpreters of both language and culture. They are essential to the nursing process, especially assessment and patient education. Therefore, every effort should be made to increase their retention and timely graduation.

Identifying the Need for a New Approach

After reviewing the literature, I became convinced of a connection between high levels of test anxiety and previous trauma. First, most of the students I had been working with were from high-risk populations, such as women, people of color, people who have experienced severe poverty, and those who were foreign-born or ESL. Second, during an exam they experienced several of the cardinal symptoms of PTSD, such as freezing, numbing, having out-of-body sensations, and loss of recall of known information. These students also described feelings of dread and the need to escape. And third, they had no insight or understanding of their intense reactions to exams, a situation that often occurs when flashbacks of previous trauma intrude. I refer to test anxiety that is linked to trauma as incapacitating test anxiety, or ITA, because both the neurophysiology and symptoms prevent or incapacitate students from getting grades that accurately reflect their command of the material.

Test Anxiety Interventions

The review of the literature identified the interventions that were most effective in decreasing test anxiety. Ergene's (2003) meta-analysis of 56 well-designed studies showed that a combination of cognitive and skill-focused activities were most effective.

McIlroy et al. (2000) determined that psychological factors, such as worry and test-irrelevant thoughts, caused the greatest decrements in test performance. He posited that interventions that addressed these would improve test performance. However, I did not find any study or program to decrease test anxiety that incorporated psychological safety. This is a significant omission because test anxiety is triggered by the perception of psychological danger. Therefore, test-anxious students need to be able to counter their perception of psychological danger, that is, they need to perceive psychological safety. According to Maslow (1968), nurturing and caring are the most effective ways to provide psychological safety. Offering care to an anxious person provides a biologically mediated and emotionally based sense of safety. Clearly, a program intended to reduce test anxiety needs to incorporate interventions that maximize a sense of psychological safety.

The Students' Test Anxiety Management Program, or STAMP, attempts to do just that—maximize a sense of psychological safety. The uniqueness of the STAMP program is the individualized intentional caring that is provided to participants, within a group setting, that gives them a sense of psychological safety. The program was piloted in the winter semester of 2005 and has continued to evolve and grow since then, guided by cycles of program evaluation and revision. It is supported and funded by the Associate Dean of Nursing and the Dean of the School of Health.

THE STUDENTS' TEST ANXIETY MANAGEMENT PROGRAM (STAMP)

Program Goals

The primary goal of the STAMP program is to create a milieu of caring that allows test-anxious students to learn and utilize new ways to decrease their incapacitating test anxiety so that they perform well on exams. In addition, there are subgoals that, according to the literature and my clinical experience, are necessary to achieve the primary goal. For example, Martin and Poorman (1991), as well as Matters and Burnett (2003), found that self-esteem and academic self-image, respectively, were the strongest predictors of exam performance. Therefore, two subgoals of the program are to improve participants' self-esteem and academic self-image.

Program Design

The pilot project was designed to reduce test anxiety, aid students to pass their last nursing class, and increase passing rates on the national licensing exam for registered nurses (NCLEX-RN).

Participants were asked to commit to attending 10, 90-minute weekly sessions. They also signed a consent form approved by the Institutional Review Board (IRB) of the college. In turn, I promised confidentiality; lunches that honored all dietary needs, both religious and health-based; a supportive and caring environment in which to learn new skills to manage their test anxiety; a workbook designed to become a personal journal of their experiences in the program; and last, but very important, opportunities to celebrate and have fun. Every session began with lunch and a check-in, during which each student could choose to share her experiences, thoughts, and feelings with the group. And each session was imbued with intentional caring. After check-in, one of the STAMP interventions (see discussion later in chapter) became the main focus for the day's meeting.

Program Evaluation

Two inventories are administered to monitor the effectiveness of STAMP interventions. The first is the Revised Test Anxiety Scale (RTAS), as shown in the Appendix, which the participants take on the first and last days of the program. The RTAS is a 4-factor, 20-item inventory that uses a Likert scale of seven, with 1 as strongly agree, and 7 as strongly disagree, for a possible range of scores from 20 to 140. The RTAS measures the intensity of each of the four components of test anxiety: worry, tension, bodily symptoms, and test-irrelevant thoughts (Sarason, 1984). A high score reflects a low level of test anxiety. Therefore, an increase in scores would reflect a decrease in test anxiety and the program's overall success. The RTAS was chosen, in part, because it has been refined and cross-culturally validated on students from Egypt, the United States, Brazil, Ireland, and Scotland (El-Zahhar & Benson, 1994; McIlroy et al., 2000). The second inventory is the STAMP Experiential Questionnaire, which students take during the last group meeting. It is composed of three open-ended questions that students respond to in writing. They are: (a) How do you feel during an exam (now, after participating in the STAMP program)? (b) What have you learned from the STAMP program? and (c) What changes would help make the STAMP program better?

PILOT PROJECT: PROGRAM PARTICIPANTS

The STAMP program was first offered in Fall 2005 as a pilot project. The first group of students were in the Associate Degree program and were in their last nursing class before graduation. The nursing class had 76 students, of which 34 expressed the intent to join STAMP and 18 actually enrolled, but only 12 attended 8 or more sessions. The reasons given for the inability to participate were: work demands, childcare limitations, and transportation restrictions—in short, financial considerations.

Students decided to participate in the program because they felt they had test anxiety that was blocking them from demonstrating their true command of nursing knowledge on multiple-choice tests. Their RTAS scores showed very high levels of test anxiety, which corroborated their self-assessments. The average RTAS score of participants was 52.1.

The 12 students were from diverse backgrounds. There were 5 U.S.-born Caucasians, 1 U.S.-born African American, 4 African-born, 1 Hmong, and 1 Vietnamese student. Of the Caucasians, 4 were first-generation college students, as were the women from Laos and Vietnam. The 4 African students were from Liberia, Nigeria, Sierra Leone, and Somalia—all places affected by years of war, drought, and famine. All 4 had received high school diplomas from schools in Africa.

The financial circumstances of the foreign-born students differed from the U.S.-born students in that they worked to support their families here and to send money to relatives in their countries of origin. Two African women were married with children, and their salary was sent to Africa while their husbands supported the family here. The obligation to support families back home was deeply felt, so much so that cutting back on work was unthinkable. Similarly, grandparents for the Laotian and Vietnamese students provided childcare. In return, the student was expected to send money to family members abroad. Although the U.S.-born students had financial concerns, they did not have this added financial burden. In addition, all participants had a minimum of two risk factors for PTSD, as discussed earlier.

Interventions

Four primary interventions of STAMP were developed based on my review of the literature and my work with traumatized clients as well as the goals of the program and the mission of the College. The four components are: intentional caring, cognitive restructuring, calming techniques, and test-taking skills for nursing students.

Intentional Caring

Intentional caring is the essential component of STAMP and, therefore, of my relationship with each participant. This relationship must be free of judgments, shame, or the threat of abandonment. Students' statements on the Experiential Questionnaire and during a transcribed meeting called by the Associate Dean of Nursing indicate that intentional caring is the most powerful antidote for incapacitating test anxiety. Intentional caring transforms students' perceptions of danger to safety, as evidenced by the following quotes from a student, the first before she participated in STAMP, the second after: "My heart pounds and my mind wanders. I think about what everyone will say if I don't pass" and "I could tell Joyce really cared about us. She proved to us that we were really smart."

A relationship based on intentional caring must also be free of the use of power of one member over another. As long as one member has power over another, trauma survivors will be unable to experiment with new ways of dealing with their perception of danger. The extensive work of Jean Baker Miller and Irene Pierce Stiver (1997) and colleagues at the Stone Center for Women, located at Wellesley College in Massachusetts, have demonstrated that a healing relationship must be based on mutuality. By mutuality they mean mutual empowerment and mutual empathy. It is particularly important to deal with power differentials when the facilitator is an instructor and the participants are students. In STAMP, power differentials are addressed to prevent relationships in which one member, usually the facilitator, has power over another. For instance, I strive to equalize the power differential by informing students that there are no grades, assignments, or evaluations of any kind in STAMP.

Even participating in the check-in is voluntary. I further equalize the power differential by engaging all participants in the ongoing evaluation and restructuring of STAMP.

Generous listening is another key characteristic of intentional caring. By this I mean listening with a single focus and without attempts at premature problem solving. I work to remain open to all aspects of the participants' experiences and to respond to difficulty or pain with rapt attention. I am aware of the fact that trauma is not known to the self or discussed with others in the same way as neutral experiences. Therefore, intentional caring for participants may consist of my tracking the snippets of trauma a student shares until the snippets form a coherent story that validates the student's intense reaction to exams. My individualized intentional caring is informed by the work of Herman (1992) and McQueen, Shelton, and Zimmerman (2004). McQueen implemented the concept of the "other mother" in her program for African American nursing students at a historically Black college. The other mother is the nurturing person within the school setting (Collins, 1980, as cited in McQueen et al., 2004).

My work with a student I will call Anna illustrates intentional caring. Anna had to fight a constant need to escape the testing room, which resulted in a sense of desperation, fear for her safety, and poor grades. One day, during a STAMP session, I asked her if anything in the testing situation was worrisome or unnerving. She responded, "I don't know," accompanied by a blank, almost numb look. I then asked her to pay attention to cues that triggered her need to escape either during class or the next test. At the next meeting she said she realized that the need to escape begins as soon as she hears the instructors who are monitoring the exam begin to whisper. I wondered out loud if she could remember a time when hearing others whisper was associated with danger. Her first reaction was a look of puzzlement, but she soon recalled that when she was 11 years old and was escaping Liberia with her father, they would often come upon gangs of soldiers who questioned her father and then went off to whisper to one another. "I knew they were deciding whether to let us go, beat us, or even kill us."

The entire group was deeply moved by Anna's situation. They responded by gathering in toward her while actively seeking ways she could feel safe during an exam. As it turns out, what helped the most was for Anna to take a picture of her father and herself on their sofa and put the picture on the desk before an exam. She rejected the idea of using ear plugs because she felt safer hearing the whispering and then glancing at the picture to remind herself that they were safe and to reorient herself to the present moment, thus to the exam. I have found that when a student can remember enough of the trauma experience to enable her to understand her intense emotional reactions to testing, she begins to regain trust in her mind and to develop a positive academic self-image. However, if Anna were unable to remember, we would have dealt with her need to escape in other ways, such as having her sit by the door or even getting permission to walk out of the classroom and immediately reenter to experience being able to leave the anxiety-provoking situation.

Intentional caring is also expressed in concrete ways, such as providing a meal that meets the religious and dietary needs of each participant. The meal reinforces my role as nurturer and creates fellowship among members. In addition, I call students just before an exam to remind them of all they have accomplished and to let them know that they are a real person to me, not a test grade.

Intentional caring is a critical characteristic of the group milieu, which must provide safety and nurture each student's ability to try different responses to her test anxiety. To create this milieu, I relate to individual members the way I hope they will come to relate to each other and to their patients (Watson, 2003). Typically, by the second meeting, members begin showing each other concern, acceptance, and support. It is also important to celebrate the personal growth and success of each participant. Too often in the beginning I am the only one who enthusiastically, even joyously, proclaims another hurdle has been scaled or another student has passed a dreaded exam. Eventually, the group celebrates the achievements of each member. Significantly, later on they begin to celebrate their own successes.

Cognitive Restructuring

Cognitive restructuring refers to the process of identifying defeatist, shaming, or derogatory self-talk and replacing it with more realistic, positive statements. For example, many students reported saying, "I am so stupid" or "I don't deserve to be a nurse" when confronted with a test question they experience as difficult. This internal dialogue increases test anxiety and is a major source of test distraction, both of which contribute to poor test performance. Their negative self-talk also erodes their sense of being a competent student. Students are asked to make a list of the things they say to themselves when they do not know the answer to a question. I then work with participants to counter their negative self-talk with individualized positive statements. However, any attempt to encourage positive and nurturing self-talk must take into consideration the fact that anxiety occurs when danger is perceived. One cannot counter the perception of danger with platitudes or false assurances. Statements like "I am sure you will do well" do not have the potency to replace "I am stupid." What has worked is to teach the students to say statements like "I am bright as evidenced by passing the science prerequisites for the nursing program." Sometimes a student cannot integrate positive self-talk even when based on hard evidence. In this situation, I ask the students to say to themselves, "Joyce has proven that I am very smart."

Another STAMP cognitive intervention—coaching students to develop a list of self-affirmations—is supported by the work of Cohen et al. (2006). They found in a randomized controlled study of African American and European American students that allowing students to reaffirm their self-integrity significantly diminishes the negative impact of racism on minority students' academic performance. An intervention that involved reflecting on and writing about personal values was found to decrease the racial academic achievement gap by 40%. A critical part of the STAMP program involves affirming the inner beauty of individuals who choose to become healers. This concept forms the basis of their list of affirmations. Nursing students use this belief to identify their values and celebrate their essential beauty.

Calming Techniques

Calming techniques are taught to quiet the bodily sensations of anxiety, such as trembling, shortness of breath, and nausea. Research findings have shown that these sensations are major distracters that cause significant decrements in test performance (McIlroy et al., 2000). However, one of the most difficult conundrums students with a history of trauma experience is the inability to relax. Several STAMP participants reported that when they try to relax, they become agitated. It feels safer to be alert and on guard. I consulted with an expert from the Holistic Health Department at the College of St. Catherine about energy-balancing work because it can create calm without focusing on relaxation per se. In subsequent sessions, I taught these techniques myself. Furthermore, energy work is beneficial for both the giver and the receiver. We discovered that the most effective way to use energy work was for participants to offer energy balancing to each other. As givers, they could relax without triggering a hyperalert, anxious state. Soon the participants were also able to relax when receiving. Participants reported being more aware of their bodies' responses to anxiety yet being calmer and more in control. As one student said, "I don't get it. Somehow I feel anxious but it doesn't bother me so much."

Test-Taking Skills

Finally, test-taking skills for nursing students are taught with an emphasis on understanding how to apply the nursing process to multiple-choice questions. I have found that nursing students have particular difficulty with "best-answer" type questions, that is, when there is more than one correct answer but one is considered the best. Understanding the steps of the nursing process helps students to avoid this type of error. Reviewing the nursing process also helps students to think critically before choosing options. Relevant chapters from Nugent and Vitale's (2004) *Test Success: Test-Taking Techniques for Beginning Nursing Students* and materials developed for ESL nursing students are used to teach test-taking strategies in the program.

EVALUATION OF PILOT PROJECT: QUANTITATIVE DATA

Data were analyzed for the 12 students who attended a minimum of 8 of the 10 sessions; 3 outcomes were intended. The first was to lower the students' level of incapacitating test anxiety. The second was for all participants to pass their last nursing class and graduate. And, the third was for everyone to pass the NCLEX. My focus with STAMP participants is that they pass the NCLEX, not that they pass on the first attempt. In the United States, great weight is given to first-time passing rates by the organizations that accredit schools of nursing. An unfortunate outcome of this emphasis is that schools seek students who will do well on the NCLEX, rather than students who will best serve populations in need of excellent nurses. This seemingly arbitrary focus on first-time passing creates intense pressure and exacerbates incapacitating test anxiety for ESL students and those with a history of test anxiety. I attempt to counter this pressure and put first-time passing in perspective, that is, it is more convenient and less costly to pass the first time. Clearly, nursing students need to master a body of professional knowledge to practice safe and effective nursing. And, they need to pass the NCLEX to become a licensed nurse. But they do not need to pass it the first time they take the exam. Reinforcing their value and self-confidence as students goes a long way to increasing their chance of a first-time pass. First-time passing rates are included in the evaluation of the STAMP program because it is currently an accepted measure for evaluating schools of nursing.

To determine if there was a significant decrease in participants' incapacitating test anxiety, the first intended outcome of the STAMP program, pre- and post-program RTAS scores were compared. The difference between mean pre- and post-scores on the RTAS was analyzed using paired t-tests. The pre-intervention RTAS mean was 52.1, and the post-intervention RTAS mean was 94.0, reflecting lower levels of test anxiety. This difference in means is a very significant difference in that it yielded a two-sample t-statistic of 6.486 with a highly significant p-value of <0.0001, strongly supporting the hypothesis that the STAMP program, with its primary focus on intentional caring, greatly reduces incapacitating test anxiety.

At the end of fall semester 2005, all STAMP and non-STAMP students passed the last nursing class and graduated, the second intended outcome of the STAMP program. This was the first time in several years that no student had to take the comprehensive final. This exam is offered to nursing students at the end of the course who are one to three percentage points below passing. Many of the STAMP participants were the very ones at high risk for having to take the comprehensive final, that is, they were one to three percentage points below passing, or 78%. One student in STAMP had taken a comprehensive final in all her previous nursing courses other than the ones she had to repeat, except this one.

The third intended outcome, for all participants to pass the NCLEX, was also achieved. All 12 students passed the NCLEX, with only 1 student having to take it twice. The student had "warned me" by saying, "I'm gonna have to take that exam lots of times just to get used to being in such a tiny room with the door closed. Oh God, what's worse is they're watching you the whole time." She was very pleased that the exam was not the ordeal she anticipated. She retook it as soon as the State Board of Nursing permitted and passed.

The first-time passing rate for STAMP participants in 2005, the year of the pilot project, was 92%, compared to 78% for the first-time pass

Table 10.1

NCLEX PASS RATES FOR AD NURSING PROGRAMS	
STAMP program	92%
College of St. Catherine	78%
Minnesota	84%
United States	87%

rate for the College's Associate Degree (AD) program in the same year. According to 2005 data sent to nursing programs from the Minnesota Board of Nursing, the first-time pass rate for all AD programs in Minnesota was 84%, and the national rate was 87% (see Table 10.1). Therefore, the first-time pass rate of STAMP participants was higher than that of their graduating class, the state of Minnesota, and the nation.

QUALITATIVE DATA: PARTICIPANT EXPERIENCES

There are two sources of qualitative data used to evaluate the effectiveness of the STAMP pilot program. The first source is students' written responses to the STAMP Experiential Questionnaire. The second source is students' statements at a meeting requested by the Associate Dean of the School of Nursing to learn more about STAMP. The STAMP participants agreed to have this meeting recorded and transcribed. During the meeting students spoke about their incapacitating test anxiety, the varied ways that faculty and staff responded to their anxiety, and how they felt about STAMP. Virtually all the participants reported feeling better about themselves and their decision to become a nurse. They reported that participating in a group in which everyone genuinely cared about each other had shown them the power of caring in the work of healing. Having experienced that power as both givers and receivers, they were eager to share it with future patients.

The STAMP participants also wrote about their experiences in the STAMP Experiential Questionnaire during the last session of the program. In response to the question, "How do you feel during an exam (now, after participating in the STAMP program)?" several students wrote about the physical symptoms of test anxiety they *used to experience* during an exam. Many experienced gastrointestinal symptoms that commanded their attention and led to a fear of loss of bowel control. Examples are: "I get diarrhea before and during the tests" and "I lose a lot of weight the day of the exam." The most disturbing symptom reported by a participant was going blind. This student wrote, "I had a bad migraine and went blind before one test." Most often their physical symptoms were accompanied by a litany of negative self-talk. Some prime examples of negative or defeatist self-talk are: "I can't breath[e], felt like failure," "I feel like a total failure before I even start to answer the test questions," and "I keep telling myself that I'm stupid." Other students described classic symptoms of PTSD, such as, "I get out-of-body experiences during a test" and "I freeze and can't answer the questions I know." Still other students experienced a sense of danger accompanied by the need to escape the testing room. One student wrote, "I feel like I just want to get out of there." Another student spoke of the heavy workload, "It makes me feel nauseated, and I get panic attacks. Especially when a test is coupled with other assignments, the anxiety brings on huge feelings of dread."

After having participated in STAMP, students now felt they had more self-control during an exam. Students commented: "This class has helped me to be in control again before a test," "After learning how to take tests better, I pulled my grade up two grades," and "Learning the test taking strategies made me feel in control again."

In response to the second question, "What have you learned from the STAMP program?" some participants' statements were poignant, even tragic. Participants wrote, "I'm still human, not perfect. When I don't know something I am still human but I am not treated that way," "It made me realize that I am not a failure," "We had a learning experience that did not have any pressure," and "I pray. I don't want to deal with this stress." Many had gained true wisdom. Examples are: "I learned that everyone is smart in a different way. I am smart," "The main thing is to respect yourself and take care of yourself," and "I learned that what I have learned can not be taken away." Many wrote of the STAMP group as a refuge from feelings of alienation, isolation, and shame: "I'm not ashamed to express my feelings. Before I thought I was the only one feeling like this, only to find out that other people felt like me. I should be proud of myself." Another student wrote, "First of all, it helps to know that other people are struggling, that you are not crazy or stupid, but it is a common problem."

The *Intentional Caring* component received many positive comments. Examples include: "I am so thankful to have someone that not only cares about students but is willing to do that extra thing to make a difference in someone else's life," "I like it [the group], I feel comfortable; you bust us up! We have confidence," and "Joyce really did care. She checked in with us one-by-one." One student who received a midsemester letter saying she was at risk for failing wrote, "Joyce called me to see how I was doing, after getting a letter that I was failing." Later the student reported, "I would have killed myself. My husband stayed at my side until her call. Then I was alright." Another student wrote, "The group has helped me talk to myself in caring, even loving ways when I feel bad." One quote confirmed that students did not feel there was a power differential between students and myself. The student wrote, "Joyce was a very good addition to the group."

Limitations of the Pilot Project

This was a small pilot project of 12 students with severe test anxiety. While their initial scores on the RTAS corroborated their self-assessments, it is possible that these students had greater internal resources as evidenced by their self-awareness and ability to reach out for help. Some of these students had come within one or two points of failing a nursing class, but none had actually failed. In addition, there was no control group in the pilot project.

CONCLUSION

The story of the STAMP pilot project has a very positive ending. All the students have become licensed nurses. Several are continuing on for a bachelor's degree in nursing. This pilot project demonstrates a way to ameliorate or to render manageable incapacitating test anxiety so that nursing students can feel the fruit of their labors, graduate, and pass the NCLEX. Intentional caring was the unique component of STAMP; it appears to benefit nursing students with incapacitating test anxiety. The Associate Dean of Nursing commented that STAMP has the potential for far-reaching benefits in that it not only decreases test anxiety for participants, but it also improves the quality of their lives and the lives of people who are part of their support system. It has also improved NCLEX pass rates. In addition, workshops for faculty on the neurophysiological basis of incapacitating test anxiety, along with the success of STAMP, have fostered a change in attitudes toward test-anxious students.

Update

The STAMP program continues to evolve. Changes in the program are informed by feedback from students and faculty who are training to lead future groups as well as my observations and reflections. First, students reported feeling stigmatized by the word *anxiety* in the title of the program. They felt it marked them as having an emotional problem and was blocking others from joining. In response, I changed the name from Students' Test Anxiety Management Program (STAMP) to Skills and Approaches to Grade Excellence, or SAGE. There was an immediate increase in enrollment, particularly of foreign-born students. At present there are 57 students who have completed the STAMP or SAGE program over the previous five semesters. And the reduction in incapacitating test anxiety remains highly significant with a p-value of <0.0001.

Second, a training program has been implemented in response to the demand for more SAGE groups. Presently, professional staff from the counseling and learning centers are preparing to lead future groups using the SAGE curriculum.

Third, a new pilot project is in progress in which SAGE is offered as a 1-credit, 7-week, fundamentals course (at 50% reduced tuition). Each SAGE course is paired with one of two nursing courses with the highest rate of failure, that is, courses with the highest numbers of students who need to resequence the course before they can proceed to the next nursing course. Students who are resequencing the class are encouraged to enroll in SAGE, whereas other students who believe they would benefit are invited to join. In the first two groups, 17 resequencers went on to pass the course, and all but one went on to pass the subsequent nursing course.

And last, a spiritual component has been added to the SAGE curriculum. I created this addition after observing and reflecting on input from students. The spiritual component is both universal and specific to many different religious beliefs. It responds to the theistic traditions of Judaism, Christianity, and Islam. It also includes the nontheistic traditions, such as Buddhism. Before an exam and during an exam when students experience incapacitating test anxiety, participants of theistic traditions are encouraged to pray; students with agnostic or atheistic beliefs are encouraged to meditate. All participants are encouraged to practice mindfulness and to recite affirmations I have created for nursing students. The focus of the spiritual component is on the interconnections between healing and spirituality.

The SAGE program continues to demonstrate success for both diverse and traditional nursing students and for the College of St. Catherine. Pass rates for the NCLEX remain higher for SAGE participants. The latest pilot project demonstrated another benefit of SAGE in that it allowed students who had failed a nursing course to continue on to graduation. The SAGE model is designed to be reproducible, measurable, and sustainable. For more information about SAGE, contact Joyce Abel at jvabel@stkate.edu.

RECOMMENDATIONS

The following recommendations are offered to enable colleges of nursing, their administrators, faculty, and students, to benefit from the findings of the SAGE program.

Deans and Program Administrators

1. Create programs to educate faculty about incapacitating test anxiety (ITA) and the negative effects it has on otherwise dedicated students.
2. Provide information to faculty regarding the neurophysiological alterations that occur in the brain when an individual is anxious; these changes impede critical thinking and recall of known information thereby making accurate assessments of students' knowledge difficult.
3. Critically evaluate how students are assessed, developing both alternative assessments to multiple-choice testing as well as ways to reduce linguistic bias in the wording of multiple-choice test items (see chapter 11 of this book.)
4. Provide guidelines for responding effectively to students with significant discrepancies between satisfactory clinical achievement and poor test results and for assessing whether ITA is a causative factor.
5. Initiate protocols to identify students who are experiencing ITA.

6. Provide support for faculty to implement strategies that reduce ITA and promote increased academic performance.
7. Engage faculty in considering how caring is valued, modeled, and incorporated into the nursing curriculum.
8. Create opportunities for these students to learn ways to create calm, clarity, and confidence while studying for and while taking exams.

Nursing Faculty

The following recommendations are offered to help reduce students' anxiety during lectures and exams.

1. Hand out a complete set of notes for lectures. This allows students to focus on the lecture itself, ask questions, and participate in discussions without worrying about taking accurate notes.
2. Begin your lecture by affirming students' intelligence and expressing your confidence in their ability to learn the material.
3. Welcome students' questions, and invite students to share areas of confusion during the lecture.
4. Use a 1-minute reflection paper after each lecture. Each student is handed a paper with three questions on it: (a) Were there any topics that you found especially confusing? Which one(s)? (b) Do you have a specific question that you would like answered? (c) Is there anything you would like me to review before the next lecture? Review students' answers after each lecture to determine topics that need further discussion, either during class or on the school's intranet system.
5. Implement strategies to reduce test anxiety just prior to an exam by offering affirmations that support your students' intelligence, recognize their dedication to becoming a nurse, and express your confidence in their ability to pass the exam and to become fine nurses.
6. During the exam, inform students in a positive and calming way of the time they have remaining to complete the exam. You can say, "You still have several minutes left, 10 to be exact." This has a different impact than "You only have 10 minutes left." The tone of the latter statement creates a sense of urgency and a need to rush through the remaining questions.

QUESTIONS FOR DIALOGUE

1. What ideas or concepts did you find most meaningful in this chapter? Identify your insights and questions to bring to a dialogue with your colleagues.
2. The author presents several exemplars of students with incapacitating test anxiety. Dialogue with colleagues about similar situations that have arisen in your program and how they were handled.
3. In your nursing program, how much emphasis is placed on passing the nursing licensure exam on the first attempt? What are the ethical implications of placing so much emphasis on first-time pass rates?
4. Dialogue with colleagues about ways to help students with incapacitating test anxiety achieve their potential. What resources in your institution could be mobilized to help in this regard?
5. Which of Abel's recommendations for faculty are you apt to implement in your teaching and assessment practices?
6. Which of Abel's recommendations for deans and program administrators are already in place in your program? Which are most needed to complement the existing resources?

APPENDIX

THE REVISED TEST ANXIETY SCALE

The following statements refer to how you feel when you take an exam. Use the scale below to rate items 1 through 20 in terms of how you feel when taking exams in general. Please respond to all items, and circle the number that most applies to you, according to the following code:

1 = Strongly Agree, 2 = Agree, 3 = Slightly Agree, 4 = Neutral,
5 = Slightly Disagree, 6 = Disagree, 7 = Strongly Disagree

1. Thinking about my grade in a course interferes with my work on exams.
2. I seem to defeat myself while taking important exams.
3. During exams I find myself thinking about the consequences of failing.

4. While taking exams I find myself thinking how much brighter other people are.
5. While taking an exam I often think about how difficult it is.
6. During an exam I think about how much I should have prepared.
7. I start feeling very uneasy just before getting an exam result.
8. During exams I feel very tense.
9. I worry a great deal before taking an exam.
10. I am anxious about exams.
11. I worry before an exam because I do not know what to expect.
12. I get a headache during an important exam.
13. My mouth feels dry during an exam.
14. I sometimes find myself trembling before or during an exam.
15. While taking an exam my muscles are very tight.
16. I have difficulty breathing during an exam.
17. During exams I find myself thinking about things unrelated to the material being tested.
18. I think about current events during an exam.
19. While taking exams I sometimes think about being somewhere else.
20. During exams I find I am distracted by thoughts of upcoming events.

Source: "Further Refinement and Validation of the Revised Test Anxiety Scale," by N. El-Zahhar & J. Benson, 1994, *Structural Equation Modeling, 1*(3), 203–221. *Structural Equation Modeling* is a publication of Taylor and Francis Group. The journal can be found on the Web at www.informaworld.com.

REFERENCES

American Psychiatric Association. (1994). Anxiety disorders. In *Diagnostic and statistical manual of mental disorders* (4th ed., pp. 429–484). Washington, DC: Author.

Bauer, K. W., Becker, E. T., & Bishop, J. (1998). A survey of counseling needs of male and female college students. *Journal of College Student Development, 39,* 205–210.

Bremmer, J. D., & Charney, D. S. (2004). The neurobiology of anxiety disorders. In D. S. Charney & E. J. Nestler (Eds.), *Neurobiology of mental illness* (2nd ed., pp. 605–627). New York: Oxford University Press.

Brewer, T. (2002). Test-taking anxiety among nursing & general college students. *Journal of Psychosocial Nursing, 40*(11), 23–29.

Cohen, G. L., Garcia, J., Apfel, N., & Master, A. (2006). Reducing the racial achievement gap: A social-psychological intervention. *Science, 313,* 1307–1310.

Davis, H., Schutz, P. A., & Schwanenflugel, P. J. (2002). Organization of concepts relevant to emotions and their regulation during test taking. *The Journal of Experimental Education, 70*(4), 316–342.

Davis, M. (2004). Functional neuroanatomy of anxiety and fear. In D. S. Charney & E. J. Nestler (Eds.), *Neurobiology of mental illness* (2nd ed., pp. 584–604). New York: Oxford University Press.

Ehlers, A., Hackman, A., & Michael, T. (2004). Intrusive re-experiencing in post traumatic stress disorder: Phenomenology, theory and therapy. *Psychology Press, 12*(4), 403–415.

El-Zahhar, N., & Benson, J. (1994). Further refinement and validation of the revised test anxiety scale. *Structural Equation Modeling, 1*(3), 203–221.

Ergene, T. (2003). Effective interventions on test anxiety reduction: A meta-analysis. *School Psychology International, 24*(3), 313–328.

Gilligan, C. (2002). *The birth of pleasure: A new map of love.* New York: Vintage Books.

Herman, J. (1992). *Trauma and recovery: The aftermath of violence from domestic abuse to political terror.* New York: Basic Books.

Hojat, M., & Lyons, K. (1998). Psychosocial characteristics of female students in the allied health and medical colleges: Psychometrics of the measures and personality profiles. *Advances in Health Sciences Education, 3*(2), 119–132.

Kaiman, C. (2003). PTSD in the World War II combat veteran. *American Journal of Nursing, 103*(11), 32–41.

Kent, J. M., & Rauch, S. L. (2004). Neuroimaging studies of anxiety disorders. In D. S. Charney & E. J. Nestler (Eds.), *Neurobiology of mental illness* (2nd ed., pp. 639–660). New York: Oxford University Press.

Keogh, E., Bond, F. W., French, C. C., Richards, A., & Davis, R. E. (2004). Test anxiety, susceptibility to distraction and examination performance. *Anxiety, Stress & Coping, 17*(3), 241–252.

Lee, J. H. (1999). Test anxiety and working memory. *The Journal of Experimental Education, 67*(3), 218–241.

Martin, J., & Poorman, S. G. (1991). The role of nonacademic variables in passing the National Council Licensure Examination. *Journal of Professional Nursing, 7*(1), 25–32.

Maslow, A. (1968). *Towards a psychology of being* (2nd ed.). New York: Van Nostrand.

Matters, G., & Burnett, P. (2003). Psychological predictors of the propensity to omit short-response items on a high-stakes achievement test. *Educational and Psychological Measurement, 63*(2), 239–256.

McIlroy, D., Adamson, G., & Bunting, B. (2000). An evaluation of the factor structure and predictive utility of a test anxiety scale with reference to student's past performance and personality indices. *British Journal of Educational Psychology, 70,* 17–33.

McQueen, L., Shelton, P., & Zimmerman, L. (2004). A collective community approach to preparing nursing students for the NCLEX RN examination. *The Association of Black Nursing Faculty Journal, 15*(3), 55–58.

Miller, J. B., & Stiver, I. P. (1997). *The healing connection: How women form relationships.* Boston: Beacon Press.

Miller, M. C. (Ed.). (2004). Women and depression: How biology and society may make women more vulnerable to mood disorders. *Harvard Mental Health Letter, 20*(11), 1–3.

Nugent, P. M., & Vitale, B. A. (2004). *Test success: Test-taking techniques for beginning nursing students* (4th ed.). Philadelphia: F. A. Davis.

Purnell, L. (1999). Youth violence and post-traumatic stress disorder: Assessment, implications, and promising school-based strategies. In C. W. Branch (Ed.), *Adolescent gangs: Old issues new approaches* (pp. 115–127). Philadelphia: Brunner/Mazel.

Sarason, L. G. (1984). Stress, anxiety and cognitive interference: Reactions to tests. *Journal of Personality and Social Psychology, 6*(4), 929–938.

Swanson, S. C., & Howell, C. (1989). The relative influence of identified components of test anxiety in baccalaureate nursing students. *Journal of Nursing Education, 28* (5), 215–219.

Watson, J. (2003). Love and caring: Ethics of face and hand—An invitation to return to the heart and soul of nursing and our deep humanity. *Nursing Administration Quarterly,* 27(3), 197–202.

Wilson, G. S. (1999). Personality variables in levels of predicted and actual test anxiety among college students. *Education Research Quarterly,* 22(3), 3–16.

11 Removing Language as a Barrier to Success on Multiple-Choice Nursing Exams

SUSAN DANDRIDGE BOSHER

Several years ago, a nursing colleague (Jeannine) contacted me about a student, "Fatima," in her first semester of the baccalaureate-degree nursing program. Fatima was having difficulty with multiple-choice (MC) exams. The student was a nonnative speaker of English, and because I teach English-as-a-Second-Language (ESL) at my college, Jeannine thought I could help. (*Note:* Students for whom English is not their native language are referred to here as ESL students regardless of their language proficiency or coursework.)

> *Hi Susan*
> *I'd like your input regarding one of my students whose first language is Somali. She is really struggling with the multiple choice format of our tests. She just barely passed one and failed another. She has one more exam a week from this Monday and I'd like to help her be successful . . .*
> *I appreciate your help. Thanks.*

In my reply, I wondered if the wording of the test items might be creating a problem for the student and asked Jeannine if she would be open to learning more about linguistic modification, a process for revising test items to reduce their linguistic complexity and increase their readability.

Jeannine—
I wonder if the student is having difficulty understanding the wording of MC test items. That's a common area of difficulty for ESL students in nursing. I would suggest meeting with the student one-on-one and going over the items that she got wrong on the most recent test she failed and have her explain why she picked the answers she did. You might find in the process that she knows the content, but had difficulty understanding the questions. Would you and your colleague be open to "linguistic modification" as a possible testing accommodation for this student? If you find that she does know the content and that it's the wording that is getting in the way of her demonstrating her nursing knowledge, there is support in the literature for using this technique as a testing accommodation for ESL students . . .

Jeannine subsequently met one-on-one with the student and reviewed the items the student had answered incorrectly on the previous exam. In the process, she realized that Fatima was having particular difficulty with "best-answer" and "all of the above" questions. Jeannine was open to learning about linguistic modification and asked that I look at the remaining tests in the course and suggest ways to improve their wording. She also gave Fatima the option of taking the remaining tests in the learning center, where ESL students are given time and a half on exams. This option of extended time for ESL students is based on research findings that students take significantly longer to process text in their second language than in their first (Donin & Silva, 1993) and that even highly fluent bilinguals take longer to read in their weaker language (Segalowitz, 1986). Thus, even if ESL students know the material, it takes them longer to read and process the test items because of the language.

A few days later I was contacted by Fatima. I knew her because she had been in two of my ESL classes that are required for students who are nonnative speakers of English who score below 80 on the in-house Michigan English Language Assessment Battery. (Her score on this test had been 65.) In my courses, Fatima had been a very diligent and hardworking student, revising her papers multiple times to strengthen their content and organization and working with a tutor in the learning center to edit her papers for errors.

Fatima had relatively strong literacy skills in her native language, often an important factor in how easily a student acquires academic literacy in another language. She had completed 10 years of schooling in her native country before immigrating to the United States at age 14. Fatima spent 2 1/2 years in the U.S. school system, starting mid-way through 10th grade. By the time she began studying at the College of St. Catherine, she had been in the United States for just 3 1/2 years, a relatively short amount of time considering it often takes ESL students as long as 6–8 years to acquire proficiency in academic reading and writing, depending on their age on arrival and years of schooling in their native country (Collier, 1987, 1989). Although some of Fatima's education in her home country had been in English, she still struggled with academic reading and writing. Because of her perseverance and hard work, however, she made good progress in her language skills and, with a GPA of 3.1, was accepted into the nursing program 2 years later.

When I met with Fatima, we talked about a number of issues, including why she thought she was having difficulty with multiple-choice testing. She talked about the confusing nature of multiple-choice test items and about the difficulty she had in choosing between two similar options. She also talked about not always being sure what the question was asking. There were other issues, too, which compounded the situation and increased her anxiety about the next test, making her efforts to study less than productive. Because Fatima had already failed a test in this class and barely passed another, she was convinced that she needed to score 90% or above on the next one to pass the course, which combined with intense pressure from her family to succeed, made her even more anxious. In addition, she had stopped studying for exams with her study group, thinking that because she hadn't done well on the previous two tests, perhaps she would be better off if she studied alone.

In fact, Fatima had a higher average in the course than she thought because of her stronger performance on a case-study exam and a group project. She also was doing well in her clinicals. So, although she did need to pass the next test, she did not need to score a 90%. Having this information seemed to reduce Fatima's anxiety considerably. Also, after finding out more about how her study group prepared for exams, I urged her to reconsider her decision to study alone. Not only was the friendship and support of her study group important for her, but the way in which they studied—by dividing up topics and presenting them to each other—offered rich opportunities for meaningful dialogue about the material, an effective way in which to learn material, as well as to develop critical literacy skills (Cummins, 1989). I also told Fatima that I would be working with her instructor on the wording of the next exam and showed Fatima some techniques for breaking down the wording of test items to make them more comprehensible.

After our meeting, Fatima sent me the following e-mail:

> *Hello,*
> *Thank you very much for all your help. It is good that you are simplifying the wording of the questions. And also I feel better now, since I don't have to worry about getting 90% or above on the exam. I'll be studying with my friends for the exam. Thanks a lot for all you do . . .*

Two weeks later I received another e-mail from Fatima:

> *Hello,*
> *I got my result for the nursing exam that I took a week ago . . . I passed it (49.5/55) I got 90% . . . thank you so much for all your help.*

Fatima received a final grade of B in the course, and the following spring she graduated from the College with a degree in nursing and a GPA of 3.2. That summer, she passed the nursing licensure exam in the United States (NCLEX) on her second attempt.

In a recent conversation with Fatima, who is now a practicing nurse, she said that what made the biggest difference for her on that next exam was the change in wording. In addition, she said that the support she had received from us, her instructor and me, had given her confidence. Fatima had studied hard for the exam and for the first time took it in the learning center, which she said was a less stressful environment than the classroom. She talked about how much it had bothered her to see other students getting up to leave when she was "still on item 10 on a 50-item exam." When she saw people leave, she would start to put herself down saying, "I don't know anything." Fatima continued to take her exams in the learning center the next semester so she wouldn't have to "see other people leaving."

This exemplar illustrates what can happen when students are given the support they need and when faculty are open to testing accommodations that create a more level playing field for linguistically diverse students. Commitment to diversity in the nursing profession requires that nurse educators look not just at what and how they teach but also at how they assess students. Without greater equity in the assessment process, some students will likely experience difficulty progressing in their program and may ultimately be unsuccessful. Too often, instructors assume that when a student fails a test, there must be something wrong with the student—she does not know the material, he didn't study enough, her

English is not good enough, or perhaps he is not smart enough to be a nurse. However, in my research, I have found that more often than not there are other issues at play that suggest the need to look critically at multiple-choice tests and the barriers they create for students, particularly students for whom English is not their native language.

LINGUISTIC BIAS IN MULTIPLE-CHOICE TESTS

In many nursing courses, multiple-choice tests are an important means for assessing students' mastery of course content. They also constitute a large percentage of students' final grades in many courses. However, ESL students often have difficulty with multiple-choice tests (Bosher, 2003; Klisch, 1994), both in their nursing courses and on the NCLEX (Cunningham, Stacciarini, & Towle, 2004). Students and faculty alike recognize multiple-choice tests as one of the most difficult and challenging issues for students, as evidenced by a growing number of articles that address this topic (see chapters 5, 10, and 17 in this book). In a needs analysis of ESL students in a baccalaureate-degree nursing program (Bosher, 2001, 2006), both students and faculty rated "taking multiple-choice tests" as the most difficult task out of 74 language and culture-related skills and tasks that students must be able to perform successfully in the nursing program.

In Fall 1999, the College of St. Catherine was awarded a 3-year grant from the U.S. Department of Health and Human Services to recruit and retain multicultural and economically disadvantaged nursing students. As part of that grant, I analyzed 19 multiple-choice exams from 6 nursing courses for 52 types of flaws. These flaws were grouped into four general categories based on a review of the literature: test-wise flaws, flaws of irrelevant difficulty, linguistic/structural bias, and cultural bias (Case & Swanson, 1985; Haladyna, 1994; Mohan, 1986). The total number of flaws identified in the 673 test items was 1,490, *an average of 2.2 flaws per item* (Bosher, 2003). Of the 52 types of flaws, 28 types occurred at least 10 times.

Test-Wise Flaws

Test-wise flaws, the first category of analysis, provide clues to the correct answer and make it easier for "test-wise" students to answer questions correctly (Case & Swanson, 1985), giving them an unfair advantage over students who are not test-wise. For example, test-wise students know that if one of the options is longer, more specific, or more complete than the others, it is also likely to be the correct answer. Other test-wise flaws include: grammatical errors in options that are not the correct answer, repetition of a key word or phrase from the stem in the correct answer, and use of "all of the above" as an option. Although much of the literature (Case & Swanson, 1985) has focused on test-wise flaws, only 3% of the flaws in this study were of this type (Bosher, 2003).

Irrelevant Difficulty

Sixty-one percent of the flaws in this study were due to irrelevant difficulty, the second category of analysis (Bosher, 2003). Flaws of irrelevant difficulty make questions difficult to understand for reasons unrelated to the content or focus of the assessment (Case & Swanson, 1985). While flaws of irrelevant difficulty can potentially affect the performance of all test-takers because they require additional processing time to resolve, they are especially problematic for ESL students, whose processing time is already slower than that of their native English-speaking peers (Donin & Silva, 1993; Segalowitz, 1986).

Completion Format

One common source of irrelevant difficulty is the use of the completion format in the lead-in rather than the question format. The completion format places greater demands on the test-taker's short-term memory (Haladyna, 1994) because the student must either retain the lead-in in his or her short-term memory or go back and forth between the lead-in and each option, in order to evaluate the truthfulness of each.

In the following example, the lead-in, "the nurse recognizes that this finding indicates that," is in completion format.

Original

1a. A patient with respiratory disease has a shift to the left in the oxygen-hemoglobin dissociation curve. The nurse recognizes that this finding indicates that:

Revision

1b. A patient has respiratory disease. He has a shift to the left in the oxygen-hemoglobin dissociation curve. What does this finding indicate?

In the revision, the lead-in uses the question format: "What does this finding indicate?" The question format, which is simpler and more direct (Haladyna, 1994), allows students to more quickly and easily discern what it is they are supposed to answer.

Other principles of test-item writing (Haladyna, 1994) include showing consistency between directions in the stem and the nature of the task and avoiding the following: negative phrasing, "none of the above" as an option, repetitious wording, and the complex multiple-choice format (which lists different combinations of right and wrong answers). When these principles are not followed, the result is flaws of irrelevant difficulty.

Best-Answer Items

Another source of irrelevant difficulty is "best-answer items." They are a common question type that require students to prioritize information, an important step in learning to think critically in clinical situations. Best-answer items are more difficult for ESL students to process than correct-answer items (Dean, 1988; Gronlund, 1976); they can also be difficult to identify. Words such as "most," "first," and "primary," which indicate an item is a "best-answer" question, should be highlighted in at least two or more ways, for example, through bold-facing, capitalizing, underlining, and/or italicizing, to help readers quickly discern the nature of the task. As Klisch (1994) argues, "Test writers should write items that can be read and comprehended easily on the first reading" (p. 36).

Compare the following two versions of the same test item:

Original

2a. Which of the following treatments for AIDS has been found to be most effective?

Revision

2b. Which treatment for AIDS is the ***MOST*** effective?

In the revision, it is easier for students to see the word "most" and therefore to discern the nature of the task at hand—that of finding more than one correct answer in the options and selecting the best answer from the correct ones.

Linguistic/Structural Bias

The third category of analysis in the study was linguistic/structural bias (Bosher, 2003), a category that includes the following: unnecessary linguistic complexity in the stem or options; lack of clarity or consistency in the wording; and errors in grammar, punctuation, and spelling. Such errors can confuse or distract the test-taker, "causing some students to lose concentration and fail to perform as they should" (Haladyna, 1994, p. 64). This category accounted for 35% of all flaws in the study (Bosher, 2003).

Embedded and Reduced Clauses

Embedded and reduced clauses are common sources of linguistic complexity in test items. Students must reread such items several times in order to understand what is being asked, a process that takes additional time and energy and may increase test anxiety (Haladyna, 1994).

In the following example there are two clauses embedded in the main clause, as indicated by the brackets.

Original

3a. An inappropriate reaction by the immune system [in which antibodies form against self-antigens] [mistaken as foreign] best describes:

Revision

3b. In the immune system, self-antigens are sometimes mistaken as foreign to the body. When this happens, antibodies form against the self-antigens. Which statement describes this inappropriate reaction by the immune system?

In the revision, the stem has been broken down into three sentences, and the two clauses have each been lengthened into a complete sentence. Although the revision is longer, it is easier to process. Students are likely to understand what is being asked after only one reading as compared to the original, which students may need to read several times to understand.

Unclear Wording

Wording that is unclear, inconsistent, inconcise, or uncommon is another common source of linguistic bias. In the following example, "high index of suspicion" is not common terminology. It is also an example of unnecessary nominalization, in which the noun form of a word ("suspicion") is used instead of the verb form ("suspect").

Original

4a. In which of the following situations should the nurse have a high index of suspicion for water intoxication?

Revision

4b. In which situation does the nurse suspect water intoxication?

In the revision, the verb *suspect* has been used rather than the noun *suspicion*. Verbs offer a more direct, concrete way of stating a point than nouns, which tend to create abstraction and distance between the action ("suspect") and the agent ("the nurse").

Cultural Bias

The last category of analysis was cultural bias, or the use of cultural content that is not equally available to all cultural groups (Mohan, 1986). Only 1% of the items in this study were found to contain this type of flaw (Bosher, 2003) perhaps because this type of flaw is less common than originally thought or is easier to recognize and therefore to avoid.

The results of this study clearly point to the need for faculty to look critically at their multiple-choice test items to ensure they follow principles of good test-item construction (see Appendix A). Faculty readily acknowledge that writing multiple-choice tests is no easy task; yet, training is often not provided by their institutions. Commercially available test banks do not offer an easy alternative because they must often be tweaked for content, as well as language. On the other hand, there are serious ethical implications of students failing tests that are poorly worded.

LINGUISTIC MODIFICATION

In addition to principles of good test-item construction, linguistic modification offers additional techniques for reducing the language load of multiple-choice test items. Linguistic modification is a procedure developed for use in high-stakes testing with English Language Learners (ELLs) in primary and secondary schools in the United States. It is based on the premise that every test is to some extent a test of language proficiency and that nonnative English speakers must process and negotiate the language of tests to a much greater extent than native English speakers. This task is made all the more difficult when there is irrelevant difficulty or linguistic bias in the test items, but even well-written test items can contain considerable syntactic and semantic complexity, which can lead to construct-irrelevant variance. Variation in test scores that is due to language, rather than knowledge of the content, introduces measurement error, such that "test results may not reflect accurately the qualities and competencies intended to be measured" (American Educational Research Association [AERA], American Psychological Association [APA], and National Council on Measurement in Education [NCME], 1999, p. 91). Therefore, test scores cannot be assumed to be a valid and reliable measure of examinees' knowledge. Within the context of nursing course exams, this means that if students fail a test, they may have failed the test because they did not understand what the questions were asking, not because they did not know the nursing content. Indeed, referring back to the exemplar at the beginning of this chapter, the nursing professor found that *the student did know the content,* but had been confused by the wording of some of the items.

Characteristics of Linguistic Modification

When linguistic modification is applied to test items, the reading load of test items is reduced while their content and integrity are maintained (Abedi & Lord, 2001). Key content area vocabulary and terms are left intact, but modifications are made to the rest of the item to reduce its semantic and syntactic complexity (Abedi, Hofstetter, Baker, & Lord, 2001).

Reducing Semantic Complexity

To reduce the semantic complexity, low frequency, uncommon words are replaced by high frequency, familiar words, and vague, abstract language is replaced by direct, concrete language (Bowles, 2004). Synonyms and pronouns are avoided as is more culturally bound language, such as idioms, colloquial language, and humor.

Reducing Syntactic Complexity

To reduce the syntactic complexity of test items, lengthy sentences are broken down into separate sentences; complex sentences are replaced by simple or compound sentences; reduced, embedded clauses and participial phrases are expanded into full clauses or sentences; compound nouns (or nouns with more than one prenoun modifier) are broken down into separate elements; the simple present and simple past tense are used instead of compound verb tenses; active verbs are used instead of passive verbs (whenever appropriate); modals (e.g., should, would, might, could, will) are avoided; and content is ordered sequentially (Bowles, 2004).

Linguistic modification reduces the language load in test items, making it easier for students to identify key concepts in test items and understand more quickly and easily what is being asked. While there is some overlap between principles of good test-item construction and linguistic modification, the former has more to do with the overall clarity and coherence of test items while the latter has to do with reducing their semantic and linguistic complexity. Both are necessary for increasing the comprehensibility of test items.

THE EFFECTS OF LINGUISTIC MODIFICATION ON ESL STUDENTS' COMPREHENSION OF NURSING COURSE TEST ITEMS

In 2003, a study was conducted to determine the effects of linguistic modification on the comprehensibility of test items for ESL nursing students (Bosher, 2004; Bosher & Bowles, 2008). The study also investigated what makes a test item difficult to understand from the perspective of ESL students. Five first-year ESL nursing students participated in the study. Each student met with the researcher three or four times, with each session lasting approximately 1 hour. After an initial interview, participants reviewed each of four multiple-choice tests they had taken earlier in the semester in their first-semester pathophysiology course. Students were asked to read aloud those items they had answered incorrectly when they had first taken the test and to explain why they had chosen the answers they had. If they could no longer remember their reasoning at the time they took the test, they were asked to answer the item again, as if it were the first time, and to verbalize their thoughts as they read and selected an answer.

Data Analysis

There was a total of 171 test items on the four tests. From the total set of test items answered by the five participants (855), 29% (or 250) were answered incorrectly by at least one of the participants and were reviewed (Bosher & Bowles, 2008). Any item that at least one of the participants considered difficult to understand because of the way it was worded or that was confusing in some way from a linguistic or cultural perspective was identified for revision. *Sixty-seven items, or 39% of the test items, that had been answered incorrectly were identified as potentially problematic from a linguistic or cultural perspective.*

These 67 items were then revised using the principles of linguistic modification (Abedi & Lord, 2001; Abedi, Lord, & Hofstetter, 1998; Abedi, Lord, & Plummer, 1995; Bowles, 2004; Rivera & Stansfield, 2004) and presented for review at a group validation meeting attended by three content experts (two instructors of the pathophysiology course and one nursing administrator), one expert in linguistic modification, one testing expert, and two ESL experts. The purpose of the meeting was to discuss and revise the test items; the nursing specialists ensured that the nursing content was not affected by the revisions, and the ESL/testing specialists ensured that the revisions resulted in decreased complexity and increased readability of the test items.

During the group validation meeting, 38 of the 67 items were discussed and revised (see Appendix B). Subsequently, a questionnaire was prepared that included both the original and modified versions of the 38 items so that the five participants could assess the overall readability and degree of difficulty of the two versions (Bosher & Bowles, 2008). Participants were asked to identify the version that was easier to understand and explain their choice. They were also asked to underline all words, phrases, and clauses in both versions that were difficult to understand or were confusing in some way. Participants were also interviewed about selected items on the questionnaire and asked to evaluate their participation in the study.

Results of Study

Participants identified modified items as more comprehensible 77% of the time and original items as more comprehensible 23% of the time (Bosher & Bowles, 2008). When the evaluations of each item were calculated as a group, rather than individually, the results were even stronger: 84% of the modified items were identified as more comprehensible than the original versions by at least three of the participants. Only six original versions (or 16%) were identified by the majority of participants as more comprehensible than the modified versions, and one of these items had been mistakenly identified as a best-answer item.

In interviews conducted at the end of the study, students were asked to comment on the reasons they found the modified versions easier to understand (Bosher & Bowles, 2008). The reasons they gave most frequently were as follows. (*Note:* Four of these characteristics coincide with principles of good test-item writing that were discussed earlier in the chapter. The examples referred to here can be found earlier in the chapter in the specified sections.)

Use of Shorter, Simpler Sentences

Shorter, simpler sentences were used in the revisions rather than longer, more complex sentences. Comparing examples 3a and 3b (see section on *Linguistic Bias*), all five students preferred the revision. One student underlined: "against self-antigens mistaken as foreign best describes," a portion of the text that includes the second embedded clause, which is also reduced, and wrote: "This is confusing."

Information Stated Directly

Information was stated directly in the revisions. rather than "hidden" in the sentence. Compare the following versions:

Original

5a. Which of the following would be the best intervention(s) for persons who may not have oral fluids and are experiencing thirst as a result of intracellular volume depletion?

Revision

5b. A patient experiences thirst because of intracellular volume depletion. The patient is ***NOT*** allowed oral fluids. What is the ***BEST*** nursing intervention?

In the original, the main point is stated at the end of the sentence. In the revision, the main point is at the beginning: "A patient is experiencing thirst because of intracellular volume depletion." The next point, that "The patient is ***NOT*** allowed oral fluids," can then be understood within the context of the first point. The question follows the information provided in the two previous sentences. In response to the original version, one student underlined: "persons who may not have oral fluids and are experiencing thirst as a result of intracellular volume depletion," indicating this part of the sentence was confusing. All five students preferred the revision.

Use of Question Format

The question format was used for the lead-in in the revisions rather than the completion format. Comparing examples 1a and 1b (see section on *Completion Format*), all five students preferred the revision. Comments on the question format include: "The question is more concise"; "It is more straightforward"; and "Easier to comprehend."

Highlighting of Key Words

Key words, such as MOST, BEST, and FIRST, were highlighted in the revisions. Comparing examples 2a and 2b (see section on *Best-Answer Items*), all five students preferred the revision. Comments on the highlighting of key words included: "The bolded & underlined word *most* helps"; "Highlight of *MOST* is effective"; and "'Most' is very helpful & it makes it easier to pick answers."

Use of Common Words

More common words were used in the revisions rather than less frequently used words. Comparing examples 4a and 4b (see section on *Unclear Wording*), three students underlined "high index of suspicion" and commented that they did not know what it meant. One student wrote: "it is not necessary [and] makes me think about what this part of the sentence has to do with the question (I get sidetracked)." The students found the revision easier to understand. One student wrote: "I know all the words in this version." Another student wrote: "This is lot easier b/c there is no big vocab. like 'index' which makes [the revised version] simplified & clear."

In the interviews at the end of the study, every student commented on the decreased amount of time it took her to read and understand the revised test items. One student commented: "When I read the revised version . . . it's broken up into facts and then finally the question, I could just picture the whole thing in my mind and [I] just read it once, whereas before, I have to read it two or three times just to get what they're asking for."

Another student commented: The original version "takes . . . time and you read it, but then there are times when you have to rush through a test, and so . . . [the revised version] would be just more straightforward and you wouldn't have to take at least a minute to think about it, but for [the original version] I think I would sometimes take at least a minute to think about it." Another student summed up why the revised versions were more understandable to her and commented as well on the decreased processing time: "If the questions were really straightforward, you'd just go think about answers and not think about [the questions]. I personally have to read questions twice or three times sometimes just because of the wording . . . I have to come up with understanding what they're asking." The student went on to talk about the differential and discriminatory effect the wording of test items has on students: "[Nursing faculty] tend to think about asking questions to people who speak English [as their native language] . . . They forget about people . . . whose first language is not English . . . I always look at the classroom to see who's left [after a test] . . . I find that most of the time it's always . . . us . . . that's always left behind . . . the minorities."

FACULTY CONCERNS ABOUT LINGUISTIC MODIFICATION AND THE NCLEX

Faculty often remark that if test items were linguistically modified for nursing course exams, then students would be at a disadvantage taking the NCLEX. One faculty member commented in a questionnaire about the value of this kind of research: "Students *also* need to be prepared for NCLEX . . . Do we do a disservice to students, especially the ESL students, if we don't . . . let them practice on poorly written NCLEX-type questions?" Another faculty member wrote: "Our items need to be modeled after NCLEX items as this is a nationally approved and recognized exam."

Faculty concerns in this regard are legitimate; they want to make sure students are prepared for the licensure exam. However, in my work with faculty on revising test items at numerous schools of nursing, I found many test items to be poorly worded, grammatically incorrect, and/or misleading, for which preparation for the NCLEX is simply not a valid excuse.

Furthermore, according to the National Council of State Boards of Nursing, the organization that oversees NCLEX test development and the testing of nursing licensure candidates in the United States, pretest items for the NCLEX are subjected to both an editorial review and a sensitivity review, in which items are reviewed for language as well as cultural bias and stereotyping. During the field testing, if any items show signs of functioning differently for individuals of the same ability from different ethnic, cultural, or gender groups, those items are reviewed for potential bias by a differential item functioning (DIF) panel, which consists of a linguist, a nurse, and a member of a focal minority group. Items that are reviewed by the panel are not necessarily thrown out if the content of the item is needed; rather, the item is revised and retained (A. Wendt, personal communication, July 2004; Wendt, Zara, & Marks, 2000).

Despite procedures that are in place in the development of NCLEX test items, the results of several studies indicate that construct-irrelevant variance is an issue with NCLEX itself. In a study comparing graduation and licensure examination pass rates of native English speakers and Mexican American nursing students who spoke English as a second language (Sims-Giddens, 2002), no significant difference was found between program completion rates, but for first-time pass rates on the NCLEX, there was a 21% difference between the two groups. Ninety-four percent of the 525 native speakers of English who successfully completed the associate degree program in nursing from 1967–1995 passed the NCLEX, compared to 73% of the 78 Mexican American students. This 21% difference was statistically significant at the .05 level.

Another study, of 142 graduates of an ethnically diverse nursing program (Johnston, 2001), found that the average pass rate on the NCLEX was 85% for students whose native language was English, regardless of their academic record, but just 45% for students whose native language was not English. Regression analysis indicated that 20% of the variance in test scores could be explained by language, a clear threat to the reliability and validity of the NCLEX.

IMPLICATIONS FOR THE NCLEX

In response to growing concern about the difference in pass rates between native and nonnative English speakers on the NCLEX, the National Council of State Boards of Nursing (NCSBN) conducted a study to determine the effect of language status on test scores (NCSBN, 2005). Researchers found that the first-time pass rate for non–English-only candidates was 10–15% lower than for candidates who indicated that "English" alone was their primary language. According to the study, there was no difference in performance between English-only and non–English-only students on 82%–83% of the items. After items were calibrated, the two groups had a similar probability of answering the test item correctly. Therefore, the researchers claim any difference in pass rates was due to a difference in *nursing ability* and *not native language status*.

Researchers did find, however, that non–English-only candidates required greater processing time to complete the test. The average item response time for non–English-only candidates was longer than for English-only candidates, and the percentage of candidates who ran out of time was also greater for non–English-only candidates. The researchers concluded: "[T]here is some relationship between lack of English language proficiency and NCLEX performance" (NCSBN, 2005, p. 245).

To determine the effects of linguistic modification on NCLEX test scores, a large-scale quantitative study is needed that would compare test scores on original and modified test items for both native speakers of English and nonnative speakers of English (Abedi & Bosher, 2006). If such a study were conducted and linguistic modification was found to promote equitable assessment of native and nonnative English speakers alike, then perhaps the use of linguistically modified language could be introduced on the NCLEX. Such a study, however, is not currently a research priority for NCSBN (T. O'Neill, personal communication, August 21, 2006).

IMPLICATIONS FOR FACULTY DEVELOPMENT

There are many ways in which the findings of the two studies described in this chapter could be applied to faculty development in the writing of test items. First, the findings may help to convince some still-skeptical nursing instructors about the need to revise test items for greater clarity and to reduce the language load. Some faculty still conflate a student's ability to perform well on multiple-choice tests with a student's ability to communicate effectively as professional nurses. Regarding the potential usefulness of this study, one nursing faculty member remarked: "The goal is laudable; however, students need to be able to deal with complex communication." However, is the language of multiple-choice tests representative of communication in general or even of communication between nurses and clients in a health care setting? Does preference for linguistically modified versions of test items mean that students are not capable of handling complex communication in other contexts? As one student stated in an interview: "During that test setting, you know, people are nervous, so they . . . lose their confiden[ce] and then the questions are [confusing] and then they cannot think like they regularly think."

In addition, faculty often assume incorrectly that linguistic modification results in simplification of content (Bosher & Bowles, 2008), as is evident in the following comment: "Yes, we need to be culturally, language aware but students need to be able to answer questions about nursing." To the students who participated in this study, however, it was clear that the content of the revised or modified test items was essentially the same as the original versions. As one student commented: "The content's not changed in any way, I mean as far as I can tell. The question, the meaning is the same. It's just that the way the question is asked, the . . . format . . . makes it much . . . easier. It makes it faster for sure and easier to comprehend, I would say." Faculty who have participated in various workshops have also realized that the content and integrity of the original items are preserved during the modification process.

Second, the study on linguistic modification offers a model for nursing and ESL faculty to collaborate on the modification of test items (Bosher & Bowles, 2008). In the United States, there has been surprisingly little input from ESL professionals in efforts to address the needs of ESL students in nursing programs, even though language is often cited in the nursing literature as the biggest barrier to success (Amaro, Abriam-Yago, & Yoder, 2006; Yoder, 1996). Although one article did call for collaboration with ESL faculty (Malu, Figlear, & Figlear, 1994), the purpose was to assist in screening applicants for their language proficiency. Other programs reported increasing the cut-off score on the TOEFL (Test of English as a Foreign Language) from 500 to 550 for admission in an effort to reduce "problems with language proficiency" in their programs (Memmer & Worth, 1991, p. 391), a response that seems counterproductive to the goal of increasing diversity in nursing. In short, the benefits for ESL nursing students and nursing faculty alike that could result from collaboration between nursing and ESL faculty remained largely unrecognized and untapped. More emphasis should be given to preparing ESL students for the language and cultural demands of nursing (Bosher, 2006, in press), rather than reducing access.

CONCLUSION

As indicated in the exemplar at the beginning of this chapter, the language of multiple-choice exams is a barrier for many ESL students in nursing. Application of the principles of good test-item construction as well as of linguistic modification creates a more equitable playing field in assessment for students who are nonnative speakers of English. It may also be helpful for students who speak a nonstandard dialect of English or for first-generation college students who are not experienced with or have not been successful with the decontextualized language of multiple-choice exams. Although linguistic modification has been found to increase the comprehensibility of test items for nonnative speakers of English, further research is needed to determine its effects on test scores for nursing students.

The demand for qualified nurses in the United States is rapidly increasing, as is the number of immigrant students enrolled in nursing programs today (Davidhizar, Dowd, & Giger, 1998; Guhde, 2003; Kataoka-Yahiro & Abriam-Yago, 1997; Malu & Figlear, 1998, Memmer & Worth, 1991). A significant barrier to the success of ESL nursing students is the difficulty they encounter doing well on multiple-choice nursing tests, including the nursing licensure exam (NCLEX). As demonstrated in these two studies, multiple-choice test items are sometimes worded in ways that prevent examinees from demonstrating their knowledge of nursing practice. Applying the principles of test-item construction and linguistic modification to make test items more readily comprehensible by students not only increases the reliability and validity of test scores but may also increase the pass rate of students who otherwise are successful in their programs. An increase in pass rates would bring much-needed cultural diversity to the nursing profession and cultural sensitivity to nursing practice, helping to reduce health care disparities.

RECOMMENDATIONS FOR NURSE EDUCATORS AND ADMINISTRATORS

The following recommendations are for nursing faculty who are responsible for assessing students' understanding of nursing knowledge and for nursing administrators whose leadership is essential in creating more equitable policies and procedures for the assessment of students.

1. Assess students in a variety of ways, including case study exams, reflective papers, group projects, and oral presentations. Some students are better able to demonstrate their nursing knowledge through tasks and activities that are more holistic, contextualized, and integrative in nature.
2. Encourage students to form study groups that are racially, culturally, and linguistically diverse. Make sure all students who want to be part of a study group have found a group or have formed their own.
3. Help students make the most out of their study groups. If your institution has a learning center, invite a study skills specialist from the center to talk with students about effective study techniques and strategies that tap into different learning styles, for example, writing marginal notes, creating flash cards, teaching topics to one another, demonstrating procedures, creating review tapes, and so forth.
4. Offer review sessions for students led by faculty, and at these sessions have students practice taking multiple-choice tests so they are familiar with the format and nature of the task. Introduce students to various multiple-choice test-taking strategies. Several books on this topic have been written especially for nursing students, including *Test success—Test-taking techniques for beginning nursing students* by Nugent and Vitale (2000), and could be used in review sessions or workshops to familiarize students with ways to think through various types of test items.
5. Provide faculty with training in the writing of multiple-choice test items.
6. When writing multiple-choice test items, use principles of good test-item construction (see Appendix A), avoiding unnecessary semantic and syntactic complexity.
7. Work with ESL/language experts at your institution to develop a procedure for reducing the language load of test items (see Appendix B for steps to follow in linguistic modification).
8. Meet one-on-one with students who are having difficulty with multiple-choice tests. Have students explain why they chose the answers that were incorrect. Look for patterns in their

responses. Did they have difficulty understanding the wording of test items or the content being assessed? Be open to students' perspectives and the possibility of flaws in the wording of your test items.

9. Create a procedure for reviewing and revising test items with differential response rates for native and nonnative speakers of English.
10. Create a procedure for reviewing test scores of students who were unfairly disadvantaged by the wording of test items or who may have failed an exam because of poorly worded test items.
11. Allow all students enough time to complete their tests. Because of the additional time it takes ESL students to process the language of tests, create a policy that allows ESL students time and a half to complete their exams.
12. Create a policy that allows ESL students to take their exams in the learning center at your institution or in some other environment that is less stressful and anxiety-provoking (see chapter 10 in this book for discussion of incapacitating test anxiety). Not all ESL students will want or need to take advantage of this option; they may also be offended if nursing faculty assume they need extra time. Rather than announce the policy in class or put it on the syllabus, send a flyer to students who have indicated on their application that English is not their native language. Contact individual students through their adviser after the results of the first exam in each course to see if students might benefit from additional time and a less stressful environment.
13. If ESL students take their exams in the learning center, a nursing faculty member should be present or available to answer questions. Otherwise, students may decide to take the test with the rest of the class so they can have access to faculty members, a choice that students should not have to make if additional time and a less stressful environment would significantly improve their test scores.
14. Explore ways in which to collaborate with ESL faculty at your institution, to create ways in which to better prepare ESL students for the language and cultural demands of nursing, as well as to support ESL students who may be having difficulty in your nursing program.

QUESTIONS FOR DIALOGUE

1. What ideas or concepts did you find most meaningful in this chapter? Identify your insights and questions to bring to a dialogue with your colleagues.
2. What percent of final course grades in your program are based on multiple-choice exams? Discuss the ethical implications of students failing multiple-choice nursing exams, and perhaps even courses, because of poorly worded test items.
3. When a student fails a multiple-choice exam, what do faculty generally assume about that student? In one-on-one conferences with students who have done poorly on multiple-choice tests, what insights have you had that challenged the assumptions you had made about the student?
4. Does your program routinely analyze test scores to determine if subpopulations of the class are disproportionately having difficulty succeeding? If so, what policies are in place to determine the reasons for inequities in assessment outcomes? If not, dialogue with colleagues about ways in which your program could respond to these inequities.
5. What common flaws discussed in this chapter could you identify in your program's test items? What kind of training is provided for nursing faculty in your program in the writing of multiple-choice test items? If none, what kind of training would you need to avoid linguistic bias in the test items you write?
6. In your opinion, which of Bosher's recommendations are most critical in rectifying the inequities in your program's assessment practices?

APPENDIX A

REDUCING LINGUISTIC BIAS IN MULTIPLE-CHOICE NURSING EXAMS: CRITERIA FOR TEST QUESTIONS

1. Options follow grammatically from the stem.
2. Options are of equal length; key is not longer, more specific, or more complete.
3. Same word is not repeated in stem and key.
4. Lead-in is in question format, not completion format.
5. Negative phrasing is avoided.

6. Best-answer wording is bolded, capitalized, and either underlined or italicized.
7. Task/content of the stem is not tricky or unnecessarily complicated.
8. Stem is clear and unambiguous.
9. "None of the above" or "All of the above" are not used as options.
10. Options are grammatically consistent or parallel in form.
11. Repetitious wording in the options is avoided.
12. Complex multiple-choice format is avoided, i.e., only one answer per option.
13. Options are logically compatible with the stem.
14. There are no reduced or implied conditionals in the stem.
15. There are no embedded or reduced clauses.
16. Questions are placed at the beginning of the sentence, not at the end.
17. Unnecessary or inconsistent use of modals (e.g., should, would, might) is avoided.
18. Active voice is used rather than passive voice.
19. Referents of pronouns are unambiguous.
20. Subjects of active verbs and recipients of passive verbs are always clear.
21. There are no dangling participles (i.e., the implied subject of an introductory phrase or clause is the same as the stated subject of the main clause).
22. Wording is clear and concise.
23. Wording is consistent between the stem and options and among the options.
24. Items do not include culturally specific information.

APPENDIX B

PROCEDURE FOR LINGUISTIC MODIFICATION

Step 1: Each person in the group reads the original item carefully, identifying any technical terms, fixed phrases, or content-specific vocabulary that is being tested in the item that needs to be maintained in the modified version. The content area specialists are key in this effort because they know what is crucial to maintaining the content validity of the item.

Step 2: Once key terms are identified, group members read the draft revision that has been prepared ahead of the meeting by an ESL/testing expert. All group members reflect on the revised item, ensuring that it tests the same content as the original item (i.e., that the revision has not altered the construct being tested). Changes are made as necessary to ensure that the validity of the item is intact.

Step 3: Additional changes are made to the draft revision to further reduce the semantic and linguistic complexity of the test item. Low frequency nontechnical vocabulary is replaced with higher frequency vocabulary. Difficult syntactic structures (e.g., long, complex sentences; reduced, embedded clauses; abstract constructions, etc.) are identified and replaced with simpler structures.

Step 4: The group reads the item again. Unnecessary synonyms (multiple words used for the same referent) are eliminated. Other difficult syntactic elements (e.g., relative clauses, passive voice, etc.) are identified, and where possible, the item is further modified to eliminate those structures. Finally, any low-frequency, nonessential technical words are glossed, with brief explanations or definitions placed in parentheses beside the word.

Step 5: The group then reads the revised item one last time, with all changes incorporated. All group members have one final opportunity to voice concerns about the item and to discuss any additional changes that need to be made. All group members need to be satisfied with the resulting modified item before moving on to the subsequent one.

Adapted from *Leveling the Assessment Playing Field in the Culturally Diverse Nursing Profession,* by M. Bowles, February 2004, PowerPoint presentation, College of St. Catherine, St. Paul, MN.

REFERENCES

Abedi, J., & Bosher, S. (2006). *The effects of linguistic modification of NCLEX® test items on test performance of non-native vs. native speakers of English.* Unpublished research proposal, submitted to National Council of State Boards of Nursing, Chicago, IL.

Abedi, J., Hofstetter, C., Baker, E., & Lord, C. (2001). *NAEP math performance and test accommodations: Interactions with student language background* (CSE Technical Report No. 536). Los Angeles: University of California, Center for the Study of Evaluation/National Center for Research on Evaluation, Standards, and Student Testing.

Abedi, J., & Lord, C. (2001). The language factor in mathematics tests. *Applied Measurement in Education, 14*(3), 219–234.

Abedi, J., Lord, C., & Hofstetter, C. (1998). *Impact of selected background variables on students' NAEP math performance* (CSE Technical Report No. 478). Los Angeles: University of California, Center for the Study of Evaluation/National Center for Research on Evaluation, Standards, and Student Testing.

Abedi, J., Lord, C., & Plummer, J. R. (1995). *Language background as a variable in NAEP mathematics performance: NAEP TRP Task 3D: Language background study.* Los Angeles: University of California, Center for the Study of Evaluation/National Center for Research on Evaluation, Standards, and Student Testing.

Amaro, D. J., Abriam-Yago, K., & Yoder, M. (2006). Perceived barriers for ethnically diverse students in nursing programs. *Journal of Nursing Education, 45*(7), 247–254.

American Educational Research Association (AERA), American Psychological Association (APA), & National Council on Measurement in Education (NCME). (1999). *Standards for educational and psychological testing.* Washington, DC: American Psychological Association.

Bosher, S. (2001). *Needs analysis of ESL nursing students.* Project RN: Opportunity and Success. Unpublished final report. College of St. Catherine, St. Paul, MN.

Bosher, S. (2003, January–February). Barriers to creating a more culturally diverse nursing profession: Linguistic bias in multiple-choice nursing exams. *Nursing Education Perspectives, 24,* 25–34.

Bosher, S. (2004, July). *The effects of linguistic simplification on NCLEX-RN test scores: A pilot study.* Unpublished final report. Center of Excellence in Women and Health. College of St. Catherine, St. Paul, MN.

Bosher, S. (2006). ESL meets nursing: Developing an English for Nursing course. In M. A. Snow & L. Kamhi-Stein (Eds.), *Developing a new course for adult learners* (pp. 63–98). Washington, DC: TESOL.

Bosher, S. (in press). English for nursing: Developing discipline-specific materials. In J. Richards (Ed.), *Materials in ELT: Theory and practice.* Cambridge: Cambridge University Press.

Bosher, S., & Bowles, M. (2008, May-June). The effects of linguistic modification on ESL students' comprehension of nursing course test items. *Nursing Education Perspectives, 29*(3), 165–172.

Bowles, M. (2004, February). *Leveling the assessment playing field in the culturally diverse nursing profession.* PowerPoint presentation, College of St. Catherine, St. Paul, MN.

Case, S. M., & Swanson, D. B. (1985). *Constructing written test questions for the basic and clinical sciences.* Philadelphia, PA: National Board of Medical Examiners.

Collier, V. (1987). Age and rate of acquisition of second language for academic purposes. *TESOL Quarterly, 21,* 617–641.

Collier, V. (1989). How long? A synthesis of research on academic achievement in a second language. *TESOL Quarterly, 23,* 509–531.

Cummins, J. (1989). *Empowering minority students.* Sacramento, CA: California Association for Bilingual Education.

Cunningham, H., Stacciarini, J. M., & Towle, S. (2004). Strategies to promote success on the NCLEX-RN for students with English as a second language. *Nurse Educator, 29*(1), 15–19.

Davidhizar, R., Dowd, S. B., & Giger, J. N. (1998). Educating the culturally diverse healthcare student. *Nurse Educator, 23,* 38–42.

Dean, B. (1988). *Going by the boards: A needs assessment of refugee practical nursing students preparing for the Board exam.* Unpublished master's thesis, University of Minnesota.

Donin, J., & Silva, M. (1993). The relationship between first-and second-language reading comprehension of occupation-specific texts. *Language Learning, 43,* 373–401.

Gronlund, N. E., (1976). *Measurement and evaluation in teaching.* New York: Macmillan.

Guhde, J. A. (2003). English-as-a-Second-Language (ESL) nursing students: Strategies for building verbal and written language skills. *Journal of Cultural Diversity, 10,* 113–118.

Haladyna, T. M. (1994). *Developing and validating multiple-choice test items.* Hillsdale, NJ: Lawrence Erlbaum.

Johnston, J. G. (2001). Influence of English language on ability to pass the NCLEX-RN. In E. Waltz & L. Jenkins (Eds.), *Measurement of nursing outcomes* (2nd ed., pp. 204–207). New York: Springer Publishing.

Kataoka-Yahiro, M., & Abriam-Yago, K. (1997). Culturally competent teaching strategies for Asian nursing students for whom English is a second language. *Journal of Cultural Diversity, 4,* 83–87.

Klisch, M. L. (1994). Guidelines for reducing bias in nursing examinations. *Nurse Educator, 19,* 35–39.

Malu, K. F., & Figlear, M. R. (1998). Enhancing the language development of immigrant ESL nursing students. *Nurse Educator, 23,* 43–46.

Malu, K. F., Figlear, M. R., & Figlear, E. A. (1994). The multicultural ESL nursing student: A prescription for admission. *The Journal of Multicultural Nursing, 1*(2), 15–20.

Memmer, M. K., & Worth, C. C. (1991). Retention of English-as-a-Second-Language (ESL) students: Approaches used by California's 21 generic baccalaureate nursing programs. *Journal of Nursing Education, 30,* 389–396.

Mohan, B. (1986). *Language and content.* Reading, MA: Addison-Wesley.

National Council of State Boards of Nursing (NCSBN). (2005). Investigated NCLEX performance differential between U.S.-educated English as a Second Language (ESL) graduates and non-ESL graduates. In *Business Book* (pp. 241–245). Washington, DC: NCSBN 2005 Annual Meeting.

Nugent, P. N., & Vitale, B. A. (2004). *Test success: Test-taking techniques for beginning nursing students.* Philadelphia: F. A. Davis.

Rivera, C., & Stansfield, C. W. (2004). The effect of linguistic simplification of science test items on score comparability. *Educational Assessment,* 9(3&4), 79–105.

Segalowitz, N. (1986). Second language reading. In J. Vaid (Ed.), *Language processing in bilinguals: Psycholinguistic and neuropsychological perspectives* (pp. 3–19). Hillsdale, NJ: Erlbaum.

Sims-Giddens, S. (2002). Graduation and success rates of Mexican-American undergraduate nursing students in an associate degree nursing program. *ERIC Document 477 418.*

Wendt, A., Zara, A., & Marks, C. (2000, August). *The NCLEX process: Serving as an anchor for the NCLEX examination.* Unpublished presentation. NCSBN Annual Meeting, Minneapolis, MN.

Yoder, M. K. (1996). Instructional responses to ethnically diverse nursing students. *Journal of Nursing Education, 35*(7), 315–321.

12

Innovation in Language Proficiency Assessment: The Canadian English Language Benchmark Assessment for Nurses (CELBAN)

LUCY EPP AND CATHERINE LEWIS

Dear Sir/Madam:

I would like to extend my gratitude to you for providing this special test for foreign nurses who would like to practice nursing in Canada. I had already tried TSE [Test of Spoken English] for six times but I was not rated more than 45. I lost 1 year of effort and expense! Above all, it consumed my emotion to a degree that I got discouraged and decided to give up and go back to my country in September. Before doing so I attended the [nursing licensing bodies'] information session on Sept. 16th, when I first heard about CELBAN. After I checked the website for CELBAN, I got the idea that it could be the best test ever.

The live, warm, and welcoming environment which was provided by the honorable supervisors [during CELBAN testing] eased my tension and the frustration of not being rated as a generally effective speaker while I had almost never had a problem speaking with nearly ten native Canadians who I was in touch with almost every day . . . Finally . . . I passed a test [CELBAN]. It is very interesting that I did answer the same way that I used to do for TSE and passed CELBAN on my first

---

Adapted with permission from "Innovation in Language Proficiency Assessment: The Canadian English Language Benchmark Assessment for Nurses (CELBAN)," by L. Epp & C. Lewis, 2007, *Red River College Forum: Applied Research and Innovation, 5,* 49–70.

attempt. Even my strengths and weaknesses are incredibly precise and I do accept them wholeheartedly.

I could write pages and pages to emphasize . . . the degree of my thankfulness for CELBAN, if time permitted. In one word I regained my lost confidence and courage and I owe this to CELBAN.

Yours truly,

The Canadian English Language Benchmark Assessment for Nurses (CELBAN) was developed from 2000–2004 following best practices for language assessment development, and it is unique in several important ways. First, it is based on an in-depth analysis of the language demands, or target language use (TLU), of the nursing profession across Canada. Second, reports to candidates include feedback on strengths and weaknesses in productive skills (speaking and writing). Thus, candidates have an indication of areas they need to work on to improve their language skills for nursing. A third unique feature of CELBAN is that the speaking assessment is carried out as a face-to-face interaction with two trained speaking assessors, allowing for a more authentic exchange. Fourth, the Canadian national standards for adult English as a Second Language, Canadian Language Benchmarks (CLB), are used as the basis for CELBAN.[1] These standards provide a common language for test developers, stakeholders, and candidates. Based on these unique features, CELBAN provides an innovative and relevant model for an occupation-specific English language assessment tool.

BACKGROUND

A large number of nursing professionals in Canada are approaching retirement age in the next few years. At the same time, it is expected that an aging population will place greater demands on the health care profession. Based on these realities, concerns have been expressed regarding projections of a critical shortage of nursing professionals in Canada (Canadian Nursing Association, 2002).[2] In 2000, the Ontario Ministry of Health and Long Term Care stated that unless solutions were found, and found soon, the country's health care system would suffer significantly (Registered Nursing Association of Ontario With Registered Practical Nurses Association of Ontario, 2000).

Internationally educated (IE) nurses entering the profession in Canada could help ease the shortage. However, IE nurses in Canada have experienced difficulty in the process of obtaining licensure. One concern has been that none of the English language assessment tools approved by Canadian licensing bodies was based on the language demands of the nursing profession. Recognition of this reality prompted the exploration of alternatives and the inception of the CELBAN project.

Best Practices

The involvement of stakeholders, from the beginning and throughout the process, has been key to the success of CELBAN. This involvement ensured that, when CELBAN was implemented, licensing bodies were aware of the process of test development and were already committed to the concept of a nursing-specific language assessment. The involvement of a wide range of stakeholders in surveys, focus groups, and interviews also provided information for test developers. This input provided direction in assigning CLB levels for the English language demands of nursing and in choosing appropriate content for the assessment tool.

Best practices were also followed through the involvement of a wide range of consultants across Canada. These included experts in second language acquisition, test development, psychometrics, and nursing. In addition, current literature related to language assessment development theory and practice was reviewed, including works by Alderson, Clapham, and Wall (1995); Bachman and Palmer (1996); Buck (2001); Cushing Weigle (2002); Douglas (2000); McNamara (2000); and Weir (1993). The test developers followed additional best practices, which included an analysis of target language use, pilot testing drafts of the new assessment tool with the target population, and the use of rigorous measures of reliability and validity through statistical analysis of results.

PROJECT DESCRIPTION

The development of CELBAN was carried out in four stages. First, a feasibility study was carried out with stakeholders. Second, researchers did an in-depth analysis of the language demands of the nursing profession across Canada (Phase I). Third, CELBAN was developed (Phase II), following "best practices" and using the data gathered in Phase I as a foundation. The fourth stage was the implementation of CELBAN (Phase III).

Feasibility Study

In 2000–2001, a feasibility study, the first stage of the project, was carried out by the Centre for Canadian Language Benchmarks (CCLB).[3] This survey of 50 nursing stakeholder organizations across Canada indicated that existing English language assessment tools (e.g., Test of English as a Foreign Language [TOEFL], Test of Spoken English [TSE], and others) were too general to adequately evaluate the ability of IE nurses to communicate effectively in the nursing profession in Canada. The results clearly indicated the need for a nursing-specific English language assessment tool. Based on these findings, the CCLB decided to undertake a multiphase project to develop what is now known as CELBAN.

Phase I: Analysis of the Language Demands of the Nursing Profession

In 2002, the CCLB initiated the second stage, a six-month project to analyze the target language use (TLU) of the nursing profession across Canada.[4] The project was carried out by two researchers from the Language Training Centre (LTC) at Red River College (RRC). Both were second language experts with excellent knowledge of the CLB and experience in applying the CLB framework to the workplace. The project team also included nationally recognized second language acquisition consultants. The significance of this national study was that, for the first time, a CLB level could be applied to describe the language proficiency standards required for nurses in speaking, listening, reading, and writing.

A mixed method approach in the research methodology was adopted for this project. The following steps were carried out in order to gather data to establish the language demands of the nursing profession: (1) Survey questionnaires were sent to 1,000 randomly selected nurses across Canada, asking them to rate the importance of language tasks described by the CLB document; (2) the CanTEST was administered to 10 internationally educated nurses in 5 provinces;[5] (3) focus groups were held with a range of stakeholders in five provinces;[6] (4) 23 nurses were interviewed across the country; and (5) nurses in a wide range of settings were observed on the job in five provinces. In addition, a National Advisory Committee (NAC) made up of nursing stakeholders was established to assist in guiding the project.

All the data were analyzed by a psychometrics expert and then compared to CLB descriptors by language experts. Based on an in-depth analysis of all data, it was determined that an IE nurse entering the profession in Canada should be able to demonstrate English language competency at the following CLB levels in each of the skill areas (see Centre for Canadian Language Benchmarks Web site: www.language.ca for descriptors of these levels):

- Speaking: CLB 8
- Listening: CLB 9
- Reading: CLB 8
- Writing: CLB 7

In addition, a great deal of valuable data was gathered regarding the types of language interactions carried out by nurses in the workplace. Some of the data gathered during the observations of nurses were analyzed and reported in pie charts. Twenty nurses were observed for a total of 80.25 hours (56.25 hours observing Registered Nurses [RNs] and 24 hours observing Licensed Practical Nurses [LPNs]). Nurses were observed in five provinces in Canada, in a wide range of settings, including hospital medical units, surgery units, subacute units, emergency, intensive care units, acute care, maternity, long-term care, home visits, a foot clinic, a community health centre, and a public health education presentation (see figure on "Situational Language Use" in Appendix A and figure on "Language Tasks" in Appendix B). The data gathered provided the underlying framework for the next stage, the development of CELBAN.

The value of using a mixed-methods approach was evident from the results of the project. In many ways, each method helped to validate the others. For example, analysis of the surveys sent to practicing nurses provided quantitative data indicating that speaking and listening were the most demanding skills for nurses. This information was supported by qualitative data gathered in focus groups and interviews. An analysis of the strengths and limitations of each method was conducted to interpret the results holistically. This approach contributed to the reliability of the outcomes.

The CELBAN is based on this in-depth analysis of the TLU (i.e., the language used in the Canadian nursing context, identified in Phase I). According to Douglas (2000), a critical feature of language for specific purposes test development is a detailed analysis of the TLU situation. The in-depth analysis carried out during Phase I of this project laid the foundation for an assessment tool that reflects the real language demands of the nursing profession in Canada.

Phase II: The Development of CELBAN

In 2002, CCLB initiated the third stage, a nine-month project for the development of an English language proficiency assessment tool for the nursing profession.[7] The test development team for CELBAN was identified in the initial planning stage of the project. Again, two language experts from the Language Training Centre (LTC) at Red River College with excellent knowledge of the CLB and experience in applying the CLB framework to the workplace led the team. In total, there were 16 participants on the team including the following: a project manager, two researchers/test developers, three project consultants, three nursing consultants, a statistics consultant, two test development consultants, a linguistics consultant, a test and measurement consultant, and two test reviewers. These individuals were all experts in their particular fields and assisted from several educational and provincial locations including the CanTEST Project Office (University of Ottawa), Red River College (Winnipeg), University of Manitoba, Ontario Institute of Studies in Education (University of Toronto), and a private consulting firm in Edmonton.

The test developers did an initial literature review in order to ensure best practices in the development of the assessment tool. This review was an important piece in obtaining background information and establishing a theoretical framework. A bibliography of the resources used for the development of the CELBAN was compiled (see Epp & Lewis, 2003). Also, a National Advisory Committee (NAC), composed of a wide range of stakeholders, was again established, primarily to provide feedback at various stages of the project.

The development of test specifications was a lengthy and ongoing process, which was seen as a circular, not linear, process. At each stage of the project, test specifications were amended, revised, and elaborated upon. In the end, CELBAN was designed as four subtests: Speaking, Listening, Reading, and Writing. Scoring methods and grids for the assessment of Speaking and Writing were also developed.

CELBAN Draft One

Draft One of CELBAN was developed following best practices, with input from consultants. The information and resources collected during

Phase I, *An Analysis of the English Language Demands of the Nursing Profession Across Canada,* were an integral part of the development of the assessment tool. The Phase I data provided authentic texts, tasks, and scenarios for designing the assessment tool, which contributed to the "face validity" of the test.[8] Verbatims from observations were used to provide a framework for speaking and listening scenarios.

Pie chart analyses of the interactions and tasks observed provided helpful information (see Appendices A and B). For example, in Chart 2 (Appendix B), *asks for information, explains,* and *gives instructions* were identified as the most frequently observed language tasks. Based on this analysis, two role-plays were developed for the CELBAN Speaking Assessment. In Role-Play One, the candidate plays the part of a nurse, asking a "patient" (role-played by one of the assessors) questions to elicit information to fill out a form. Using this format, it is possible to assess candidates' ability to ask questions, as well as their ability to take initiative for an interaction. In Role-Play Two, the candidate plays the part of a nurse, giving instructions to a "patient" (role-played by the other assessor). In this role-play it is possible to assess candidates' ability to give information, explain, and respond to objections.

Feedback from stakeholders was also considered. For example, stakeholders identified talking on the telephone as a critical skill for nurses. As a result, a range of phone interactions is included in the CELBAN Listening Assessment. Samples of reading and writing collected during observations provided authentic text models. The nursing consultants provided excellent feedback and support in ensuring the authenticity of test items and tasks.

The assessment tool was designed as four separate subtests to assess each aspect of language: Speaking, Listening, Reading, and Writing. The test development team members provided feedback on the overall framework for the test, individual components, and specific items. Current testing methodology was incorporated into the design of the assessment tool.

The development of Speaking and Writing grids was a complex process requiring extensive familiarity with the CLB document. The consultants with expertise in test development were an important resource during this part of the development process. These grids were revised on an ongoing basis throughout the process as descriptors and performance indicators were clarified and more clearly articulated.

Once a complete draft for each subtest was developed, it was sent to the test reviewers. (The language and test-development experts provided input throughout the development time; however, the reviewers critiqued the completed draft.) Revisions to the test were made based on feedback from the reviewers.

Pilot testing of Draft One was conducted in Toronto, Ontario (CARE for Nurses Project) and Winnipeg, Manitoba (Red River College). The candidates included:

- 80 L2 IE nurses in the field (in the process of having credentials recognized).[9]
- 40 L1 students who had completed some field experience in the profession.[10]
- 5 L1 and L2 professionals presently practicing (within 5 years) in Canada.

  Total number of candidates: 125

Data obtained from Draft One piloting provided the test developers with both qualitative and quantitative data on which to base revisions. In terms of quantitative data, crucial indicators were alpha reliabilities of each component of the test (see "Analysis of Reliability Scores"), indicators of validity (see "Analysis of Validity"), and item discrimination. Qualitative data were gathered through surveys completed by candidates and feedback from interviews and focus groups. The data informed the test developers about the strengths and weaknesses of the assessment tool and its delivery, both through statistical analysis and anecdotal reports.

Another means of testing language proficiency of the candidates was conducted for a comparative analysis. During pilot testing of CELBAN, the candidates were assessed using the Canadian Language Benchmarks Placement Test (CLBPT) to establish comparisons.[11] Correlations between candidates' results on these two tests informed the test-developers of the validity and reliability of the new assessment (for results see "Construct Validity").

Researchers also conducted focus groups with a wide range of stakeholders to obtain feedback and provide an opportunity for stakeholders to hear different perspectives and discuss their concerns. As with Phase I, the focus groups in Phase II were important because they also provided an opportunity for stakeholders to network with each other in ways that perhaps were not previously experienced. Focus groups were conducted during the time frame in which pilot-testing occurred in specific cities.

Once the first round of pilot-testing was completed, revisions were made to Draft One based on analysis of the statistics and feedback from consultants and participants. Having a team of experts representing a wide range of relevant perspectives was extremely helpful in revising, rewriting, and adding or deleting specific test-items or complete sections. For example, when statistical analysis identified low alpha reliabilities on questions, those specific test-items were reviewed and revised or removed if necessary. Also, when qualitative data in the form of surveys from participants identified unclear instructions or inadequate time allotted, this feedback was considered when making revisions.

CELBAN Draft Two

Pilot testing of Draft Two was carried out in Ottawa, Ontario (Algonquin College); Edmonton, Alberta (Grant MacEwan College); Calgary, Alberta (Grant MacEwan College); and Vancouver, British Columbia (Vancouver Community College). The participants included:

- 83 L2 internationally educated professionals in the field (in the process of having credentials recognized).
- 58 L1 students who had completed some field experience in the profession.
- 4 L1 and L2 professionals presently practicing (within 5 years) in Canada.

  Total number of candidates: 145

Pilot testing of Draft Two followed the same format as with Draft One, and the same type of data was collected and analyzed. A summary of the results of the final analysis is reported later.

Analysis of Reliability Scores

Reliability scores (coefficient alpha) on Draft Two of CELBAN, covering all assessment criteria were as follows:[12]

- Speaking: 0.944
- Listening: 0.939
- Reading: 0.965
- Writing: 0.905

These results indicate that the CELBAN clearly exceeds reliability criteria.[13]

Analysis of Validity

According to the American Psychological Association (APA, as quoted by Bachman, 1990), "The most important quality of test interpretation or use is validity, the extent to which the inferences or decisions we make on the basis of test scores are meaningful, appropriate and useful" (p. 25).[14] As Douglas (2000) points out, the key question is not whether a test is valid, but rather, for what purposes is it valid?

The validity of any test, including the CELBAN, is most often determined by analyzing data that relate to one of the following validity types:

- *content validity* (the extent to which the questions on a test are representative of the behavior that is being measured)
- *construct validity* (the extent to which a test measures some theoretical construct)
- *face validity* (how stakeholders perceive the attractiveness and appropriateness of a test)

The analysis of the CELBAN illustrates that best practices were followed to address each of these categories of validity.

Content Validity

There are minimal statistical procedures to show that content validity exists. Content validity is typically established before the test is administered. The generally accepted procedure involves defining the testing universe (the sample of all possible behaviours of the attribute being measured) and developing questions that map onto the particular testing universe. Once developed, the questions are rated by experts who determine the appropriateness of each question to the testing universe.

In the case of the CELBAN, both these steps (mapping questions to the testing universe and expert rating of items) were carried out, ensuring that the CELBAN is content-valid—it representatively samples the nursing language-testing universe.

Construct Validity

While there are many different methods that can be used to provide evidence of construct validity, two of the most common methods involve:

- Correlating the test with other established tests that measure a similar construct, referred to as convergent validity.

- Showing that different populations of participants, who theoretically should perform differently on the test, do perform differently on the test.

As part of the pilot testing of Draft One and Two, 78 candidates were tested on both the CELBAN and the Canadian Language Benchmarks Placement Test (CLBPT). The CLBPT is a test that measures similar constructs (e.g., speaking, listening, reading and writing) to those measured by CELBAN. Psychometric analysis of like constructs on the CELBAN and CLBPT produced good convergent validity values (i.e., correlations between similar constructs should be positive, and higher [see bold values in table below] than correlations between dissimilar constructs [discriminate validity in table below]). In Table 12.1, it is evident that the highest correlations are between similar constructs (e.g., speaking and speaking), and the lowest are between dissimilar constructs (e.g., listening and writing). Together, these values provide us with another measure of construct validity.

In addition, comparisons were made between Canadian-educated nurses and nurses educated outside Canada. Of the Canadian-educated nurses, 73% were native English speakers, and all were educated in English. (The other 27% of Canadian-educated nurses were nonnative speakers of English, although most had come to Canada as children or

Table 12.1

CORRELATIONS BETWEEN CANADIAN LANGUAGE BENCHMARK PLACEMENT TEST (CLBPT) AND CELBAN

	CLBPT			
CELBAN	LISTENING	READING	SPEAKING	WRITING
Listening	**0.495** n = 61	0.444 n = 61	0.607 n = 61	0.327 n = 61
Reading	0.406 n = 74	**0.625** n = 74	0.281 n = 73	0.438 n = 74
Speaking	0.687 n = 61	0.484 n = 61	**0.741** n = 61	0.541 n = 61
Writing	0.376 n = 74	0.417 n = 74	0.342 n = 73	**0.533** n = 74

teenagers, predominately from the Philippines or China.) Construct validity was demonstrated through the differences in performance of Canadian-educated (both native and nonnative speakers of English) versus internationally educated nurses. Differences in the scores of Canadian-educated vs. internationally educated nurses were analyzed and significant differences, at the alpha = 0.05 level, were found.[15] These results indicate that CELBAN has construct validity.

Face Validity

Face validity involves the stakeholders' perception of the test. That is, do the stakeholders believe that the test measures what it is supposed to measure? Bachman (1990) states that "in examining validity, we must also be concerned with the appropriateness and usefulness of the test score for a given purpose" (p. 25).

After each section of the test, the candidates (test-takers) involved in pilot-testing in Phase II were asked a series of questions about the test. Results from this feedback were as indicated in Table 12.2.

Based on both statistical evidence and feedback from candidates, CELBAN demonstrates high validity, showing that the scores are inherently appropriate and useful in terms of providing scores for the given purpose, the evaluation of English language proficiency for the nursing profession in Canada.

At this point, more fine-tuning of the assessment tool was carried out as a result of analysis of the data gathered during the pilot testing. Changes were based on an analysis of both qualitative and quantitative data. Qualitative data provided by feedback from candidates and observations by proctors resulted in adjustments to the time provided for candidates in each section of the test. Also, instructions given to candidates were slightly modified or clarified. The quantitative data provided by statistical analysis (alpha reliabilities and item discrimination) resulted in changes in the wording of stems or distracters and the elimination of several multiple-choice questions in Listening and Reading.

Final Draft

Final revisions to the assessment tool were made once the results of the qualitative and quantitative data obtained during pilot-testing had been analyzed. These revisions included content, time frames, and instructions for administration, as well as the final test specifications document.

Table 12.2

CANDIDATE RESPONSES TO SURVEY QUESTIONS RELATED TO CELBAN LISTENING

QUESTIONS REGARDING: CELBAN LISTENING	ANSWERS (% OF RESPONDENTS)		
The test length was . . .	too short 22.1%	just right 62.9%	too long 15.0%
The questions were . . .	too easy 9.1%	just right 83.9%	too hard 7.0%
The time allowed for the test was . . .	too much 3.5%	enough 54.2%	not enough 42.4%
Was the content familiar?	very familiar 55.5%	somewhat familiar 35.2%	not familiar 9.2%
Overall impression of CELBAN Listening	very good 27.5%	good 50.0%	fair[a] 22.5%

QUESTIONS REGARDING FORMAT AND CONTENT OF CELBAN LISTENING	ANSWERS (% OF RESPONDENTS)	
What did you think of the nursing content?	effective 99.3%	not effective 0.7%
What did you think of the multiple choice format?	effective 94.3%	not effective 5.7%
What did you think of the chart format?	effective 95.0%	not effective 4.3%
What did you think of the video section?	effective 91.3%	not effective 8.7%
What did you think of the audio section?	effective 90.0%	not effective 10.0%

[a]In retrospect, we realized that some candidates interpreted "fair" to mean "equitable," which has a very different connotation than "fair" as in "mediocre." This may have affected the results, especially because it was noted that candidates had very positive feedback on other aspects of the test, and then responded with "fair" on overall impressions of the test components.

Note: Similar questions were asked for each section of CELBAN (i.e., Reading, Writing, Speaking). For details on this feedback, see Phase II report.

Format and Content of Final Version of CELBAN

The context and content of all tasks in the speaking, listening, reading, and writing assessment are based on data collected from Phase I. Tasks were created with input from nursing instructors and consultants to ensure authenticity.

CELBAN Speaking Assessment

- The speaking assessment includes an oral interview and two role-plays.
- Two assessors carry out the assessment.
- Speaking assessment is tape-recorded for future reference if needed by assessors to verify score.
- The speaking assessment includes two role-plays in which the candidate is asked to interact with the "patient" (one of the assessors), first by asking questions to obtain information and second by giving instructions, collecting information, offering explanations, and responding to objections. In addition, during the interview the candidate is asked to answer questions to demonstrate the ability to narrate, describe, summarize, synthesize, state and support opinion, and persuade.
- Total time: 30 minutes
- Criteria for scoring speaking tasks is based on CLB descriptors:
  - General use of language
  - Intelligibility
  - Organization
  - Fluency
  - Use of cohesive devices
  - Adequacy of vocabulary for purpose
  - Grammar
  - Use of strategies
  - Speaking tasks demonstrated
- Scores are assigned as CLB levels.
- Feedback on strengths and weaknesses in Speaking is provided.

CELBAN Listening Assessment

- There are five video scenarios (in various settings including hospital, home, clinic, and medical office; these scenarios include a representative sample of ages, genders, and visible minorities in nurses, patients, family members, and other health care professionals).

- There are four audio scenarios (phone calls and shift-to-shift reports).
- Scenarios include interactions between nurses and patients, family members, and other professionals.
- Question format: multiple-choice (some in chart format)
- Total time: 45 minutes
- Scores are assigned as CLB levels.

CELBAN Reading Assessment

- The reading assessment includes two sections:
  - skimming and scanning (10 minutes)
  - reading comprehension (40 minutes)
- Text includes various formats such as charts, patient notes, manuals, and information texts related to health issues.
- Question format:
  - short-answer questions (skimming and scanning)
  - multiple-choice questions (reading comprehension), including a cloze exercise (in a cloze exercise, test-takers choose the correct option to fill in the blanks in a text)
- Scores are assigned as CLB levels.

CELBAN Writing Assessment

- The writing assessment includes two sections:
  - form-filling (10 minutes)
  - report-writing (20 minutes)
- Criteria for scoring writing tasks is based on CLB descriptors:
  - Criteria for form-filling:
    - conventions of form-filling (spelling, legibility, point form)
    - necessary information included (main points and supporting details)
  - Criteria for report-writing:
    - effectiveness

- grammar
- discourse/fluency
- vocabulary for purpose/content

- Scores are assigned as CLB levels.
- Feedback on strengths and weaknesses in Writing is provided.

CELBAN ADMINISTRATION

CELBAN can be administered in three ways: (a) complete CELBAN (Listening, Writing, Reading, and Speaking); (b) group test only (Listening, Writing, and Reading only); or (c) Speaking assessment only. Some provincial nursing licensing bodies accept a combination of scores from two tests (e.g., a TOEFL Listening, Reading, and Writing and a CELBAN Speaking Assessment). It is the prerogative of the licensing bodies to accept a combination of scores because they have officially endorsed CELBAN as an acceptable alternative to previously endorsed tests. If a candidate chooses CELBAN, he/she must achieve the following CELBAN scores, reported as CLB levels, to pass and satisfy the English language proficiency requirements of the nursing licensing bodies: (a) Speaking–CLB Level 8, (b) Listening–CLB Level 9, (c) Reading–CLB Level 8, and (d) Writing–CLB Level 7.

Phase III: Implementation of CELBAN

In 2003–2004, the fourth stage, the implementation of CELBAN, began. A national administrative centre was established to be responsible for national CELBAN administration and implementation. This office is the Canadian English Language Assessment Services (CELAS) Centre, located at Red River College's Language Training Centre in Winnipeg, Manitoba. The CELAS Centre is responsible for the selection, set-up, and training of the administration team, and support of official CELBAN Administration Sites.

To date, eight CELBAN Administration Sites have been set up across Canada (Vancouver and Surrey, British Columbia; Edmonton and Calgary, Alberta; Winnipeg, Manitoba; Toronto, Ontario; Scarborough, Ontario; and Hamilton, Ontario). In addition, all licensing bodies for registered nurses and practical nurses across Canada have recognized CELBAN as one of the options available for IE nurses to demonstrate their English language requirement for licensure.

To accompany the implementation of CELBAN, resources have recently been made available to support internationally educated nurses seeking information about and assistance in preparing for CELBAN. First, in 2004–2005, a Web site www.celban.org was established to provide information regarding CELBAN. Second, both an online and offline CELBAN Readiness Self-Assessment (CRSA) have been made available to candidates who wish to familiarize themselves with CELBAN and self-assess their readiness to attempt CELBAN. The online CRSA is now available free of charge on the Web site. The offline CRSA is available to candidates in the form of a kit for a nominal fee. The offline kit includes a video (VHS, DVD, or CD) and four booklets: *Test-taking Strategies Booklet, General Information & Test Booklet, Answer Booklet,* and *Answer Key Booklet.* Also, in early 2006, the CELAS Centre developed an institutional version of the CRSA for use by educational institutions that provide programs and services for internationally educated nurses. This resource was designed to provide an *Orientation to CELBAN* and exposure to CELBAN through the CRSA, including a guidebook for the facilitator of a CELBAN Orientation workshop or course. The kit includes all the components of the candidate kit, with the added supports for an instructor in an educational setting. Both the candidate kit and the institutional kit are available for purchase through the CELAS Centre, and order forms are available on the Web site: www.celban.org.

During the initial implementation of CELBAN, additional feedback from candidates was collected and analyzed. Approximately 50 candidates provided feedback to statements that compared CELBAN with other English language assessment tools recognized by nursing licensing bodies in Canada. (*Note:* Candidates identify on their CELBAN registration form which recognized tests they have previously taken, including date and scores. The recognized tests identified are: TOEFL, TSE, the International English Language Testing System [IELTS], the Michigan English Language Assessment Battery [MELAB], the Canadian Academic English Language Assessment [CAEL], and the Test of English for International Communication [TOEIC]). In completing the short questionnaire, candidates reflect about their experience on other tests compared to CELBAN. The responses were analyzed with the results as indicated in Table 12.3.

These statistics again indicate strong face validity from the perspective of candidates when they compare CELBAN to other English language assessment tools.

Table 12.3

CANDIDATE RESPONSES TO SURVEY QUESTIONS COMPARING CELBAN WITH OTHER TESTS

STATEMENT	STRONGLY DISAGREE	DISAGREE	NOT SURE	AGREE	STRONGLY AGREE
The CELBAN *more accurately* assesses my English abilities.	7.7%	4.1%	11.5%	36.7%	38.8%
The CELBAN is a *more relevant* test of the English skills needed for nursing in Canada.	7.7%	4.1%	12.2%	28.6%	46.9%
It is beneficial to me that upon receiving my CELBAN test results (scores), I will also be receiving *feedback on my strengths and weaknesses* in both Speaking and Writing.	8.3%	2.1%	0%	26%	63%

As implementation of CELBAN continued, in 2005–2006, two new versions of CELBAN (Versions 2 and 3) were developed. Each new version was modeled after the original CELBAN with new content. New video and audio segments were produced for the CELBAN Listening assessment; new passages and tasks for CELBAN Reading (skimming/scanning and reading comprehension) and CELBAN Writing were developed; and new role-plays for CELBAN Speaking assessment were developed. As with the original CELBAN, these new versions were piloted extensively with 150 IE nurses in several cities across Canada to ensure validity and reliability.

Although no data are currently available regarding any change in the number of IE nurses who have been licensed in Canada since the implementation of CELBAN, feedback from IE nurses who were having difficulty gaining licensure using previous tests has been quite positive, as evident in the following quotes:

- "All I can say about CELBAN is that it is a good idea and I'm glad you gave us the chance to take it."

- "Thanks so much for implementing this exam. I have been waiting for this. (I took the pilot back in 2003.) Thanks again."
- "CELBAN assessment is great."
- "I'm glad to take CELBAN test and I think this test is suitable for an applicant who wants to work as a nurse in Canada. . . . It's more suitable than TOEFL or TSE."

RECOMMENDATIONS FOR NURSE EDUCATORS

The development of CELBAN provides several lessons for nurse educators. First, it is important for nurse educators to be aware not only of the language used in a nursing context but also of the unique culture of nursing in a specific country or region. For example, in North America nurses may be expected to participate in decision-making regarding patient care, while in some other countries, they may be required to follow physicians' orders. The analysis of the language demands in nursing carried out in the development of CELBAN provides information about English language use in nursing in a North American context, and this analysis has been very helpful to nurse educators who teach second-language (L2) nurses.

Also, collaboration between nurse educators, nursing bridge program providers, and ESL instructors is recommended to assist internationally educated nurses to reach their goal of practicing nursing. For example, nurse educators can share with ESL instructors the language challenges that nurses face during practicums to help guide development of program content for internationally educated nurses. Several colleges in Canada (e.g., Algonquin College, Ottawa, Ontario; Mohawk College, Hamilton, Ontario; Kwantlen University College, Surrey, British Columbia; and Red River College, Manitoba) provide excellent models of how this type of collaboration can work.

In addition, ESL students need to be provided with opportunities to practice interactions in the clinical setting. In this regard, CELBAN-related products and services can provide unique resources to nurse educators. A new assessment tool, the Institutional CELBAN, has recently been developed and offers two complete versions that are available to institutions. These new assessment tools are modeled after the official CELBAN. They are designed to be a nonofficial assessment, used by institutions with IE nurses as an English proficiency entry and/or exit test, or as a diagnostic tool for use within a program.

Two versions of the Institutional CELBAN were developed and piloted simultaneously between March and July 2007. As with the development of the official CELBAN, institutions and pilot candidates contributed significantly during the piloting process and provided a rich source of qualitative data. In addition, quantitative data were collected, and statistical analysis was conducted, which informed revisions to the tool. As of October 2007, the Institutional CELBAN (Version 1 or Version 2) in a self-guided format is available for institutions to use for educational purposes and can be purchased in a kit format from the CELAS Centre.[16]

The CELBAN Web site (www.celban.org) also provides helpful information for nurse educators. It offers an online *CELBAN Readiness Self-Assessment (CRSA), Test-Taking Strategies for CELBAN, Information for Candidates,* and a range of other resources. An offline CRSA kit is also available for purchase.

CONCLUSION

The attributes of CELBAN make it unique and relevant. First, the development of CELBAN has been a rigorous, comprehensive, and collaborative effort with input from a wide range of stakeholders and experts from across the country. Second, the content of CELBAN reflects the language tasks of the nursing profession in Canada, as identified through extensive research across Canada during Phase I of the project. Third, CELBAN has been developed according to current methodology of test development based on best practices. Fourth, the reliability of CELBAN is based on pilot testing with the specific target population (internationally educated nurses), a unique feature to CELBAN when compared with the other most commonly accepted English language proficiency assessments used by internationally educated nurses, such as TOEFL, IELTS, and so forth. Fifth, CELBAN results include individualized feedback regarding candidates' strengths and weaknesses in speaking and writing. Again, this is a unique feature of CELBAN when compared with the other most commonly accepted English language proficiency assessments used by internationally educated nurses. Finally, ongoing feedback from many stakeholders has guided each stage in the process of test development and implementation of CELBAN and CELBAN-related products and services.

Based on the rigorous methodology followed in its development and implementation, CELBAN is proving to be a more reliable, valid, and relevant assessment of the English language proficiency of nurses in Canada than any other assessment tool currently available. Access to CELBAN may help to ease the nursing shortage in Canada as internationally educated nurses now have access to a more viable alternative as they seek to demonstrate their English language proficiency as part of licensure requirements to practice nursing in Canada.

Acknowledgements

Each phase of the CELBAN project was completed through the dedication and effort of the following members of the Research and Test Development Team:

- Lucy Epp (Principal Investigator and Test Developer, Red River College)
- Catherine Lewis (Co-Investigator and Test Developer, Red River College)
- Audrey Bonham (Project Manager, Red River College)
- Shelley Bates (Test Development Consultant, Red River College)
- Mary Stawychny (Consultant, ACCESS Program, Red River College)
- Liz Polakoff, Sandra Romano, Kathy Kirkman (Nursing Instructors, Faculty of Nursing, Red River College)
- Tom Harrigan (Statistician and Psychometric Consultant, Faculty of Nursing, Red River College/University of Manitoba)
- eTV Staff, CELBAN Listening Video/Audio Production Team, Red River College
- Alister Cumming (Test Development Consultant, Ontario Institute for Studies in Education, University of Toronto)
- Philip Nagy (Psychometrics Consultant, Ontario Institute for Studies in Education, University of Toronto)
- Margaret Des Brisay (Test Development Consultant, CanTEST Project Office, University of Ottawa)
- Amelia Hope (Test Development Consultant, CanTEST Project Office, University of Ottawa)

- Gail Stewart (Test Reviewer, University of Toronto)
- Grazyna P. Smith (Test Reviewer, Independent Consultant, Edmonton, Alberta)

The test developers also wish to acknowledge the following individuals and groups who contributed time and expertise to the project:

- Centre for Canadian Language Benchmarks (CCLB) Board Members, CCLB Nursing Committee, and CELBAN National Advisory Committee (NAC): Rob Boldt (chair), Jim Jones, Peggy Frederikse, Carolyn Dieleman, Margaret Pidlaski, Pauline McNaughton (CCLB Executive Director), and Marianne Kayed (CCLB Project Manager)
- Nursing College administrators and ESL program providers from the following locations: Care for Nurses (Toronto), Algonquin College (Ottawa), Grant MacEwan College (Edmonton & Calgary), Vancouver Community College
- Internationally educated nurses, nursing students, and newly practising nurses (both internationally educated and Canadian-educated) who participated in piloting
- Stakeholders who participated in focus groups in four provinces

QUESTIONS FOR DIALOGUE

1. What ideas or concepts did you find most meaningful in this chapter? Identify your insights and questions to bring to a dialogue with your colleagues.
2. In your country, are immigrant nurses for whom English is not their first language assessed for language proficiency as part of their nursing reentry certification process? If so, what language proficiency tests are used?
3. Discuss the ethical implications of using general language proficiency tests as a criterion for reentry into professional nursing practice, given that these tests are not specific to the context of nursing practice.
4. Look at Appendix B "Language Tasks." Is this breakdown representative of the language tasks used in the clinical settings in

which your students are learning to practice nursing? If not, how does culture contribute to the differences?

5. If you live outside of Canada, discuss the likelihood of a nursing-specific language proficiency test being developed in your country.
6. Discuss the importance of assessing spoken proficiency as part of the overall assessment of an immigrant nurse's language proficiency.

APPENDIX A

SITUATIONAL LANGUAGE USE

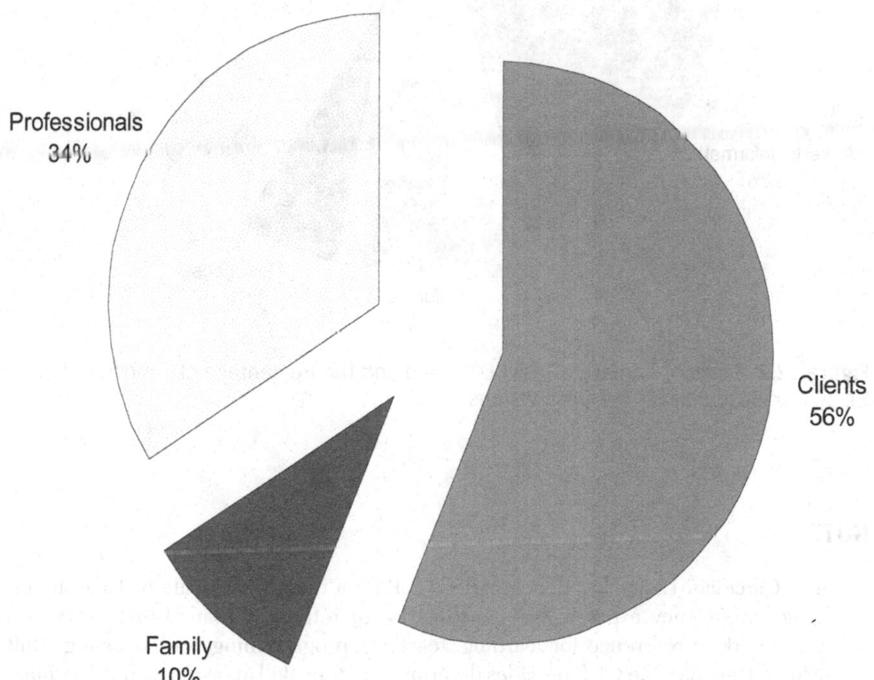

Figure 12.1 Situational Use of Language by Nurses During Observations

APPENDIX B

LANGUAGE TASKS

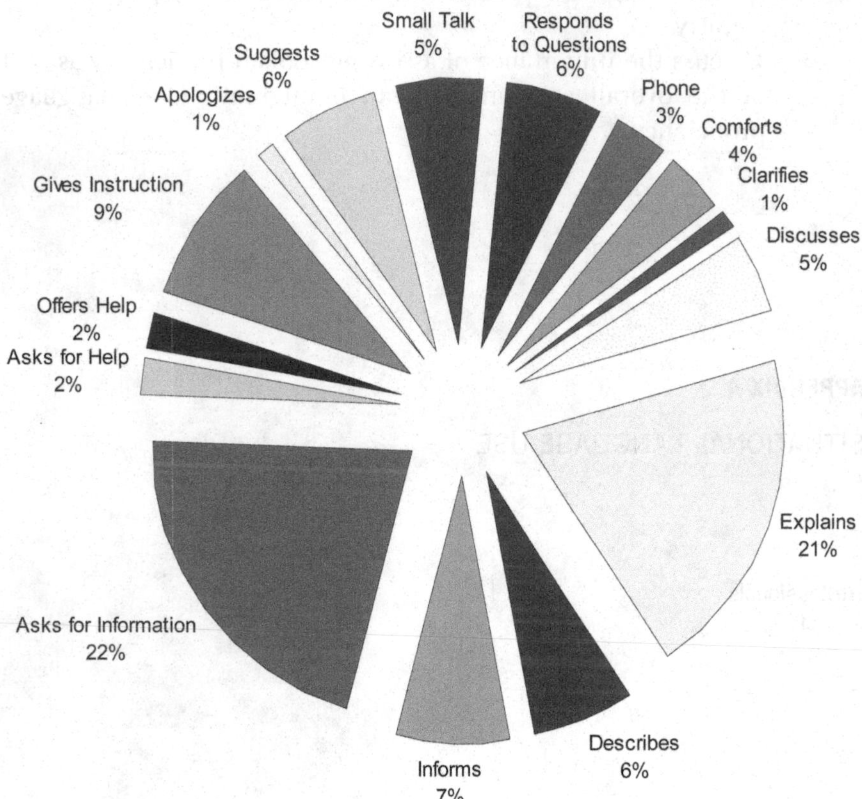

Figure 12.2 Types of Language Tasks Observed and the Percentage of Time Spent on Each Task Based on All the Observations

NOTES

1. The Canadian Language Benchmarks (CLB) is a descriptive scale of English language proficiency expressed as benchmarks (or reference points) that provides a framework of reference for learning, teaching, programming, and assessing adult ESL in Canada. The CLB provides descriptors in four skill areas: speaking, listening, reading, and writing. Language proficiency is measured on a scale of twelve levels, from CLB Level 1 to 12 divided into three stages: Stage One (Basic—Levels 1–4), Stage Two (Intermediate—Levels 5–8), Stage Three (Advanced—Levels 9–12).

2. In 2002, the Canadian Nursing Association report *Planning for the Future: Nursing Human Resource Projections* projected a shortage of 78,000 RNs by 2011 and a shortage of 113,000 RNS by 2016.
3. The CCLB is a national, not-for-profit organization primarily serving the adult English as a Second Language (ESL) community in Canada including learners, teachers, program administrators, and materials, curriculum and test developers. A Canada-wide combination of language training specialists, assessment service providers, and both federal and provincial government members forms the CCLB Board of Directors, and staff of the CCLB are committed to maintaining and promoting language proficiency standards based on the Canadian Language Benchmarks. The CCLB Web site is: www.language.ca.
4. For more detailed information regarding this project, a report by Epp and Stawychny (2002) titled *Phase I, Benchmarking the English Language Demands of the Nursing Profession Across Canada* can be downloaded from the CCLB Web site: www.language.ca.
5. The CanTEST is an English language proficiency test developed by the University of Ottawa and used by some Canadian postsecondary institutions to ensure that candidates meet the English language requirements for admission into programs. CanTEST band scores have been aligned with CLB levels. For more information, contact the CanTEST Project Office: cantest@uottawa.ca.
6. Stakeholders included representatives from nursing licensing bodies, nursing instructors, immigrant-serving agencies, employers, nurses (including IE nurses), and nursing unions.
7. For more detailed information regarding this project, a report by Epp and Lewis (2003) titled *Phase II, The Development of CELBAN* can be downloaded from the CCLB Web site: www.language.ca.
8. *Face validity* is the extent to which a test meets the expectations of those involved in its use, for example, administrators, teachers, candidates, and test score users; it is the acceptability of a test to its stakeholders.
9. L2 refers to candidates whose native language *is not* English.
10. L1 refers to candidates whose native language *is* English.
11. The CLBPT is a task-based assessment tool referenced to the CLB 2000. It is designed to determine the English language proficiency of newcomers to Canada who speak English as a Second Language. Results are provided in listening, speaking, reading and writing. The proficiency levels are based upon the competencies described in CLB 2000 covering CLB Levels 1–8. For more information contact the CCLB at www.language.ca.
12. Reliability is the consistency of measurements of individuals by a test, usually expressed as a "reliability coefficient" or "coefficient alpha." A reliability coefficient is expressed as a number on a scale from 0 to 1, where higher values express greater consistency of a test. Minimal acceptable reliability ranges from 0.7–0.9 on this 0 to 1 scale.
13. A more in-depth analysis of the pilot testing statistics is included in the Phase II report (available at the CCLB Web site: www.language.ca).
14. Test validity is evidence that a test is being used appropriately and measures what it sets out to measure.
15. For more details, see the Phase II report.

16. To obtain further information about CELBAN, or CELBAN-related products or services, contact: Canadian English Language Assessment Services (CELAS) Centre, Red River College, Language Training Centre, Suite 400-123 Main Street, Winnipeg, Manitoba, Canada, R3C 1A3. Phone: (204) 945–0588. E-mail: celas@rrc.mb.ca.

REFERENCES

Alderson, C., Clapman, C., & Wall, D. (1995). *Language test construction and evaluation.* Cambridge: Cambridge University Press.

Bachman, L. (1990). *Fundamental considerations in language testing.* Oxford: Oxford University Press.

Bachman, L., & Palmer, A. S. (1996). *Language testing in practice.* Oxford: Oxford University Press.

Buck, G. (2001). *Assessing listening.* Cambridge: Cambridge University Press.

Canadian Nursing Association. (2002). *Planning for the future: Nursing human resource projections.* Toronto: Author.

Cushing Weigle, S. (2002). *Assessing writing.* Cambridge: Cambridge University Press.

Douglas, D. (2000). *Assessing languages for specific purposes.* Cambridge: Cambridge University Press.

Epp, L., & Lewis, C. (2003). *The development of CELBAN (Canadian English Language Benchmark Assessment for Nurses): A nursing-specific language assessment tool. (Phase II report).* Centre for Canadian Language Benchmarks, Ottawa, ON, Canada (Report available for download at http://www.language.ca).

Epp, L., & Stawychny, M. (2002). *Benchmarking the English language demands of the nursing profession across Canada (Phase I report).* Centre for Canadian Language Benchmarks, Ottawa, ON, Canada. (Report available for download at http://www.language.ca).

McNamara, T. (2000). *Language testing.* Oxford: Oxford University Press.

Registered Nursing Association of Ontario With Registered Practical Nurses Association of Ontario. (2000). *Ensuring the care will be there.* Toronto: Registered Nursing Association of Ontario and Registered Practical Nurses Association of Ontario.

Weir, C. (1993). *Understanding and developing language tests.* London: Prentice Hall International.

Programs That Model Structural Change

PART IV

13 Latino Nursing Career Opportunity Program: A Project Designed to Increase the Number of Latino Nurses

CARMEN RAMIREZ

My parents don't have any idea what it is like to go to school or to have a dream about going to college and becoming a nurse. My teachers don't have any idea of what goes on in my life outside of school, in my home, with my friends, or even here at school. I have friends who came here when they were babies, they do not have documents and will not be able to work or go to school when they finish high school, but they only know this country; they have never lived anywhere else. I am lucky because I was born here. My parents never went to school because they came from the country and there was a war going on, it was too dangerous to walk to the little town where there was a school. They have not learned English because there is no time to go to school, they both work two jobs. I am lucky because I can help my mother at her second job and then we can be together in the evening. I get my little brother after school and we go home to do house work and start cooking and wash the breakfast dishes. When my mother gets home she eats and then we go to her second job, but with my help we finish in 3 hours. It is late by the time I can do my homework and sometimes I fall asleep. My mother wants me to be a nurse, but she doesn't know that you have to go to college and have money and make good grades. My teachers don't understand why I don't finish my homework or stay after school for tutoring. They think that Latinos are not smart and don't care about school. My school has lots of clubs and sports, but I have to go home and help with my little brother and with all the work. I still feel lucky, because at least I know I will be able to go to school somehow and I will be able to get a job. I am happy this program meets at lunch time or I would never learn about what I have to do to become a nurse. Even my parents have come to a parent meeting and they were happy to learn about my dream.

The Latino Nursing Career Opportunity Program (LNCOP) at the Catholic University of America (CUA) is designed to serve the most educationally and economically disadvantaged ethnic and racially diverse groups and specifically to increase the number of Hispanic nurses, the most underrepresented group among registered nurses in the United States. The terms *Hispanic* and *Latino* are used interchangeably by the LNCOP, recognizing that the term *Hispanic* is used in a more global sense to denote language ancestry, and the term *Latino* is used more often to denote ancestry from Latin American countries including Mexico, Central and South America, and the Caribbean. It should also be noted that North Americans of Latin American ancestry often identify themselves as Latino or Hispanic.

The reasons for choosing to implement the Latino Nursing Career Opportunity Program in the District of Columbia and Montgomery County, Maryland, were related to both need and location. Mirroring the United States, the Washington, DC metropolitan area contains a fast growing, largely immigrant Latino population and a shortage of health care providers who adequately meet their specific access and language needs. Educational attainment in the local Hispanic community trails that of other groups. The area is complex, transitory, and struggles with all the attendant challenges of extremes in income, education, and health status, particularly within its minority population. Although the Latino Nursing Career Opportunity Program operates primarily in the District of Columbia and Montgomery County, Maryland, individual students who contact the program from other surrounding counties in both Maryland and Virginia are welcome to participate.

The Catholic University of America School of Nursing (CUA SON) is located in the District of Columbia and borders Montgomery County, Maryland. It is a dense urban area with a large and rapidly growing Hispanic population, and the area is geographically manageable for the administration and implementation of LNCOP activities. The CUA SON, consistently ranked among the top nursing schools in the nation, has a long history of clinical partnerships with health care providers in these jurisdictions. The SON offers baccalaureate, masters, and doctoral degree programs. Although CUA has few enrolled Latino students (5% of the total student body), the University has a strong history of support for and participation in the Latino community and in Latin American countries. The CUA SON initiated a summer nursing camp in 2002 that served as the pilot project for the LNCOP and continues to bring Latino and other diverse high school students interested in nursing to the CUA campus. The LNCOP project seeks to extend that effort as well as to address the pressing nursing shortage.

THE NURSING SHORTAGE AND BARRIERS FOR LATINOS

As the Latino population soars, the nursing shortage continues unabated. Estimates vary for the number of new and replacement nurses who will be needed within the coming 15 years, but the number is staggering. In November 2005, the U.S. Department of Labor Bureau of Labor Statistics estimated 1.2 million additional nurses will be needed by 2014. Auerbach, Buerhaus, and Staiger (2007) recalculated the projected RN shortage, adding increased RN education efforts into the equation, and still projected a shortage of approximately 340,000 registered nurses by the year 2020.

A number of factors contribute to the nursing shortage. A shortage of nursing school faculty restricts enrollments, so nursing schools have had to turn away thousands of qualified prospective students. High turnover rates and job dissatisfaction exacerbate the problem, with the shortage contributing to nursing burnout. Additionally, changing demographics require more nurses to care for the aging U.S. population (American Association of Colleges of Nursing, 2007).

The LNCOP was designed to address the nursing shortage while at the same time meeting the community need for more Latino nurses. Hispanics constitute 14% of the U.S. population, yet, they represent only 1.8% of registered nurses (Anders, Edmonds, Monreal, & Galvan, 2007). The disparity between percentage of the population and percentage of the RN workforce in the United States is greatest for Hispanics (Health Resources and Services Administration [HRSA], 2004) of all groups in society. Despite their underrepresentation in nursing, Hispanic nurses make a strong contribution to the profession. HRSA (2004) reported that 88% of Hispanic nurses are employed in nursing positions, and

75.2% work full time. Villarruel (2002) points out that "minority nurses are more likely to be younger, to stay in nursing longer, to work full time, and to work in health care shortage areas" (p. 11). She advocates addressing the nursing shortage through increasing minority representation in the nursing profession. The Institute of Medicine (IOM, 2004) concluded that minority health care professionals are significantly more likely than Whites to serve minority and medically underserved communities; minority patients, if given a choice, prefer professionals from their own backgrounds; and interaction in health professions training among diverse students broadens the perspectives of all. In order to increase diverse professional representation, promote diverse professional perspectives, and meet the needs of an increasingly diverse population, numerous barriers must be overcome.

Prospective Latino nursing students often encounter barriers in high school to attending college, and as demonstrated in the literature, barriers may also be encountered in the earlier school years (Anders et al., 2007; Canales, 2000; Cantu & Rogers, 2007; Schmidt, 2003; Schwartz, 2001; Taxis, 2002; Villarruel, Canales, & Torres, 2001). The Latino middle and high school students of Washington, DC, and Montgomery County, Maryland, represent varying parent educational and economic levels, racial and ethnic identity, religious affiliation, language capability, and national origin. The Council of Latino Agencies of DC, the DC Public School System, and the Montgomery County Public School System have also reported many students come from recent immigrant families, are limited English proficient (LEP), and are enrolled in English as a Second Language (ESL) classes; many come from homes in which one or both parents never attended school; and many will be the first in their family to graduate from high school or attend college. Washington, DC and Montgomery County Hispanic students report the lowest standardized scores, graduation rates, math and English proficiency, and progression to college of all groups in high school.

When Latino students do make it to college, they have the greatest need for financial and academic support of all groups and will need to learn skills to navigate the academic and social challenges of the university. Hispanic women, in particular, will be challenged to balance personal, academic, and professional goals with familial interdependence. They will need to know that academic success is valued, expected, and achievable; they will require support systems that respond to their academic, health, and social needs; and they will need family and parent involvement and support to ensure their success.

Montgomery County's Latino Health Initiative reported that obtaining a nursing license is a complex and costly process. Barriers include lack of English proficiency, lack of information about the licensing process, cost of licensure (especially for those who must pass English tests), and cost of the NCLEX certification exam. However, Latino nurses bring considerable assets to the health care system. Their motivation is very high, and they have strong roots in the community (Carmen Saenz, Nurses Pilot Program Coordinator, Latino Health Initiative, Montgomery County Department of Health and Human Services, personal communication, October 6, 2005).

The Latino population is increasing rapidly; yet, the nursing workforce does not reflect this demographic, locally or nationally. The status of Latino public school students trails behind their counterparts of all races and ethnicities. Schools at every level disproportionately lack Latino teachers. Nursing faculties at postsecondary nursing schools do not reflect the makeup of the U.S. population as a whole, and many more ethnically and racially diverse professors are needed. In order to achieve proportionate racial and ethnic representation among health professionals, specifically nurses, that reflects the population at large and the patient population, more professional Latino nurses must be educated. This is well-documented in the literature and equally apparent from observation of practice in the local health services arena. The LNCOP is designed to pursue this goal. The following section outlines some of the inroads that this project has made to increase the number of Latino students who are preparing to become registered nurses.

PROGRAM DESCRIPTION: THE LATINO NURSING CAREER OPPORTUNITY PROGRAM

The LNCOP of the CUA SON was designed to meet the following objectives:

1. Design, implement, and evaluate a structured pre-entry nursing program primarily for Hispanic 7–12 grade students attending selected Washington, DC, and Montgomery County, Maryland, middle, junior high, and high schools. Design summer camp and academic year activities for students from all underrepresented groups in nursing to increase the visibility of nursing as

a career, build academic and social supports, and help students learn health promotion skills.

2. Design, implement, and evaluate a faculty development program to build and update cultural competencies and enhance skills in mentoring, advising, and teaching students from racial and ethnic minorities with a focus on Latino students. Conduct a series of faculty development workshops based on a needs assessment survey of area nursing school faculty open to CUA and local area nursing school faculty.
3. Design, implement, and evaluate a comprehensive retention program in the baccalaureate nursing degree program at CUA to increase the retention of Hispanic students. Explore several strategies to provide students with academic, social, and financial resources throughout their undergraduate education, including financial aid support, by providing students with instruction and support in the research, application, and procurement of stipends, scholarships, grants, loans, and other sources of funding.

Although the LNCOP welcomes all interested students to participate in program activities, only those students who meet the definition of having an educationally or economically disadvantaged background, including students who are racial/ethnic minorities underrepresented among nurses, and who express an interest in becoming a registered nurse are eligible for participation in the scholarship and stipend component of the program.

The LNCOP employs four teaching assistants, who are graduate students in the SON, to help with recruitment and retention activities. To date, the program has supported a total of six Spanish-speaking graduate teaching assistants, including four Latinas and one African American, with a monthly stipend. Catholic University provides each with full tuition, an in-kind value of $25,000+ per student/per academic year. The program also provides a work-study position for a Latina undergraduate nursing student supported by non-HRSA federal work-study funds.

Pre-Entry Nursing Activities

Each year, the Latino program director and four program teaching assistants meet weekly during 1–2 hour sessions with approximately 150 students in 11 area high schools with high Latino populations. The weekly sessions with students who self-identify as having an interest in nursing are conducted throughout the school year and consist of predesigned modules on numerous topics, such as: selecting a school of nursing, researching specialties of interest, writing college essays, developing effective study skills, applying for financial aid, attending college open houses, visiting clinical sites, and shadowing nurses in specialties of interest. In addition, the four Latino program teaching assistants are assigned to participating high schools and work one-on-one with students interested in nursing careers.

College and career presentations are also made to "feeder schools," middle schools whose students go on to attend the high schools participating in the Latino program, sometimes in conjunction with career and college fairs that are held in the high schools and middle schools participating in the Latino program.

In addition, the program director, often accompanied by program staff and teaching assistants, meets with and makes presentations to community-based organizations, foundations, boards, hospital and health facilities, professional organizations, and elected leaders active in the Latino community. In the first 3 years of the project, 30 such presentations were made.

The week-long summer camps, piloted at CUA, have become a part of the Latino program. At these camps, students learn academic skills along with health promotion skills and experience working in the nursing practice lab with patient simulation models. The most popular and awe-inspiring of all camp activities has been a tour and observation experience in the neonatal intensive care unit of a local hospital. Observation of open heart surgery is scheduled for the next summer camp experience. The students in the summer camp represent all races and ethnicities: African American; Africans from French- and English-speaking countries; Hispanics from Mexico, Central and South America; Asians from the Indian subcontinent and the Far East; and Whites. To evaluate the experience, students fill out Likert-style satisfaction surveys and provide qualitative comments. Satisfaction among the students has been very high, and several students elected to return the following summer.

Faculty Development Activities

Faculty development workshops are offered to CUA faculty and faculty from other schools of nursing in the mid-Atlantic region. During 2004–2005, three such workshops were held. Approximately 50 faculty members attended each workshop, and a core group of approximately 35 participants attended all three. Workshops focused on understanding the challenges of increasing the number of Hispanic nurses, the recruitment and retention process among high school and college students in order to increase the number of Hispanic nurses, and the faculty role in creating an environment of success for Hispanic and other diverse nursing students. Conferences are evaluated using Likert-style satisfaction scales and qualitative comments. Satisfaction for the programs has been high with participants indicating high interest in continued dialogue and active efforts for recruitment of Latinos into their nursing programs.

The program director has also presented workshops at the American Nurses Association annual convention, the National Association of Hispanic Nurses (NAHN) annual convention, and the National Hispanic Medical Association annual convention. Presentations have also been made to individual schools of nursing, and plans to present a faculty workshop in the Boston area during the 2008 NAHN annual conference are underway.

Recruitment and Retention Activities

The university is working to establish a year-long program of student support services for incoming freshman at CUA to enhance recruitment, achievement, and retention of Latino students in nursing. Faculty and staff of the school of nursing participate in orientation activities for first-year students, during which diverse students are invited to the school of nursing to explore careers in nursing and experience a day in the life of a nursing student. Students visit nursing classes, libraries, computer and skills labs; tour the campus; meet nurses in various specialties; learn about financial aid opportunities; learn about academic support services and academic skills development; and have the opportunity for discussions with nursing students, nursing faculty, and nurse presenters.

The LNCOP has supported 21 eligible minority students, both Latino and African American, with stipends and awarded six undergraduate scholarships to five Latinos and one African American who were enrolled full time in a school of nursing of their choice.

Prior to enrolling in the CUA school of nursing and while enrolled in the school of nursing, students work closely with the program director and teaching assistants to secure funding for tuition and other college expenses, participate in internships, attend professional meetings, obtain tutoring and other academic support, attend leadership camps and workshops, and participate in community health and service experiences. Three Latina students currently have National Institutes of Health internships and will present their research at the next NAHN annual conference.

COLLABORATION WITH COMMUNITY PARTNERS

During the first year of the grant, it took considerable effort to identify faculty, administrators, and counselors at each high school who had an interest in the work of the Latino program and who were willing to support the work of the project. However, the LNCOP is now well established in the partner high schools that have a high number of Latino students. Strong relations with the participating high schools have resulted in large numbers of students participating in the program. To date, program staff have worked with and compiled data on approximately 290 school visits per year, including approximately 1,000 students and 100 parent and 75 teacher/counselor/administrator contacts. These inroads into the schools, as well as contacts that have been developed with Latino parents and Latino community-based youth-serving organizations, extra-curricular future nurses clubs, Latino clubs, Latino parent groups, and international student organizations have allowed us to both continue and increase support to students.

Strong connections with area nursing schools and community colleges have also been established. In fact, three members of the program's advisory board are from other schools of nursing, including the dean of health sciences at Montgomery College and faculty from Prince George's Community College and the 4-year Bowie State program. These connections augment the Latino program and support recruitment and retention of Latino and other diverse nursing students.

There is ongoing collaboration with schools, colleges, student groups, community-based organizations, parent groups, and health facilities and "linking" of these groups so that collaboration and pre-entry preparation will continue after project completion. In addition, there is ongoing systematic effort and collaboration with counselors, teachers, school nurses, administrators, and parent groups in the partner schools to ensure structured access to information on nursing careers presently and in the future.

PROGRAM PARTICIPANT DATA

To date, data have been assessed for 226 high school students who have participated in the program. While a third of the students enrolled in the program during their senior year, over 50% joined between 9th and 11th grade; of these, 117 were referred by a teacher, 22 by a mentor, and 83 by a school counselor. Approximately 60% of the student participants are Hispanic/Latino. Other ethnicities include: Black/African American (22%), Asian (8%), Caucasian (2%), and mixed heritage (5%). Of note, 75% of students reported that they work either full or part time, and at least 33% have childcare responsibilities in addition to school requirements. On entry to the program, almost 60% reported a specific interest in nursing or other health-related field as a career with another 11% stating their intent to pursue a college education following high school. Fifty-four percent of the students met with program staff between 1–8 times in individual, small group, or large group sessions. Contacts ranged in frequency from 1–32 in number with an average duration of an hour per session, with a range of 20 minutes to 3 hours per contact across the past year. Purposes for the student contacts included: general information sessions, counseling, and study modules.

Of importance to note is that most of the high school students who participated in the Latino program and who graduated from high school are currently enrolled in 2-year community and 4-year colleges. At least seven who graduated from partner high schools are attending nursing schools, and several others are enrolled in prenursing courses or pursuing careers in health care.

Qualitative data confirm the important role that the LNCOP has played in recruiting and retaining Latino and other underrepresented students in nursing, as evidenced by the following texts of e-mails received from seven stipend and scholarship recipients:

> *I thank you for greeting me for my first semester at college. I must say it was a big challenge for me, never thought it could be this hard. But as the days pass I improve in my college classes and realize I must keep going. Hopefully, I will be getting my final grades soon by this or the next week. I will e-mail it to you otherwise can I mail it to you?*
>
> *My summer internship was a success; I really enjoyed working at NIH. I was able to run PCR's and Gels as well as many other things. It's one summer experience I won't forget. I am back in school now and I am taking Microbiology with a Lab, Chemistry with a lab, Ecological Theology, Philosophy and Modern Dance (This fulfills my physical education*

requirement). Classes seem like they will be tough but I feel like I'm on a good start. Labs seem like they will be a lot of fun. I will soon be sending my midterm grades and I hope all is well. Thank you for your kindness and I will continue to stay in touch.

I know it's been a long time. Just wanted to let you guys know I'm doing well . . . this semester has been really crazy. It is really hard compared to last semester, but I'm getting closer to the real nursing courses so I'm really excited. Hope all is good!!

The funds are in my account. Thank you so much for everything! God Bless.

Yes, I'm attending Columbia Union College (4-years, fulltime) next year and I will be staying on campus. And I plan on pursuing nursing as a career. Thanks for everything.

The Latino Nursing Scholarship has made it possible for me to afford to go to Nursing School. I am indeed grateful to have this help. Being a recipient of the scholarship is also motivational because it lets me know people do care; moreover it fuels the desire for me to keep good grades.

Thank you so much for your offer. I have definitely not thanked you enough for all the opportunities you have given me for the past 2 years. I've definitely learned so much, and enjoyed working with you. Thanks for thinking of me and caring.

CONCLUSION

The LNCOP is designed to improve access to quality health care through appropriate preparation, composition, and distribution of the health professions workforce, to improve access to a diverse and culturally competent and sensitive health professions workforce by increasing the number of bilingual Latino nurses, and to further prepare culturally competent and sensitive nursing faculty and students.

The program has been encouraged and supported by the dean of the school of nursing and by the highest levels of administration of the Catholic University of America. The CUA SON faculty members have responded in a positive and supportive manner to the Latino program initiatives and the diverse students who have enrolled in the school of nursing.

Introducing new initiatives, even in supportive environments, can be challenging, however. Faculty members from throughout the mid-Atlantic attending diversity workshops have revealed that even when diversity is encouraged, faculty members often experience conflict between acknowledging the importance of the recruitment and retention of diverse students in nursing and the lack of time and recognition allotted for work done on such projects. Tenure-track faculty are focused on the "hoops" already in their path, and nontenure-track faculty are either in part-time positions that already require too many preparation hours for the hours actually reimbursed or in clinical positions in which faculty see students only in the clinical area with little, if any, opportunity to mentor or advise students or be involved with recruitment and retention activities.

Other faculty have reported a lack of faculty interest in their schools and the belief by some faculty that recruitment and retention of students is not their responsibility. One workshop participant reported being told that diversity was welcome as long as it did not entail "dumbing down" the curriculum. Workshop participants have reported experiences as varied as schools offering courses in Spanish for Health Professionals and establishing discussion groups to increase Spanish conversational skills, to schools in which faculty openly stated that it was not their job to cater to diversity and foreign languages. If diversity is not already an important issue to school administrators, it may be difficult, but not impossible, to implement programs that seek to increase diversity in nursing.

RECOMMENDATIONS FOR NURSING EDUCATION ADMINISTRATORS

The recommendations that follow for nursing education administrators and nursing educators are based on the work of the LNCOP to foster commitment to higher education among diverse students and a belief that it is the innate responsibility of every teacher and professor to link students with the specific services that nurture academic, social, cultural, and spiritual development and the responsibility of every administrator to support such involvement of teachers and administrators.

- Support faculty and staff in doing in-depth work with students and their parents. It is critical to introduce high school graduates who plan to go on to college to the exciting and varied careers in nursing and to support them through their transition from high school into college.
- Bring together educators who are researching and publishing in the area of mentoring and advising students and who impact the retention of underrepresented students in nursing.

- Encourage faculty to participate in workshops and conferences to update cultural competencies and enhance their skills in mentoring, advising, and teaching students from disadvantaged backgrounds underrepresented in nursing.
- Establish a peer mentoring project and develop peer mentoring education.
- Develop courses in Spanish for health professionals.
- Establish summer camps for minority youth to become familiar with the campus culture and become enthused and knowledgeable about the nursing profession.
- Host health facility and college visits for middle and high school students each semester.
- Explore sources of funding and procure stipends and scholarships for Latino students. Potential sources are: private foundations, financial assistance programs, scholarships, reduced tuition arrangements, School of Nursing funding, and tuition payback agreements with prospective employers.
- Establish an advisory board of Latino nurse leaders to assure community participation, continuous improvement, and achievement of project objectives.
- Sponsor faculty recognition and/or reward events to honor the work faculty have done on recruitment and retention projects. This would both encourage faculty participation and recognize the increased workload required by these projects.

RECOMMENDATIONS FOR NURSE EDUCATORS

- Research diversity topics and issues and bring them to the attention of administration and faculty.
- Attend diversity workshops and conferences to augment your knowledge and sustain your beliefs and interest.
- Seek external funding for project implementation.
- Integrate your interest in diversity in nursing into requirements for publication, community service, continuing education, clinical practice, and tenure-track requirements.
- Work with hospitals and other clinical sites and schools that are supportive of a diverse nursing workforce.
- Attend mentoring workshops, and learn the difference between mentoring and advising.

- Familiarize yourself with academic support services and other student service offices in the university. In much the same way that a nurse investigates services and referrals for clients, educators should be able to "refer" students to academic, health, and social services; cultural activities; and spiritual support groups. Follow-up with students just as you would with a client.
- Establish contacts that you can call directly in each student support and service area.

For those nursing faculty and administrators who are willing to become involved in projects such as the LNCOP, the rewards are great. The past 5 years of work that I have been involved in as project director for the Latino program have included some of the most rewarding work I have ever done in nursing, in education, and in the community with adolescents and college students, with parent groups, and among fellow professionals.

QUESTIONS FOR DIALOGUE

1. What ideas or concepts did you find most meaningful in this chapter? Identify your insights and questions to bring to a dialogue with your colleagues.
2. Is there a fast growing Latino population in your community? If there is a growing Latino population in your community, what specific barriers exist that are unique to this population? If no, what is the fastest growing minority population in your community, and what specific barriers do they face in attending your institution? What is your institution doing to minimize these barriers?
3. For faculty involved in efforts to recruit and retain minority students at your institution, what recognition and compensation is and/or should administration make available to encourage faculty and staff to do this important work?
4. What initiatives are in place in your institution to reach out to minority students at the middle and high school level? Dialogue with colleagues about the unique obstacles and opportunities for developing productive relationships with faculty, administrators, and counselors in local schools.

5. In addition to middle schools and high schools, what other community-based youth-serving organizations could you partner with to increase the visibility of and interest in nursing as a profession? What resources could you mobilize to do this work? How might your students serve as role models in the community?
6. What can you do in your school of nursing to mentor nurse leaders from minority communities—for example, through graduate assistantships, teaching assistantships, work study positions, collaboration on research projects, coauthorship of publications, and internships in your institution as well as in research institutions in the surrounding community. Dialogue with colleagues about how you can set up these and/or other opportunities for minority nurse leadership development.

REFERENCES

American Association of Colleges of Nursing. (2007). *Nursing shortage fact sheet.* Retrieved May 20, 2008, from http://www.aacn.nche.edu/Media/FactSheets/NursingShortage.htm

Anders, R. L., Edmonds, V. M., Monreal, H., & Galvan, M. R. (2007). *Hispanic Health Care International, 5*(3), 128–135.

Auerbach, D. I., Buerhaus, P. I., & Staiger, D. O. (2007). Better late than never: Workforce supply implications of later entry into nursing. *Health Affairs, 26*(1), 178–185.

Canales, M. (2000). Othering: Toward an understanding of difference. *Advances in Nursing Science, 22*(4), 16–31.

Cantu, A. G., & Rogers, N. M. (2007). Creating a mentoring and community culture in nursing. *Hispanic Health Care International, 5*(3), 124–127.

Health Resources and Services Administration (HRSA). (2004). *The Registered Nurse population: Findings from the National Sample Survey of Registered Nurses.* Retrieved May 20, 2008, from http://bhpr.hrsa.gov/healthworkforce/reports/rnsurvey

Institute of Medicine (IOM). (2004). *In The Nation's Compelling Interest: Ensuring Diversity in the Healthcare Workforce, Executive Summary.* Washington, DC: National Academies Press.

Schmidt, P. (2003, November 28). Academe's Hispanic future. *The Chronicle of Higher Education, 50*(14), A8.

Schwartz, W. (2001). *Strategies for improving the educational outcomes of Latinas.* Retrieved May 20, 2008, from http://www.ericdigests.org/2002-2/latinas.htm

Taxis, J. C. (2002). The underrepresentation of Hispanics/Latinos in nursing education: A deafening silence. *Research and Theory for Nursing Practice: An International Journal, 16*(4), 249–261.

Villarruel, A. (2002). Recruiting minority nurses: We're asking ourselves the wrong questions. *American Journal of Nursing, 102*(5), 11.

Villarruel, A. M., Canales, M., & Torres, S. (2001). Bridges and barriers: Educational mobility of Hispanic nurses. *Journal of Nursing Education, 40*(6), 245–251.

14 Barriers to Success: American Indian Students in Nursing

JUDY JACOBY
MONTANA LITTLE SHELL TRIBE OF CHIPPEWA

A 30-year-old American Indian student is enrolled in a competitive bachelor of nursing program. As a single parent with three children under the age of six, she has succeeded in her personal goal of pursuing her college education. She is in the last semester of her junior year. This last year has been a hard one. Even though financially it has been hard to make ends meet, she has continued in her nursing program. She does not feel comfortable with communicating with her advisor or nursing faculty about the problems that are occurring in her personal life or that she is American Indian (her mother is an enrolled member of a tribe and her deceased father was Caucasian). School rumors are that American Indian students do not get through this program.

A year before, she had failed one of the nursing courses due to health problems. The fear of failure to progress in the program raises her stress. Her mother reminds her that she can do this, "Look how far you have come. You made it through high school, and I know you can do this." Her mother's support has been an impetus to keep on going. She will be the first in her family with a college education. Neither of her parents graduated from high school.

In gratitude to my mother, Theresa Doney Erickson, who continues to support me and guide me with her wisdom and prayers.

Sitting in class, she is given a note by one of the nursing site directors to come to her office after class. In the meeting, she is told that she has failed her second course and will need to drop out of the nursing program. Awe-stricken and shaken about the news, she packs up her books and heads for home.

She calls her mother who is living out of state and tells her the depressing news that she is no longer in the program. She reminds herself that she is a licensed practical nurse and is glad she has something to fall back on.

Later on in the week there is a knock at the door; it's her mother. She has decided to move in and states she will not let her daughter give up the idea of a college degree. Her mother tells her, "There are other nursing schools in this state. You need to keep on trying and don't give up." She throws some of her daughter's clothes into a small suitcase and tells her to drive to the other nursing college over a hundred miles away and check out the program. The young mother of three drives over 2 hours and meets with the dean of a 2-year program. After reviewing her transcripts, the dean states she is willing to accept her and then explains to her what is expected and that she can start classes in four weeks. Overwhelmed with relief, the Indian woman accepts the guidance from the Dean and enrolls into a new program. The Indian woman explains to the Dean her background and the hardships she has encountered. The Dean explains to the Indian student, "We have many Indian students throughout the state that attend here; you will not be alone."

One year later, the young Indian woman is standing with her mother at her nurse pinning ceremony along with her three small children. Tears of joy come from both the Indian woman and her mother. She has completed her associate degree in nursing.

Eight years later, the same nursing program opens up a bachelor's program and contacts the Indian nurse. She applies to the program and graduates with a bachelor's degree in nursing.

This story illustrates the need for nursing programs that reach out to American Indian students and help them be successful despite other obstacles in their lives. Once this student found a program that was welcoming and supportive, she succeeded in accomplishing her goal of becoming a nurse and graduating with a baccalaureate degree. Similar to this college, the University of North Dakota (UND) has created a welcoming and supportive environment for Native American students in nursing. Indeed, since the creation of the Recruitment/Retention of

American Indians Into Nursing (RAIN) program in 2000, the number of baccalaureate-prepared Native American nursing students has increased seven-fold, and the recruitment and retention of Native American students into nursing at the UND continues to thrive. Many schools of nursing have inquired about UND's RAIN program and its effective strategies for success (University of North Dakota College of Nursing, 2005). This chapter begins with a description of the mentorship model that is used in the RAIN program, followed by the history of the RAIN program, and then discusses what has helped American Indian students obtain their degrees, as well as some of the obstacles that make it difficult for them to complete their studies. Oral traditions, storytelling, and other aspects of American Indian culture, such as humor, are also described and explained, as well as how they influence the world view of American Indian students.

A MENTORSHIP MODEL FOR NATIVE AMERICAN NURSING STUDENTS

Nugent, Childs, Jones, and Cook (2004) describe the challenges that Indian students face in education. Indian students must deal with a change in culture when they leave their homes to go to college. In addition, the adjustment to college life can be difficult. The cultural shock that Indian students face can affect their study habits, test-taking skills, reading comprehension, and writing, along with their communication skills. Differences in communicative style between American Indian students and non-Native instructors make it difficult for American Indians to analyze and synthesize information they encounter in their classes. Indian students often learn by visual or tactile demonstrations and practice; therefore, lectures that explain skills or ideas without demonstrating those skills and allowing students to redemonstrate them can hinder the Indian students' ability to learn the material.

In response to these challenges, Nugent et al. (2004) propose a mentorship model. This model creates an educational learning environment supporting the needs of all students regardless of their cultural, ethnic, or gender background. This model uses concepts of mentorship, faculty and institutional support, and academic support, including providing financial support and opportunities for self-development and professional and leadership development. First, academic support is provided in the form of tutoring and remedial support for students. In addition, mentors provide students with an introduction to what the experience of nursing school will be like before they begin the program. Second, students are provided with personal and emotional support. This support helps them adjust to the new environment of college life and be successful in their academics, and as a result, students experience self-development. Third, students are introduced to the concept of professionalism and strategies for achieving their career goals. Fourth, there is support for the recruitment and retention of minority students. This initiative includes providing educational workshops that teach nursing faculty the importance of understanding differences in cultural ways with minority students.

The RAIN program and other Indian educational programs that exist at the University of North Dakota address the problems described by Nugent et al. (2004) and incorporate a mentorship model into their programs and services. In addition, to increase the role of faculty as mentors, in the fall of 2006, RAIN implemented Faculty Involved in RAIN Efforts (FIRE), a committee that involves nursing faculty in the education of Indian students. The hope is that by faculty being involved in RAIN and thereby gaining knowledge of American Indian culture, their ability to reach out to Indian students and become mentors will be enhanced. Faculty who have been immersed in Indian Country, who have visited or lived among American Indians on reservations or in urban areas, have an emic or inside view of Indian culture and, as a result, are able to communicate to Indian students effectively and help other faculty develop an emic view of the culture. In addition, RAIN students have become mentors for American Indian students who are new in the program. Such mentorship has empowered students to succeed.

HISTORY OF THE RAIN PROGRAM

In the 20 years prior to the RAIN program, from 1973 to 1993, only 19 American Indians graduated with their bachelor of science in nursing (BSN) from the University of North Dakota. The RAIN program began in the early 1990s when the Indian Health Service (IHS) began to strongly support the need to increase the number of American Indian nurses. In 2005, over 300 registered nurse positions were vacant within the IHS (2006). UND's College of Nursing started the RAIN program because Indian nurses were needed throughout Indian Country to assist Indian populations with culturally appropriate care. The

UND Medical School has had a successful medical school program for Native Americans in place since 1973.

Between 1990, when RAIN was established, and 2007, 129 American Indian nurses have graduated with a baccalaureate degree in nursing; since 1995, 30 American Indian nurses have graduated with a master's degree, 20% of whom have continued on to pursue their doctoral degree. According to a recent study (Moss et al., 2005), only 12 American Indian nurses hold a doctorate in the United States. At the time of this writing, the first American Indian PhD student enrolled in RAIN was in the second cohort of PhD courses at UND. Currently, 95% of American Indian BSN graduates of RAIN work with Indian people, and 90% of the master's-prepared nurse graduates of RAIN work with Indian populations. Of significant interest is that 63% of the nursing staff on one reservation in North Dakota graduated from RAIN.

The RAIN program is part of the Quentin N. Burdick Indian Health Programs at the University of North Dakota, which includes other Indian programs, such as Indian Students into Medical School (INMED) and Indians into Psychology Doctoral Education (INPSYDE). In 2004, a nursing workforce diversity grant was received from the Department of Health and Human Services for Working for Indian Nurse Development (WIND) and is part of the RAIN program, providing partial financial support for recruitment and retention.

DESCRIPTION OF THE RAIN PROGRAM

The Dean of the UND's College of Nursing administers the RAIN program. The RAIN personnel consist of five people: the Coordinator, who has a counseling degree and is from one of North Dakota's tribes; a nurse mentor; a science mentor; an English and writing mentor; and a secretary. The RAIN office area includes a study room and five computers for students to use. This close arrangement of office and study areas makes it easy for students to access needed services within the program.

The coordinator and mentors of RAIN complete annual trips throughout several states and multiple reservations. On these trips, the coordinator and mentors of RAIN attend American Indian conferences and give presentations explaining the RAIN program to tribal colleges and other interested parties. The coordinator position, however, involves more than recruitment; she is also involved in counseling and mentoring. She is readily available to students when they encounter obstacles to their education. In her role as coordinator, she creates an atmosphere in the RAIN program that builds trust and camaraderie among the students. An open door policy has been implemented since the beginning of the RAIN program, which means that the coordinator and mentors of RAIN are easily accessible. For example, RAIN students can have access to the computer labs and mentors anytime the offices are open.

The nurse mentor helps students with planning and doing primary research and finding secondary resources, teaches study skills to students, and guides them in preparing for presentations and exams. She also provides one-to-one help for students with learning disabilities. Nursing texts, dictionaries, and several professional journals are available in the RAIN office for students. If students are having difficulties getting their financial aid on time, textbooks are provided to them until their funding comes in.

The science mentor is in continuous contact with RAIN students who are taking science courses, helping each student develop a study plan, providing supplemental instruction and learning materials, and assisting students in improving study skills and in developing collegial rapport with their science instructors. Such mentoring support helps students accomplish the challenging professional and personal goals they have set for themselves.

The primary role of the English and writing mentor is to assist students with the extensive writing requirements at UND's College of Nursing. Each student has a writing assessment completed on initial entry into the program. During the course of the program the mentor helps students develop writing skills through workshops and handouts. The writing mentor also assists with teaching the students how to draft their papers.

In addition to mentors and computer labs, scholarships, financial aid assistance, and tuition waivers are made available to RAIN students through the UND's financial aid programs. RAIN mentors assist students in applying for these scholarships. Assistance in selecting appropriate prenursing courses at tribal colleges in preparation for admission to the College of Nursing at UND is provided by RAIN personnel in conjunction with tribal college personnel. Cooperation and communication between tribal colleges and the RAIN program contribute to the success of students in completing the appropriate prenursing courses necessary for admission to the RAIN program.

The RAIN staff provides an orientation program for their students a week before fall semester begins. This orientation introduces the student to resources available to help them succeed on campus, including tutoring, childcare, transportation, and counseling services. The orientation builds a supportive network, assisting the students and giving them the tools they need to stay focused on their studies. Because many of the RAIN students have children, families are included in the orientation. The amount of studying required for classes is explained to the spouses and family members so they understand what is expected of the RAIN student.

The RAIN program has encouraged American Indian students to act as mentors for each other. Through mentorship and camaraderie, Indian students build a culture of learning; resilience is created and strengthened among students to overcome obstacles and to achieve their goal of completing the nursing program. The University of North Dakota has more than one program for Indian students, and if the nursing student is not able to find the right mentor in his or her area of study, Native American faculty in other departments have participated in helping Native American nursing students succeed.

RAIN has clearly been successful in increasing the number of Native American nurses. In the 17 years since RAIN was established, 129 American Indian students have graduated with a baccalaureate degree in nursing, compared to 19 in the previous 20 years. The retention and graduation rate for RAIN students is greater than 88%.

BARRIERS TO SUCCESS FOR AMERICAN INDIAN STUDENTS

One barrier that makes it difficult for American Indian students to succeed is faculty who lack understanding of historical laws that have impacted Indian people and who have little knowledge about the culture of Indian people. Many knowledgeable, insightful non-Native and American Indian authors (Cohen, 1988; Deloria, 1969; Getches, Wilkinson, & Williams, 1998; Lopach, Brown, & Clow, 1998; O'Brien, 1993; Pevar, 2002; Wilkins, 1997) have published books regarding the historical relationship between the federal government and Indian people and the effects these laws have had on Indian populations of the United States. Especially valuable is Pevar's *Rights of Indians and Tribes* (2002), which explains the federal laws affecting American Indians from the time of their implementation to today and the influence they have had on Indian populations. Another essential text is O'Brien's *American Indian Tribal Governments* (1993), which explains how the sovereignty of American Indian communities functions in today's societies. In order to serve Indian students effectively, faculty should be familiar with the issues addressed in these books. Many Indian people believe in the influence of the past on the present. Barton (2004) describes the aboriginal epistemology, including the sacredness of the medicine wheel and the circular connections that American Indian people live by. Past processes that have occurred with American Indian people continue to influence current processes. The importance of the past reaffirms the need for nursing faculty to know about and understand the historical relationship that Indian populations have had with the federal government and the effect federal laws that were implemented to address Native American issues have had on Native American people.

Another barrier American Indian students face is having teachers with no familiarity with, or understanding of, Indian culture and the way of life on the reservation. One important cultural factor faculty need to be aware of is the strength of family ties among American Indian people—ties that extend to distant relatives and friends. For example, one student in the RAIN program had a friend in the family who was considered to be her "grandmother." This honored family friend was not blood-related but in Indian culture had strong ties to the student's family and was considered a "grandmother." This grandmother became seriously ill. The student had just arrived as a new student at the university to start classes. She was extremely upset and felt the need to return home to be with her "grandmother." In the U.S. culture and in many U.S. companies, this person would not be considered a close relative, and this situation would not be viewed as serious enough for the student to be excused from class or from work. The student's parents understood how non-Indians would view the situation and explained to the student that it would be best if she stayed at school in the nursing program. The student, however, was extremely distraught and unable to concentrate on her studies in a very rigorous nursing program. She felt uneasy being so far away from the one who was ill because in Indian cultures families gather in situations like this. Staying away was not her tradition, and she felt guilty about not being at home. After counseling with mentors at RAIN, the student took time off and went home to see her "grandmother" for the last time. When she returned, she was ready to continue with her education because she had met her family needs and her own personal needs.

Establishing family-like ties with other Native American students, many of whom are in the RAIN program, provides support for Native American students away from home. Students find it hard to adjust to college when some of them live more than 10 to 15 hours away from their families. One student, who is a mother, commented: "I came here from another state because there were nurses at my reservation who had graduated from this program. They told me that it is here that there would be support for me to get started in a nursing program and help me over obstacles that I would encounter. I have partnered with other Indian students to study; we have shared babysitting for our children and provided transportation. There is networking that is like at home (on the reservation). It is like a big family at times supporting each other."

Another student returned for her master's degree because she had completed her bachelor's degree at this university. This time, she came as a single parent with four children and one grandchild. She received a scholarship, which gave her financial resources so she could focus on completing her master's degree in nursing without worrying about money to support her family. She had worked over 8 years on her reservation as a community health nurse. She said: "I came back because I want to do more on the reservation at the grassroots level. I know that if I increase my education, I can be more than a nurse. I will be able to do management and initiate Indian programs that can be run by our own people." She also spoke of the difficulties she and her family faced living away from home:

> Life on the reservation is extremely different; there families support each other. When we leave the reservation, which is over 10 hours away, it's hard to be without that support. It's hard on my children this time because they are older. At home they were at the top of their class, but when we came here, their roles changed. They were leaders in their class and in sports. My children do not have the support they did at home and are having difficulty with the culture of the school system here. (Indian children find it hard to compete when there are no support programs for them within the school.) I know I have made a good choice to return to school, but I also see that my children have had to suffer somewhat with my decision. They are finding school more difficult and are not at the top of their class. They are looked down upon and are not asked to be on the basketball team. But they have met other Native American friends and have connected with other families on campus.

Authors Gardner (2005), Labun (2002), and Weaver (1999) give insight regarding some of the barriers that Native American students face and their failures and successes in overcoming these barriers. Gardner completed in-depth interviews that mirror what American

Indian nursing students in the RAIN program have voiced about feeling isolated because of the distance from their families of support. Knowledgeable faculty who are well versed in what life is like living on the reservation or living with Native American culture have a greater insight into the culture of the Indian student. Gardner gives a strong voice for the need to have nurse educators who are racial and ethnic minorities for the benefit of all nursing students.

Labun (2002) describes the process of recruiting several groups of minorities for the College of Nursing in Red River in Manitoba, Canada, and the development of a nursing program to address the needs of minorities in particular. Labun stresses the importance of addressing cross-cultural concerns of minority students. Labun describes how faculty questioned their students about what the students wanted or did not want to hear during classes about their culture or what was appropriate to discuss with regard to Indian culture and other cultures alike. Labun discusses the importance of building cross-cultural relationships, along with focusing on similarities among cultures rather than differences.

NATIVE AMERICAN CULTURAL TRADITIONS: STORYTELLING, NARRATIVE EPISTEMOLOGY, AND HUMOR

Storytelling, oral traditions, humor, and the culture of Native American communities are closely tied together. Indian communities learn by listening to elders tell stories of why certain cultural traditions are done the way they are. Children learn, or are educated, through storytelling. Barton (2004) describes the epistemology of aboriginal storytelling. She explains stories or the narratives she heard while working with aboriginal populations and the importance of listening to stories to learn the ways of knowing in the Indian culture: "The meanings derived from hidden phenomena demonstrate knowledge and reflective hermeneutic thinking, a process requiring no clear method with procedural steps" (p. 521). An example of this kind of storytelling and how it relates to health care is as follows:

An elderly Native American Indian woman had been on dialysis for 3 years. One day, a Native nurse asked the woman what dietary teaching she and her husband had received since she began dialysis. The husband pulled out of his bag a handful of reading material regarding dialysis and proceeded to explain that this was what had been given to him and his wife. When asked if he had read the material, he shook his head no.

The couple's primary language was their Native language, making English their second language. Though both had a sixth grade level of education, these elders were revered in their Indian community and well respected by their own people and other Indian communities. When asked what would be the right way to teach about foods, the elder replied: "As a child I was told to use all of my senses: vision to see, ears to hear, nose to smell, and hands to feel. Watching the birth of a new bird is with all of my senses. The egg is from the mother bird. I can see and touch the egg. I wait to see the new bird crack out of its shell. This is the way I can learn."

At their next meeting, the Native nurse and a dietician brought examples of foods of the right consistency and amounts of fluids, carbohydrates, protein, and calories, and proceeded to teach nutrition and make dietary recommendations for the dialysis patient and her husband. At the end of the dietary teaching, the elder looked at the plastic models of food and replied: "Pretty tasty food." The dietician and Native nurse had addressed the seeing and feeling part of learning for the couple, but had ignored taste and smell.

As illustrated in this story, humor is very much a part of Indian culture, just as storytelling is part of Indian teaching. Humor is used in many tribal entities to make a point, especially a political point. Indian artists and cartoonists have used their humor to illustrate the relationship that federally recognized tribes have had with the federal government. One cartoon that comes to mind was printed in the *Spokesman's Review* (a local newspaper in Spokane, Washington) when the legislature was pushing for the regulation of Indian casinos. The Indian cartoonist drew an Indian chief standing in line for a lotto ticket asking, "Is this where the money is?" On his shirt was the name of his tribal casino.

Dean (2003) eloquently writes: "Despite individual differences in humor appreciation, tribal variations, and continued exposure to the dominant culture, distinctive humor persists within the tribes" (p. 63). Deloria (1969) regards Native American humor as being sometimes punctuated with the frustration, anger, and shame of past circumstances of oppression and forced values. The truth is that humor has been used to make life bearable and has helped with the resilience in Indian people.

This humor exists today with Native American nursing students. To help endure the hard work and to sustain themselves in nursing programs miles from home, students use humor and laugh with each other. This does not mean nursing programs or lessons are viewed as insignificant. Laughter is used as a coping mechanism to deal with the stresses that come from a rigorous training program. In addition, the sharing of humor creates strong trusting ties and builds kindred relationships between faculty and American Indian students.

COMPLETING THE EDUCATIONAL JOURNEY

After American Indian nursing students in the RAIN program have completed their nursing studies, students participate in a traditional Indian meal and blanket ceremony. A Pendleton blanket is given to each RAIN graduate of the University of North Dakota in recognition of the successful completion of his or her degree. The students in RAIN bring traditional dishes to the meal where they engage in a blessing along with traditional drum music. This is a time when the congratulated students are able to thank professors and instructors for assisting them in obtaining their degree and for families to celebrate the graduates' success. A "give away" is done from the students to their families, friends, professors, or instructors who have assisted them along their educational journey; this is when the student gives something away to show their appreciation. This is the end of the educational journey and the beginning for a new quest to care for our Indian people who possess increased health care disparities (Parker, Haldane, Keltner, Strickland, & Tom-Orme, 2002). We know that with our education, we will make a difference. We will positively impact the future health and survival of American Indians.

RECOMMENDATIONS FOR NURSE EDUCATORS

To teach Native Americans more effectively, it would be helpful for nursing faculty to know about Indian history and culture. Faculty could gain this knowledge by taking classes in Indian studies or by having a general understanding of federal laws that affect Native Americans. Traditional Native American culture could be shared with non-Native faculty through workshops or weekend seminars developed by Native American facilitators. Such education should include discussion of differences in communication styles, such as nonverbal cues or body language. By learning about American Indian culture and differences in communication style, faculty will be able to communicate more effectively with American Indian students and, thus, help to establish relationships of mutual trust and respect.

The second recommendation is to have non–Native American nurses work within the IHS for a summer to gain experience in Native American health issues and health care delivery systems, both federal health care and tribal health care systems. Another possibility is to implement an exchange program between Indian nurses working in IHS and non-Indian nurses working in larger community hospitals off the reservation. Such an exchange program could also be implemented for nursing students, similar to the international exchange student programs of many universities, except this exchange would be within the United States. This would enhance the cultural understanding between non–Native Americans and Native Americans involved in the exchange programs and help to reduce disparities in health care for American Indians.

QUESTIONS FOR DIALOGUE

1. What ideas or concepts did you find most meaningful in this chapter? Identify your insights and questions to bring to a dialogue with your colleagues.
2. Review the exemplar at the beginning of Jacoby's chapter. Are stories like this common in your nursing program? What were you feeling as you read this story? What helped this student succeed? What prevents faculty and administrators from compassionately and personally reaching out and meeting individual students at their point of need?
3. To what extent should faculty take into consideration family and community demands on students' time? What are the programmatic and ethical implications of these considerations?
4. What are some of the most important historical events in the history of indigenous people in your country that nurse educators should know about and weave into their teaching?
5. Jacoby states, "Faculty who have been immersed in Indian Country, who have visited or lived among American Indians on reservations or in urban areas, have an emic or inside view of Indian culture and, as a result, are able to communicate to Indian students effectively and help other faculty develop an emic view of the culture." What are faculty in your program

doing to develop knowledge and understanding of other cultures through immersion experiences? Discuss the value of immersion experiences over and above simply reading about cultures different from your own. Why might these experiences be especially important for faculty members who are from the dominant culture?

6. Reread Dr. Smith's foreword in which she recommends we think beyond the typical paradigm of majority versus minority groups in society and consider the capacity of minority nurses to both discriminate against and support each other across cultures. What kind of immersion experiences and opportunities could be offered across minority cultures to strengthen solidarity, cultural understanding, and the ability to reduce health disparities?

REFERENCES

Barton, S. (2004). Narrative inquiry: Locating Aboriginal epistemology in a relational methodology. *Journal of Advanced Nursing, 45*(5), 519–526.

Cohen, F. (1988). *Handbook of Federal Indian Law.* Buffalo, NY: William S. Hein.

Dean, R. (2003). Native American humor: Implications for transcultural care. *Journal of Transcultural Nursing, 14*(1), 62–65.

Deloria, V. (1969). *Custer died for your sins.* New York: Macmillan.

Gardner, J. (2005). Barriers influencing the success of racial and ethnic minority students in nursing programs. *Journal of Transcultural Nursing, 16*(2), 155–162.

Getches, D., Wilkinson, C., & Williams, R. (1998). *Cases and materials on Federal Indian Law* (4th ed.). St. Paul, MN: West Group.

Indian Health Service (IHS) (2006). Retrieved December 1, 2006, from http://www.ihs.gov/MedicalPrograms/ncona/documents/NursingUpdate2006-SandyHaldane.pdf

Labun, E. (2002). The Red River College model: Enhancing success for Native Canadian and other nursing students from disenfranchised groups. *Journal of Transcultural Nursing, 13*(4), 311–317.

Lopach, J., Brown, M., & Clow, R. (1998). *Tribal government today.* Niwot, CO: University Press of Colorado.

Moss, M., Tibbetts, L., Henly, S., Dahlen, B., Patchel, B., & Struthers, R. (2005). Strengthening American Indian nurse scientist training through tradition: Partnering with elders. *Journal of Cultural Diversity, 12*(2), 50–55.

Nugent, K., Childs, G., Jones, R., & Cook, P. (2004). A mentorship model for the retention of minority students. *Nursing Outlook, 52,* 89–94.

O'Brien, S. (1993). *American Indian tribal governments.* Norman: University of Oklahoma Press.

Parker, J., Haldane, S., Keltner, B., Strickland, J., & Tom-Orme, L. (2002). National Alaska Native American Indian Nurses Association: Reducing health disparities within American Indian and Alaska Native populations. *Nursing Outlook, 50*(1), 16–23.

Pevar, S. (2002). *Rights of Indians and tribes.* Carbonville: Southern Illinois University Press.

University of North Dakota College of Nursing. (2005). *RAIN program recruitment and retention of American Indians into nursing* [Brochure]. Grand Forks, ND: College of Nursing.

Weaver, H. (1999). Transcultural nursing with Native Americans: Critical knowledge, skills, and attitudes. *Journal of Transcultural Nursing, 10*(3), 197–202.

Wilkins, D. (1997). *American Indian sovereignty and the U.S. Supreme Court: The masking of justice.* Austin: University of Texas Press.

15 It Takes a Village to Raise a Nurse

LORRIE R. DAVIS-DICK

Dance Professor Dance

Professor you don't know me but I am sure that you have seen me around.
Who am I? What do I look like? Well that's not important right now
I am truly amazed by all of your certifications and nursing degrees.
I see you each day as I sit and listen attentively to you speak.
Boldly I begin to think, that may be me someday.
A prolific nurse educator with diverse knowledge, flare, and no-nonsense ways.

Professor you don't know me but I am sure that you have seen me around.
Who am I? What do I look like? Well that's not important right now.
At first it seems that you wanted me here but as time passed it became crystal clear.
Today when I approach you I feel instantly rejected.
I start to think no, this cannot be true of all of you.

Professor you don't know me but I am sure that you have seen me around.
Who am I? What do I look like? Well that's not important right now.
I sit in your class day to day and we have even stood side-by-side.
I make no excuse for my silky caramel complexion,

Dedicated to my father, whose spirit of academia will push me throughout my stride to become a leader in nursing education.

long black wavy hair or even my urban style.
The grades I earn speak for themselves
and my nursing skills are always above the rest.
It's true I know what you see in me
is not your vision of the trailblazing nurse of the 21st century.

Professor you don't know me but I am sure that you have seen me around.
Who am I? What do I look like? Well that's not important right now.
Please remember that I not only see you as a disseminator of nursing knowledge.
Unfortunately what you cannot see is that you truly are the mentor and I the mentee.
Together we dance invisibly.

Professor you don't know me but I am sure that you have seen me around.
Who am I? What do I look like? Well that's not important right now.
I too represent the future and plan to become
the new Nightingale, Peplau, Roy, or the prolific Wykle.
Now please do not be ashamed that you overlooked my talent, worth, and skill.
Do not look back at the past.
Look ahead to change your perspective this academic year.
Once again there I will sit in your class listening to you teach.
Professor let's not again begin our mentor-mentee dance invisibly.

—Lorrie Davis-Dick

RECEIVING THE SEED OF MENTORSHIP

It was no surprise to my parents that I would be working on a PhD before I turned 30 years old. My parents sent me to a prestigious private school in town, and every day from the age of six until I left home my father would walk into my room, stand at the doorway, and say, "You will get your PhD . . . you have no other option in this life." As a third-generation nurse, I think that it was part of my genetic make-up to become a registered nurse and work in health care. Growing up, my parents would tell me that I always had to be better and have more education than nonminorities in this society.

In 1996, when I entered nursing school at North Carolina A & T State University, a historically Black university, I never doubted that I was making the best career choice. Since my freshman year, I knew that one of my future goals would be to positively impact the profession of nursing. As an undergraduate nursing student, I felt supported by the faculty, and with consistent dedication to my studies, I obtained a total of 19 academic honors, recognitions, and scholarships before graduating Magna Cum Laude in spring 2000.

THE MARRIAGE OF MENTORSHIP AND ACADEMIA

My travels along the lifelong road toward mentorship began during my senior year in nursing school when I received the letter of invitation from the Mu Tau Chapter of Sigma Theta Tau International Nursing Honor Society. Reading the letter of invitation served as validation that as a young Black woman I had achieved academic success as a future baccalaureate-prepared registered nurse. As any new inductee to Sigma Theta Tau, I was charged with understanding the guiding principles and expectations that make this, the only honor society in nursing, so outstanding. As I read about the organization's purpose on their Web site, I expected to see the promotion of academic excellence and the suggestion that nurses push toward a healthy global society. What I did not expect to see was a link on mentoring and mentoring-related committees and activities. I thought to myself, "What does mentoring have to do with getting good grades?" As I reflect back on that day, I realize now the important role that mentorship can play in the academic success of nursing students.

On a warm April night in spring of 2000, I attended the induction ceremony with the faculty, my parents, and peers. That evening, I realized that nursing school is more than succeeding academically; it involves making sure that others are able to succeed and make their mark on the profession of nursing, as well. Annually, the School of Nursing at North Carolina A & T State University inducts junior and senior nursing students in high academic standing into Sigma Theta Tau. That year, for the first time, the program coordinators highlighted Sigma Theta Tau's connection to mentorship by linking each inductee with a professional nursing mentor, preferably an alumnus from the university. The mentorship programs supported nationally by Sigma Theta Tau focus on creating professional nursing leaders in diverse health care settings, in particular in nursing education.

First Impressions Can Last a Lifetime

It was not until my senior year in college, at the Sigma Theta Tau induction, that I was introduced to my first professional nursing mentor. When my mentor approached me that evening, she immediately gave me the warmest hug and congratulated me on this special evening and positive academic recognition. My first impression of this African American nursing mentor was that she was approachable, caring, and excited about this networking opportunity. As my mentor asked me questions, I was curious to know where she had gone to school, where she worked, and as the mentee, what I could expect over the next year as a novice in nursing. It was obvious that I wanted to know about my mentor's professional nursing career, but she made it clear that this was my night and that she wanted me to tell her how nursing school was going and what my plans were postgraduation. When I returned home that night, my mother, who had been at the induction ceremony, told me that my mentor had wanted me to have her business card, which she then handed to me. I read the white card with the royal blue writing that revealed to me that my nursing mentor was not just a registered nurse but a nurse practitioner who held a doctoral degree in nursing. She was also a nurse educator and an established nursing professor at one of the most prestigious universities in the United States. Although her credentials certainly impressed me, it was her commitment to the mentoring relationship and her interest in my quest for a baccalaureate degree in nursing that had the greatest impact on me that evening.

Over the last 10 years, we have had a long-distance mentor–mentee relationship due to our geographical locations. We have communicated via telephone, mail, and e-mail, discussing everything from applying to graduate school, current research in nursing, the paradigm shifts in nursing education, nursing research goals, and ways to handle the stress of the nursing profession as an African American advanced practice nurse. Early in our mentor–mentee journey I would talk about how challenging it was being an African American nursing student, and the difficulties of talking with nonminority nurses about being in nursing school, and later the challenges of feeling invisible to professors in graduate school at a predominantly White university. Whenever I talked about my experiences with racism, my mentor would simply redirect my focus and ask where I saw myself in the next 5 to 10 years, keeping me focused on my dream and vision to leave a shining imprint on the nursing profession. She would often elaborate on her pursuit of her own dreams, encouraging me to focus on tomorrow and to move from a perspective of what is impacting "me" to how "I" can impact the profession of nursing.

In addition, she encouraged me to seek out opportunities, such as entering a graduate program in nursing because it was the best way I could control the outcome of my future. At times it was easy to imagine that I would be an advanced practice nurse and have a great nursing career, but my ears also heard the voice of my mentor say, "For us it will never be easy and that is why, as a Black nurse, you must put on your mental armor and be prepared for the unexpected." It was not until I began practicing as a nurse that I truly realized what she meant. I can vividly remember being hired for my first nursing job on an adult psychiatric in-patient unit. Prior to graduation, I was employed by this organization for 1 year as a certified nursing assistant before transitioning into the role of a registered nurse. Becoming a registered nurse did not level the playing field but instead made it seem as if I was one strike away from being out of the game. I soon learned that a Black registered nurse with equal or more education in the field of nursing was a bitter pill to swallow for some of the Caucasian nursing staff.

Even today, at the age of 29 with all my certifications and advanced degrees, I know that the Black registered nurse has more racially linked obstacles to tackle. When similar issues challenge me today, my mentor still helps me to see the forest despite the trees. Our generational gap of almost 30 years has been a blessing in disguise because through our conversations she has encouraged me to take a broader perspective and to understand my true purpose as an African American nurse. It has become crystal clear that my mission and purpose in nursing is to fight the battle of the attrition of Black students who are seeking baccalaureate degrees in nursing. As the complexion of the United States begins to shift to shades of brown, I envision Black registered nurses encouraging and helping nonminority registered nurses to look past race in order to provide ethnically appropriate nursing care.

At times our mentor–mentee relationship was transparent; I felt my mentor knew my day-to-day struggles even when we were engaged in little conversation. For instance, about 1 year after graduating from nursing school, I was contemplating starting graduate school and getting married. My mentor was very adamant that I wait for marriage until after graduate school and explained how this decision could solidify my financial future. She encouraged me to prioritize my professional and personal life by helping me envision what tomorrow could bring and what I could control. With hesitation and some anger, I took her advice and began to pursue an advanced education in nursing. I did not marry my high school sweetheart until I was more than halfway through the program.

In 2000, when I was introduced to my mentor, the seed of mentorship was planted in my mind, heart, and soul. After a decade of being in a mentoring relationship, I have developed and matured professionally and understand the responsibility I have as a nurse educator to encourage other African American nursing students to complete a baccalaureate degree in nursing. Since creating my personal nursing motto in 2001, I have not changed my vision, which is to "Learn, Mentor, and Empower Nurses of the 21st Century."

Turning Lemons Into Lemonade

In 2004, I enrolled in a traditional on-ground majority graduate nursing program in North Carolina. As one of the few Black nurses in my class, I often felt overlooked, misunderstood, and simply belittled. In the early weeks of my classes my emotions were positive, but as I attended class each week, it became clear that I would not get the support I needed from faculty to complete the program. When discussing graduate nursing programs with my mentor, she encouraged me to consider distance education programs. So, I decided to find out about online programs in nursing. When I first contacted the University of Phoenix, which is an online university, the academic advisor was friendly and honest about the expectations of the graduate program's faculty. In many ways, an online program met my needs and the needs of my family. As a member of Generation X, it was to my advantage that I had been using the computer since the age of three. I was able to study from my home and complete an advanced degree in nursing in about 18 months. But most importantly, my work, not the color of my skin and not the number of years I had been a nurse, spoke to the instructor and my online peers. The factor of institutional racism was instantly eliminated, and I was graded only on the quality of my postings, papers, exams, and graduate project. In 2005, I successfully completed my master's degree in nursing through the University of Phoenix's graduate school of nursing.

Because of my own experience with having a mentor, I chose to focus on mentoring African American nursing students in baccalaureate nursing programs (BSN) for my graduate project as one way to address the diversity gap in nursing.

ADDRESSING THE DIVERSITY GAP IN NURSING: MENTORING AND EVIDENCE-BASED PRACTICE

Projections from the U.S. Health Resources and Services Administration (HRSA, 2004) suggest that by the year 2020 over one million new registered nurses will be needed to support the demand for nursing care in the United States alone. In addition, there is a need for a large pool of nursing faculty from diverse specialties and backgrounds to connect to the growing student nurse population (Spratley, Johnson, Sochalski, Fritz, & Spencer, 2001).

African American nursing students in entry-level baccalaureate nursing programs are exiting nursing schools without their degrees at a disproportionate rate. This attrition contributes to the poor representation of African Americans in the nursing workforce and graduate nursing programs. The American Association of Colleges of Nursing (AACN) suggests racial/ethnic minority representation remains solid in entry-level baccalaureate nursing programs; yet, the question remains whether African American students, who represent 11.2% of the enrollment, will successfully remain in their nursing program and complete the requirements for graduation (AACN, 2002).

The shortage of African American registered nurses is troublesome; recent studies highlight that Blacks represent only 4.6% of registered nurses in the United States. This disappointing figure from the National Sample Survey of Registered Nurses (HRSA, 2004) indicates that current recruitment and retention strategies aimed at retaining African American nursing students have failed and that there is a need for a national initiative targeted to develop not only short-term but also long-term recruitment and retention of this student population. Further complicating the situation, a significant number of qualified students are currently being turned away from baccalaureate entry-level programs due to an insufficient number of nurse educators (AACN, 2006).

Research studies suggest African Americans do not pursue nursing or complete nursing programs for a variety of reasons, such as: role stereotypes, economic barriers, lack of mentors, lack of direction from early authority figures, misunderstanding about the practice of nursing, and increased opportunities in other fields (Washington, Erickson, & Ditomassi, 2004). Williams (1999) suggests that the attrition rate of African American nursing students has increased and that failure to retain Black students is associated with the lack of mentoring relationships with persons they feel comfortable with and can relate to, learn from, and emulate.

LACK OF DIVERSITY IN THE NURSING EDUCATION PIPELINE

The harsh environment minority students face in the educational pipeline leads to a lack of diversity in the nursing workforce, which has implications for culturally competent care of diverse populations. According to the National Advisory Council on Nursing Education and Practice (2000), it is critical that the nursing workforce be culturally diverse and competent in order to meet the complex health care needs of today's patient population. Lack of diversity is also reflected in the field of nursing education. African American faculty represent only 8.7% of nursing instructors and 6.8% of nursing deans (AACN, 2005). In turn, the compounding lack of diversity in faculty and among nursing students negatively impacts the efforts to recruit minorities into the nursing profession.

Research studies have revealed the power of positive mentoring relationships between mentors and nursing students to improve minority nursing student retention (Nugent, Childs, Jones, & Cook, 2004). Burnard (1987) found that students who learn from experienced nurse mentors have enhanced reflective abilities in the learning process. According to Scott (2005), mentoring is relevant for both the nursing student and the experienced nurse. Mentoring helps nursing students to successfully navigate the complex world of nursing and faculty to become better teachers. The literature also suggests that mentorship can be made more flexible and fluid through the use of technology for communication and exchange, in particular, the Internet (Knouse & Webb, 2001).

Gray and Smith (2000) looked at mentorship from the students' perspective. Interviews with students took place over a 3-year period and focused on the students' opinions of a good mentor versus a poor mentor. "Students described a good mentor as being enthusiastic, friendly, approachable, patient and understanding and having a sense of humour" (p. 1546).

Other studies of mentoring indicate that there is an apparent lack of understanding about the concept of mentoring and its implications for nurses acting as mentors (Anforth, 1992; Burnard, 1990; Morle, 1990). Mentoring is often confused with or used interchangeably with tutoring.

Tutoring is only one aspect of mentoring and is not expected to occur in each mentor–mentee relationship. A nursing tutor is someone who primarily assists in helping a student perform well with essays, term papers, tests, and improving nursing skills (Gray & Smith, 2000). On the other hand, mentors, as defined by the English National Board of Nursing, are "appropriately qualified and experienced first level practitioners, who by example and facilitation guide, assist, and support students in learning new skills, adopting new behaviors, and acquiring new attitudes . . . Mentors are there to assist, befriend, guide, advise and counsel students" (ENBN, as quoted in Suen & Chow, 2001 p. 507). It is important that mentors and mentees understand the difference between the role of a mentor and that of a tutor. Otherwise, nursing students may have a negative experience with mentoring if they were expecting a private tutor.

Researchers Atkins and Williams (1995) explored individual nurses' perceptions and experiences of mentoring undergraduate nursing students. The purpose of their research was to accurately describe and analyze mentors' perceptions of their experiences and identify issues important to them. The study focused on identifying critical features within the mentor–mentee relationship from the mentors' perspectives. Also, the study described ways in which mentoring affected the mentors' working lives and their other professional roles and responsibilities. Data were collected through interviews that were transcribed and coded according to participants' experiences. Research findings suggest that mentors require formal preparation for their role and that the activity of role modeling needs to be addressed in the preparation. Other findings include: the time for mentoring needs to be included within the working day, the role of the mentor is complex, high levels of commitment are necessary, and organized peer support groups may be valuable for mentors.

DESCRIPTION OF ENSC MENTORING PROGRAM

As a result of my graduate project for my master's degree in nursing, I developed the program Empowering Nursing Students in the Carolinas (ENSC), a mentoring program for African American nursing students attending baccalaureate nursing programs (BSN) at either majority, or primarily White, schools of nursing or historically Black colleges and universities (HBCU). The purpose of the program is to decrease the attrition rates of Black nursing students in BSN programs and to increase the number of African American advanced practice nurses, such as nurse educators and nurse practitioners, in North Carolina. Students in the program are connected with baccalaureate-prepared African American registered nurses in their community through Black nursing organizations, such as Chi Eta Phi and the National Black Nurses Association.

Nurse mentors who participate in the program must meet certain criteria. They must have a minimum of a BSN degree, be a graduate of the mentee's school or live or have lived in the community of the nursing school, and be employed full-time or part-time as a nurse. It is preferred that the mentor be an African American male or female registered nurse working in the community and that the nurse mentor have at least 1 year of nursing experience and preferably experience as a preceptor or mentor within the organization where they are currently employed or have been employed in the past. The option to mentor a nursing student who is enrolled in a distance education nursing program is also available.

Mentees who are interested in participating in the mentoring program are required to be upcoming junior or senior nursing students in a BSN nursing program. The potential mentees are asked about their academic standing. This information helps the on-site program coordinator guide the focus of the mentoring relationship. Knowledge of academic status also assists mentors to identify at-risk African American nursing students. Finally, the program coordinator should know the nursing students' reasons for wanting to build a relationship with a nurse mentor. The initial information obtained from the application process is very important; it creates a starting point on the mentor–mentee's path to a solid relationship.

The mentor and mentee are expected to participate in the program for one full academic year. They are required to meet at least once a month to discuss the student's academic standing, professional nursing issues, and any challenges the mentee may be experiencing in his or her academic, professional, and/or personal life. Communication can take place in person, on the telephone, or via the Internet. Distance should not be a barrier to establishing a mentor–mentee relationship.

The ENSC site coordinator or program director reviews the applications and selects and matches the mentors and mentees for the academic year. At the meet-and-greet night, held on the campus of the hosting BSN nursing program, the program director educates the mentors and mentees about the dynamics of a healthy mentorship. The mentee is taught that the mentor is not a counselor but a professional support system or safety net for the nursing student. Both the mentor and mentee are given a packet of information describing suggested topics of discussion during their monthly meetings, including helping mentees make the grade, find their voice, and map out their 5-year plan. Guidelines are also provided to address student crises, such as financial issues and feelings of hopelessness.

There is no financial commitment involved for the mentor or mentee, and mentors are only required to share knowledge, show compassion, and promote self-esteem in their student nurse mentee. With reference to program finances, the mentorship program can be implemented in a nursing program for a small cost for supplies such as meeting materials and refreshments. The mentor and mentee can meet in available classrooms on campus, and the meet-and-greet night can also take place at the school of nursing. The mentors and mentees are expected to stay in touch with the mentorship program director by filling out and returning by e-mail a checklist each month.

The overall success of the mentorship program is determined by an evaluation survey that the participants complete at the end of each academic year. Because the lives of students and mentors can be hectic, this survey can be administered to project participants via e-mail, mail, or telephone. The survey measures program outcomes by the following:

- A rating of 95% or > by the program mentor–mentee as "Very Good" or "Excellent" in response to the efficacy of the interpersonal relationship developed and the productivity of the interaction.
- An increase in the retention rate of African American nursing students who participate in the program in contrast to students enrolled in the same BSN program who do not participate.

At the end of each academic year, the mentors and mentees meet for a night of closure and receive certificates of appreciation for participating in the program. Graduating seniors who would like to be mentors in the future are recruited at this time. The long-term success of the mentoring program depends on whether participating mentees agree to be future mentors to subsequent generations of African American nursing students.

Student Voices: The Nursing Students' Trail of Tears

In October 2005, I was invited to attend the Sigma Theta Tau Research Day by my alma mater, North Carolina A & T State University School of Nursing, to promote the ENSC mentorship program. The event was held in the conference center of one of the city's local hospitals. When I entered the newly renovated building, I saw current nursing students preregistering for the conference; they were smiling, laughing, and standing in small groups discussing their upcoming nursing exams. I said to myself, "Less than 7 years ago, that was me, excited about Research Day, my senior year, and the upcoming graduation."

As a relatively recent graduate, I thought it would be great for African American upper-division nursing students to see and talk with a young, Black nurse who was on the verge of completing her graduate degree in nursing. I was also looking forward to talking with students about my graduate project on mentoring African American nursing students in baccalaureate programs. As I nervously set up my poster board and arranged my handouts, I wondered if any of the students would even stop at my table. Around 10 A.M. there was a break between research sessions, and students began to enter the lobby where my table and several other poster session presenters were located. I began to have doubts and thought to myself, "What if the students see my project as worthless or completely miss the potential impact this program could have on their lives?"

To my surprise, a student approached and asked, "What is this supposed to be about?"

I answered, "Empowering Nursing Students in the Carolinas (ENSC) is a mentoring program that connects African American students in upper-division courses with an African American registered nurse in the community." I continued, "Let's be honest, nursing is hard. Positive and negative challenges, such as academic stress, financial distractions, and obligations to family, not to mention the pressure to pass the nursing boards, may affect your ability to successfully graduate or graduate at all from the program." I talked about my literature review and the numerous reasons for the continued lack of diversity in nursing.

As I continued to talk with the student, the crowd around my table grew larger and larger, and before I knew it, more than 15 traditional and nontraditional Black nursing students were standing quietly in the chatter-filled room listening to me talk. At this point, I knew it was time to invite those who were interested in the program to ask questions. Instead of questions, I received thanks and praise for offering a program such as this to Black professional nursing students such as themselves. Over the next few minutes, almost 30 nursing students hurriedly filled out the ENSC application as if they were not going to see me again that day. The students dropped off their forms at my table one-by-one or in groups of two or three.

On the application, students were asked the reasons they would like to participate in the ENSC mentoring program. Students wrote comments, such as:

- "Thank you so much, it is challenging dealing with school and family. I cannot always talk with my professors or peers. This program will help me to get things off my chest."
- "Where has this program been? I needed a mentor since my freshman year."
- "It will be exciting to connect with a professional Black nurse in the community."
- "I have prayed for something or someone to help me through the stress of my senior year, thank you."
- "A mentor will complete me and make me whole."

One student who approached the table alone had a tissue to her face, and as she began to talk, soft tears ran down her mocha cheeks. The student said, "I want to thank you for what you have done."

I replied, "What did I do?"

She explained to me in her trembling voice, "I feel like I have no one to talk to. I am stressed out right now because of nursing school, how I am treated by Caucasian nurses when I am in clinical, and the pressure I am feeling from my family to graduate is just too much."

As I listened to the student reveal such sensitive information, I immediately gave her a hug and prayed to myself for this student and thought, "Oh God, they are crying out for my help."

As she walked away, I knew that her tears represented the trail of tears that these African American nursing students have shed since their freshman year. My heart was overwhelmed, and I knew at this moment the importance of a positive and effective mentoring program that would have a lasting impact on its participants.

Ever since that eventful Research Day in October, I have never doubted the purpose of the mentoring project, the power of mentoring, and the significant impact nursing mentors can have in the life of a student. Eventually Research Day came to an end, but in my heart I knew that this was just the beginning for the ENSC mentoring project.

RECOMMENDATIONS FOR MENTORING AFRICAN AMERICAN AND OTHER MINORITY NURSING STUDENTS FROM A HOLISTIC PERSPECTIVE

The mentoring experience touches both the mind and heart and embraces and stimulates thoughts about what we know to be our future. Beyond the formality of the mentoring relationship, the vulnerable spirit of the nursing student must be nurtured. At the heart of mentoring is the mentor–mentee interpersonal relationship. The foundation of this relationship is the connection that they share. Recommendations for developing a strong and effective mentor–mentee relationship that is nurturing and holistic are as follows:

1. Mentoring requires dedication from the mentor and commitment to participate in the mentoring project throughout the academic school year. Mentors and mentees may find that the process of mentorship extends far beyond the suggested time frame of the individualized mentoring program. The mentor–mentee relationship may last for several years, or even a lifetime. There is no price tag that can be placed on such an invaluable relationship.
2. A significant part of the mentoring relationship is based on the honesty and truth that the mentor and mentee share with one another, and it is critical that both the mentor and mentee recognize this. For example, if nurse mentors tell their mentees that the senior year in nursing will be a breeze and that no challenges will get in their way, they may unknowingly instill false hope. It would be more appropriate to support the student by saying that the senior year will be filled with positive challenges but that the student should see them as positive, rather than negative, issues in their academic career.
3. The next critical component of the relationship between the mentor and mentee is respect. Mentors and mentees must treat one another as equals in this relationship. Mentors who belittle their mentee or have low expectations for their mentee will indeed lose the vision of the mentoring process.
4. Next, mentors should reflect a positive and caring attitude toward their mentee at all times. A positive attitude is contagious and so are negative behaviors. Mentors may be one of the few lights shining in a dark place; they should keep in mind that

nursing students are under a tremendous amount of stress and pressure to do well in their courses.

5. The last component of the mentor–mentee relationship is appreciation for the mentor and mentee as whole persons. A mentee should recognize and appreciate that the nurse mentor may also be a graduate student, parent, and/or nurse manager. In turn, the mentor should recognize and appreciate that the mentee may also participate in student nurse organizations, volunteer at a local hospital on weekends, or work as a student research assistant to school of nursing faculty.

A DREAM OF DIVERSITY IN NURSING: WAKING UP TO MENTORSHIP

The process of mentorship is complex; however, if the mentor and mentee consistently follow these guidelines, they will establish a relationship that can have a lasting impact on the individual mentees as well as on the future of Black registered nurses. If the retention rate of participants in the program is increased, there will be more baccalaureate-prepared African American registered nurses to care for our expanding and changing society. The hope is that more African American registered nurses will decide to obtain an advanced degree under the umbrella of nursing.

As a successful African American advanced practice nurse, member of Sigma Theta Tau International, a nurse educator, and a recipient of the gift of mentorship, I feel that I have an obligation to reach out to future African American registered nurses by creating a village to help other African American students achieve their goal to become a registered nurse of the twenty-first century. Through my own experiences, I have realized that what African American nursing students need and deserve is to be connected to an African American registered nurse mentor in their community who can spend a relatively small but rewarding amount of time empowering a student nurse. Developing this program has been a humbling experience, and it has changed my perspective on obstacles that African American nurses face. The future of the African American registered nurse is bright if adequate resources and support, such as the ENSC Mentoring Program, are made available to African American nursing students.

Remember that diversity in nursing is not a dream; it is essential. Learn, mentor, and always empower the future African American registered nurses of the 21st century!

QUESTIONS FOR DIALOGUE

1. What ideas or concepts did you find most meaningful in this chapter? Identify your insights and questions to bring to a dialogue with your colleagues.
2. Read the poem at the beginning of this chapter. What is the student asking of the professor? From your perspective, what could be going on in the professor's mind?
3. Describe a mentor–mentee dance at its best—one that is both visible and intentional in its support of the student.
4. For both Hill-Cill (see chapter 4) and Davis-Dick, induction into Sigma Theta Tau International (STTI), the Honor Society of Nursing, was extremely important. How is induction into STTI determined at your institution? If there is no STTI chapter in your country, are there other honor societies or prestigious organizations to which membership is a mark of distinction? To what extent do these organizations also have a gatekeeper role? Would you describe them as culturally exclusive in nature or inclusive? In what ways?
5. In her review of the literature on mentoring, what does Davis-Dick portray as essential aspects of a professional nurse mentor? How did her mentor reflect these characteristics? Dialogue with colleagues about what changes you would like to implement to better mentor students in your program.
6. Discuss Davis-Dick's decision to pursue a graduate degree through an online university program. To what extent is this a viable or necessary alternative for graduate nursing students of color in your country? What changes do you recommend for your program to create a more inclusive environment?

REFERENCES

American Association of Colleges of Nursing (AACN). (2002). *American Association of Colleges of Nursing Annual State of the Schools.* Washington, DC: Author.

American Association of Colleges of Nursing (AACN). (2005). *Nursing shortage fact sheet.* Retrieved August 2, 2005, from http://www.aacn.nche.edu/Media/Backgrounders/shortagefacts.htm

American Association of Colleges of Nursing (AACN). (2006). *Student enrollment rises in U.S. nursing colleges and universities for the 6th consecutive year.* Retrieved December 6, 2007, from http://www.aacn.nche.edu/Media/NewsReleases/06Survey.htm

Anforth, P. (1992). Mentors, not assessors. *Nurse Education Today, 12,* 299–302.

Atkins, S., & Williams, A. (1995). Registered nurses' experiences of mentoring undergraduate nursing students. *Journal of Advanced Nursing, 21,* 1006–1015.

Burnard, P. (1987). Towards an epistemological basis for experiential learning in nurse education. *Journal of Advanced Nursing, 12,* 197–202.

Burnard, P. (1990). The student experience: Adult learning and mentorship revisited. *Nurse Education Today, 10,* 349–354.

Gray, M. A., & Smith, L. N. (2000). The qualities of an effective mentor from the student nurse's perspective: Findings from a longitudinal qualitative study. *Journal of Advanced Nursing, 32*(6), 1542–1549.

Health Resources and Services Administration (HRSA). (2004). *The registered nurse population: National sample survey of registered nurses, March, 2004.* Washington, DC: Author.

Knouse, S. B., & Webb, S. C. (2001). Mentors, substitute mentors, or virtual mentors: Alternative mentoring approaches for the military. In M. Dansby, J. Stewart, & S. Webb (Eds.), *Managing diversity in the military: Research perspectives* (pp. 145–162). New Brunswick, NJ: Transaction Publishers.

Morle, K. M. (1990). Mentorship—Is it a case of the emperor's new clothes or a rose by any other name? *Nurse Education Today, 10,* 66–69.

National Advisory Council on Nursing Education and Practice. (2000). *A national agenda for nursing workforce racial/ethnic diversity.* Washington, DC: Author.

Nugent, K. E., Childs, G., Jones, R., & Cook, P. (2004). A mentorship model for the retention of minority students. *Nursing Outlook, 52*(2), 89–94.

Scott, E. (2005). Peer-to-peer mentoring: Teaching collegiality. *Nurse Education, 30*(2), 52–56.

Spratley, E., Johnson, A., Sochalski, J., Fritz, M., & Spencer, W. (2001). *Findings from the National Sample Survey of Registered Nurses, March 2000.* Washington, DC: United States Department of Health and Human Services, Health Resources and Service Administration.

Suen, L., & Chow, F. (2001). Students' perceptions of the effectiveness of mentors in an undergraduate nursing programme in Hong Kong. *Journal of Advanced Nursing, 36*(4), 505–511.

Washington, D., Erickson, J., & Ditomassi, M. (2004). Mentoring the minority nurse leader of tomorrow. *Nursing Administration Quarterly, 28*(3), 165–169.

Williams, B. (1999). A mentoring pyramid for African American nursing students. *ABNF Journal, 10*(3), 68–70.

16 Facilitating Success for ESL Nursing Students in the Clinical Setting: Models of Learning Support

VIRGINIA HUSSIN

"Priyani" was a third-year nursing student of Indian background who had migrated to Australia a year before starting her course. Priyani was very quiet and reserved, and although she had no obvious problems communicating with patients on her practicum, there were two issues of concern that had been identified with regard to her interactions with staff. Her preceptor reported that Priyani was sometimes slow to respond to instructions. Furthermore, Priyani did not participate in "clinical problem solving" in case or team meetings, that is, she did not contribute important information about her patients even when it was pertinent to the discussion at hand.

On observing Priyani, it was clear that she understood instructions that were given directly, for example, when an imperative was used, such as, "Give Mr. Davis his medication now." However, she was slow to respond to more subtle forms of "implicit" instructions where the intent was implied or suggested, such as, "Mr. Davis looks like he needs some help with ambulation." Consequently, in my role as learning adviser, I spent time elucidating some common sentence structures used to give implicit instructions incorporating modals, such as: you could do this . . . /it might be an idea to . . . /it's time something happened . . .

Detailed questioning by the supervising university lecturer revealed that, in general, Priyani had a firm knowledge base about the diagnoses, treatment, and care given to her patients. In discussions with the supervisor and myself, Priyani said that she often had something to say in a team meeting; however, she had trouble coming up with the correct words to express herself, and more importantly, she was unsure about when or how to interrupt. These discussions were followed up with role-plays where Priyani was coached in ways to interrupt politely but assertively, in order to "get into" the discussion. After eight sessions of coaching over four weeks, Priyani successfully completed her practicum.

Priyani's case serves to reinforce the notion that many ESL students do not automatically pick up the finer points of communication behaviour simply by being exposed to them. This is because such students are culturally excluded by a lack of sociocultural knowledge underpinning the rules of sociolinguistic behaviour in a Western culture. To be successful in their placements, students often need overt instruction in areas of sociolinguistics, such as "unpacking" implicit instructions to actually make them explicit, as well as coaching and situated practice in the microskills of turn-taking and interrupting politely in conversations.

BACKGROUND

The difficulties that English as a Second Language (ESL) university students in the Health Sciences experience during the course of their clinical placements are usually associated with language, culture, a non-supportive learning environment, or a combination of these factors. In 1999, the School of Nursing at the University of South Australia identified a number of students experiencing difficulty or failing to meet the requirements of the clinical placement and subsequently negotiated with student learning support staff to improve the learning outcomes for ESL students through program development and implementation. This chapter reports on five levels of this support initiative: professional development of staff, workshops for students prior to and following their placements, individual consultations with students, on-site supervision of "at risk" students within their placements, and provision of Web-based learning support materials. The chapter then briefly outlines a subsequent program that was designed in response to increased enrolments of ESL nursing students. Finally, the chapter suggests areas of future research and makes recommendations for nurse educators who want to create a culture of inclusion for ESL students, including improving their clinical placement outcomes.

Students in the Health Sciences may be required to undertake anywhere from 2–15 weeks of clinical placement (or practicum) every year in clinics or hospitals. Within their placements, students are expected to learn and perform new clinical skills and communication tasks that they will be required after graduation. As graduate nurses, they will be professionals practising in hospitals and clinics where the safety of human life is paramount. Therefore, students need to develop cross-cultural communication strategies and an understanding both of the culture of the workplace and language used in interactions that require a range of different registers and literacies within a new discourse community. Literacy is interpreted as "mastery of a new Discourse" (Gee, 1996) where a discourse refers to: "ways of using language . . . of thinking, feeling, believing . . . that can be used to identify oneself as a member of a socially meaningful group" (p. 130).

The problems that ESL students encounter in their clinical placements are quite different from problems experienced in more traditional academic study contexts. In university courses, students are likely to have difficulty coping with the amount and complexity both of material they are expected to read and of assignments they are expected to write. Most university courses do not focus on developing students' aural and oral skills; yet, these are the very skills that are in fact tested on the clinical placement. In hospitals and clinics, students will need to understand patients and colleagues when they speak, as well as make themselves understood by others. Patients and health professionals themselves will come from a range of different cultures that affect their language production and their expectations of health care. Therefore, the students need to be able to operate in this multicultural environment where they themselves may not be familiar with culturally based beliefs and practices of the dominant Anglo-Saxon culture or of other cultures represented among the staff and clients. In addition, hospitals are usually busy places where background noise can make it more difficult for students to understand what people are saying and where staff and patients may not always have the time and patience needed to clarify meaning.

Ladyshewsky (1996) conducted a research project where he interviewed nine Asian-background International Physiotherapy students and their Western-background Clinical Instructors (CI), concluding that culturally based concepts of authority and respect as well as English language proficiency directly influenced clinical placement outcomes. Ladyshewsky found that while the CIs expected high levels of self-directedness and assertiveness from the students, the students themselves viewed assertive behaviour, such as expressing one's own ideas, as transgressing the concept of harmony. Students commented that to justify one's own opinions would show a lack of respect for teachers and their experience.

The students identified a lack of knowledge of Australian culture and idiomatic language as presenting difficulties for them on placement. They also recognised that their lack of sophistication in English made it harder for them to build rapport with a patient or to discuss theoretical issues with their CIs. Another issue was "wait time" in conversation. Most of the International Physiotherapy students reported that they often took longer than local students to choose the correct word during problem-solving discussions with their CIs. This often leads to a negative perception of the students, as Ladyshewsky (1996) points out: "In Western culture, significant delays in conversation may be interpreted as a lack of interest or a lack of knowledge. Therefore, in a cross-cultural teaching and learning situation, these wait time expectations can lead to assumptions about a student's competency" (p. 291).

A study carried out by Stewart, McAllister, Rosenthal, and Chan (1996) involved 73 Health Sciences students, including those from Nursing and Physiotherapy. In this group, 65 were international students with the remaining 7 from migrant backgrounds. The students were asked to identify difficulties faced in the clinical placement and to suggest strategies to overcome them. The results showed that 56% of students perceived that their accents were a problem. This study supported Ladyshewsky's (1996) findings in that 32% of students reported that difficulty in expressing themselves clearly in English was a negative factor, and 36% identified a lack of knowledge of Australian culture as a problem. Of the students, 27% said that they were reluctant to express their views to their supervisors, which also supported the findings in Ladyshewsky's study.

There were further findings of concern in the study conducted by Stewart et al. (1996) that suggested that the students had encountered racism on their placements and that this was attributed to the staff, not the patients. Of the students, 21% said that they had been discriminated against while on placement, 20% were uncertain as to whether or not the staff were helpful, and 24% said that their supervisors were negative toward their racial/cultural background. Respondents then selected the three most important and urgent activities needed to prepare students for placements. The three chosen were a combined workshop on cross-cultural communication for supervisors and students, learning activities on English language use in work situations, and a workshop on coping with cross-cultural conflict. The need for strategies that focus on clinical communication for ESL nursing students and cross-cultural awareness for their supervisors is echoed in work done by Brown (1996) and Hussin (2002).

THE ISSUES

Nursing is a 3-year program at the University of South Australia. In the first year students undertake two-week blocks of practicum twice a year; in the second year there are four-week blocks twice a year; and in the third year there are seven-week blocks twice a year. In 1999, the School of Nursing identified 16 ESL students experiencing difficulty in or failing to meet the requirements of their placements. This represented approximately one-third of the total number of ESL students in the program. Students undertake two placements in an academic year, one in the first semester and one in the second. These students were identified after the first practicum, and an intervention was recommended before the commencement of the following one.

The school subsequently negotiated for the development of programs to enhance the learning outcomes of these students through a service contract process with Learning Connection, the university's centralised student support unit. Within Learning Connection, learning advisers work to develop language and learning skills of students. Three learning advisers have specialisations in supporting international and ESL students, and part of their work involves English for Specific Purposes (ESP) teaching in a variety of modes, including content-based adjunct language instruction (Brinton, Snow, & Wesche, 1989).

One of these learning advisers with expertise in the area of supporting student learning in practicum began by conducting initial interviews with three nursing staff involved in the clinical supervision of ESL students, which revealed four broad categories of concern:

1. Students were not spending enough time communicating with patients, for example, they were not explaining procedures and offering reassurance to patients *while* performing a nursing task.
2. It was not always clear if students were understanding instructions; for example, they tended to "nod and smile" when asked to perform a task rather than respond verbally.

3. The students' productive communication was often unclear; for example, pronunciation of medical terminology during a "hand-over" (a verbal report given at the end of each shift) was often difficult to understand.
4. Students were not taking enough verbal initiative with team members; for example, they were not taking an active role in team meetings or "engaging in clinical reasoning."

THE SUPPORT INITIATIVE

Given the time and staffing constraints, it was decided to try to address each of the first three concerns to some extent, by providing five levels of initial support: (a) professional development of school staff, (b) workshops for first- and second-year ESL students prior to and following their placements, (c) individual consultations with the second-year students who needed pronunciation practice, (d) on-site supervision of "at risk" third-year students within their placements, and (e) provision of Web-based learning support materials. This work led to recommendations about future support and also revealed areas of cross cultural communication requiring research in order to further improve placement outcomes for ESL students.

Professional Development of Staff

The first level of support entailed providing professional development of school staff. At the School of Nursing's Teaching and Learning Day, the learning adviser contributed to a session on "The needs of ESL students on clinical placements." This session began with a presentation of some of the findings of Ladyshewsky (1996) and Stewart et al. (1996). It covered culturally based learning styles and students' attitudes toward authority, as identified by Ladyshewsky, and students' perceptions of their clinical experience: the factors they believed negatively affected their assessment and those preparatory activities they believed would improve their outcomes, as reported by Stewart et al.

Staff explored how the literature related to their own experience of supervising students on practicum. For example, university staff had worked with many ESL students who were reluctant to express their opinions to them as part of their "respect for them as teachers," as identified by Ladyshewsky (1996). Staff had found ESL students, particularly those from Asian countries, to be more deferent toward authority, and they believed that the students' lack of assertiveness in questioning their supervisors inhibited their ability to demonstrate problem-solving skills. Furthermore, many ESL students that the staff had worked with perceived their language proficiency as a negative factor affecting their clinical placement assessments, as found in the Stewart et al. (1996) study.

The learning adviser presented some specific areas of difficulty in language use, such as making and receiving phone calls and dealing with colloquial language, as outlined in Gonda, Blackman, Hussin, and Gaston (1995) and Hussin (2002). The group examined some strategies to help students overcome difficulties such as building in support mechanisms at the placement site and encouraging students to reflect on their communication within particular interactions during the placement debriefing sessions. This included working through the handout "18 Ways to Enhance the Clinical Learning Experience of ESL Nursing Students" written for clinical supervisors (see Appendix A). The session ended with an overview of the kinds of ongoing support that could be offered to School of Nursing staff by Learning Connection staff.

Workshops for Students Prior to Clinical Placements

The second level of support consisted of workshops for first- and second-year students prior to and following their clinical placements. The workshops were designed to build a safe environment where students could learn and practise communication skills before having to perform them on their placements and then to debrief the experience afterwards. Preparing for the clinical placement was a half-day workshop attended by 14 ESL nursing students in the week prior to their second clinical placement. The group comprised ten students in their first year and four in their second year. The student's backgrounds were Vietnamese, Malaysian, and Chinese. They were referred to the workshops by their lecturers, and though attendance was voluntary, all of the students attended.

After introductions, the students wrote down their main areas of concern. Of the 10 students who recorded their responses, 8 predictably identified making mistakes in their communication and misunderstanding instructions. Five responses focused on "knowing what to do" or the expectations of the clinical setting, including knowing how to handle a "rude" patient and working with equipment. Three students alluded to issues around racism, such as one student who mentioned "nasty stuff"; the fact that the students meant racism was made clear later in discussion.

Another student was concerned in case a patient was not happy to be cared for by her because of her cultural background ("racism—patients choose nurses . . ."). She wondered how she would cope with such a patient: "If patient is so uncomfortable having me as a nurs[ing] student . . . if patient is being rude [racist], how to handle it."

The four-hour workshop was divided into two parts: communicating with patients and communicating with staff, and each part included role-plays to simulate the clinical environment. Gee (1996) stresses that if we are trying to help our students achieve mastery of a secondary discourse, then we need to engage them in realistic learning situations that employ authentic tasks or, what Cope (2000) calls, "situated practice."

The workshop was designed with Fairclough's (1989) concept of "orders of discourse" in mind. These orders of discourse can be seen as a structured set of conventions associated with a communicative activity in a given place. These conventions relate not only to language use and nonverbal behaviour but also to visual signs and systems, for example, a thermometer used by the nurse to take a patient's temperature or a vase of flowers on a patient's bedside table.

Within these orders of discourse are conventions associated with language use, in particular activities that can be identified as oral genres, for example, the way that nurses talk to patients while taking their blood pressure or that doctors talk to nurses during a ward round. In the first section of the face-to-face workshop, the students were introduced to the stages of the oral genre "Taking Vital Signs," which was divided into the following staged speech functions: (a) giving information to patients, (b) explaining procedure to patients, (c) seeking cooperation from patients, (d) offering encouragement to patients, (e) offering reassurance to patients, and (f) giving feedback to patients.

The students were encouraged to firstly establish rapport with patients through engaging in social conversation. They identified topics of conversation they could discuss with patients and also how to use visual cues, such as patients' cards, photos, flowers, and books, to initiate conversation. This was followed by extensive paired role-plays where half the group of students role-playing the patients were given prepared questions to ask and concerns to express. The students role-playing nurses were required to take vital signs using the staged speech functions outlined previously, *while* initiating a social conversation by responding to visual cues (props) placed at the "bedside" by the learning adviser.

The nurses then needed to respond spontaneously to the patient's question and then to a complaint or problem, at the same time as taking their blood pressure. For example, during the role-play, one of the patients was cued to ask: "Which country are you from?" This is a question often asked particularly by older patients and generally reflects a genuine interest in the student. Therefore, students are encouraged to answer by telling the patient a little about themselves and their country of origin. Another question: "Can I have my shower now before my visitors come?" might be answered by "yes" and an offer to assist with the shower or perhaps "no" but an offer of a bed wash instead. A later problem: "I'm really concerned because my wife said that she was coming to see me an hour ago and she's still not here" would often be responded to by an offer to ring the wife.

The second section of the workshop started with an overview of students' concerns with regard to communicating with supervisors in clinical placements. The learning adviser presented information on communication strategies drawing on the work of Faerch and Kasper (1983) and Tarone (1983). These covered ways to clarify meaning, such as asking for repetition and asking clarification questions, for example, "*What* did you say we need to order from the pharmacy?" as well as a range of ways to demonstrate understanding including: (a) repetition of key words, (b) confirmation statements that paraphrase information, (c) expansion statements that add information, and (d) elaboration questions that ask for more information.

For example, in response to the instruction, "Could you ring the kitchen and order a low-fat, low-salt diet for Mrs. Green?" students are advised that they could respond with a repetition of key words: for example, ". . . a low-fat, low-salt diet" or a confirmation statement: "Okay, I'll call the kitchen and ask if Mrs. Green can have meals that are low in salt and fat." Alternatively, they could respond with an expansion statement, for example, "Yes, Mrs. Green said that she needed to lose some weight before her next operation—I'll ring the kitchen now" or an elaboration question: "Okay, I'll ring the kitchen. Should I ask them to change her next lunch menu straight away?"

The students were then presented with four case studies of patients in which the learning adviser took the role of the clinical preceptor and issued instructions and asked questions that required students to use these communication strategies to clarify meaning, check understanding, and demonstrate understanding. Students then reflected on their performance and received feedback from the learning adviser. The workshop ended with a presentation of "15 Hot Tips for Your Clinical Placement," a document that addresses some of the language, learning, and sociocultural needs of students (see Appendix B).

The workshop received favourable evaluation, with all of the students identifying the role-plays as being the most useful aspect of the workshop. Half of the students specifically mentioned practising communicating with supervisory staff as being useful, and four of the students wanted more sessions and more information. When asked for suggestions for the follow-up session after the placement, half of the students responded that they wanted to discuss their experiences of the placement, including any difficulties or problems they may have had.

Debriefing the Clinical Placement

Debriefing the clinical placement was a half-day workshop held in the week following the completion of the second clinical placement. This workshop began with a paired discussion, followed by a group discussion of each participant's positive and negative experiences of the placement. Negative experiences tended to focus around misunderstanding in interactions.

Students were then asked to describe these problematic interactions in more detail; then three from the whole group were chosen by the adviser for analysis on the basis of the richness of learning opportunities they presented. An analysis incorporating "playback" technique was applied to each of the three interactions. This technique involved describing the situation, identifying the antecedents, scripting the interaction, and identifying the result and the probable cause of the miscommunication. Alternative approaches and linguistic choices that could be used to avoid the difficulties were discussed. Then the revised script was re-enacted by the students with microskill coaching from the learning adviser.

An issue that kept surfacing in the session was the need to develop assertion skills, so the workshop ended with a discussion of some ways that assertive responses could be generated. These included the use of "I" statements such as: "I feel anxious if I don't get early feedback in the placement." Then, as a group, the students suggested areas they would like addressed in workshops before their next placement the following year: (a) more role-plays of clinical situations; (b) assertiveness and negotiation training; (c) phone conversation practice; and (d) practice on how to give a verbal "handover," that is, a report on each patient given by nurses at the end of one shift to nurses coming on duty for the next shift.

The result of these interventions was that the nursing staff reported an overall improvement in the students' communication skills with patients and with staff in the following practicum. All 14 first- and second-year students who had been referred to Learning Connection subsequently completed their practicums successfully.

Individual Consultations for Pronunciation Practice

The third level of support consisted of individual consultations with second-year students who needed pronunciation practice. The four second-year students from the original group had been identified as having pronunciation that was considered problematic during the course of their previous placement; these students were referred to the learning adviser for individual consultations. The consultations provided pronunciation practice of medical terminology, that is, for diagnoses and procedures in the context of handovers and phone calls. Students presented verbal reports about patients they were caring for, and the reports were audio-taped. Feedback tended to focus on areas such as syllable stress, sounding final consonants, and common prefixes and suffixes. After the students had had time to incorporate the feedback into practice, the reports were retaped so that they could hear their progress and note areas still requiring practice.

Using the same patients, the learning adviser set up scenarios requiring the student to make and receive phone calls using internal phones in different rooms. These calls were also taped so that feedback could be given and then incorporated into practice. The main areas of pronunciation difficulty were the names of patients, the names of drugs, and distinguishing between numbers, for example, nineteen and ninety. Students were encouraged to use communication strategies, such as repetition, clarification questions, and checking devices, for example, "Was that 's' for Sam or 'f' for Fred?" "Was that one nine or nine zero?"

On-Site Supervision of "At-Risk" Students

The fourth level of support provided on-site supervision of "at-risk" third-year students within their placements. In addition to the 14 students from the original group, 2 students from third year (including Priyani) were referred to the Learning Connection. These students were identified as being at-risk during their placement and were about to be placed on a "clinical challenge" due to their language performance on their practicum. The learning adviser held discussions to clarify perceptions of language difficulties with both the students and the clinical preceptors and then arranged to visit the students at their hospital placements. Once at the hospital, the learning adviser observed the students interacting with a patient and with a staff member. The students were given structured feedback about their performance and then on-site "coaching" in a private room. This coaching was comprised of four one-hour sessions over four weeks and took the form of role-plays that reproduced some of the interactions that had been observed. Subsequently, one of the students successfully completed her practicum, and the other student was offered a third placement later in the year, which she then passed.

Web-Based Learning Support Materials

The fifth level of support provided Web-based learning support materials. An interactive online workshop titled *Communication Skills for the Clinical Placement: A Workshop for First-Year English as a Second Language Nursing Students* was developed by the learning adviser and is available at the following Web address: http://www.unisanet.unisa.edu/learn/LearningConnection/?PATH-/Resources/la/Clinical+communication/&default-Welcome.htm. This workshop incorporates material from the face-to-face workshops with an additional section on responding to implicit instructions. It also provides language exercises that can be submitted to the learning adviser for feedback. The online workshop has been Web-linked to the first- and second-year practicum-based courses, and staff encourage all ESL students to access it before their placements. Informal feedback from students indicates that using the workshop made them feel less anxious about undertaking their clinical placement.

The provision of online support also meets the needs of various cohorts of ESL students across year levels that enter their nursing programs at different points and that undertake their practicum at different times of the academic year, requiring to an increasing extent flexibly delivered modes of support. For example, these cohorts include students who have already done some tertiary nursing study at other institutions in Australia or in other countries and so receive credit for some or all of the first-year courses, thereby entering our university at the second-year level of the program. An obvious shortcoming of the online workshop is the inherent problem of using a *written* medium to develop *oracy* in students. For example, in the online version there is no possibility for role-plays and for the immediate checking of students' responses to tasks or cues, including feedback on body language and paralinguistic features, that is available in the face-to-face version. If the students submit exercises, then they are a written form of how they *think* they might respond verbally, rather than the spoken response itself.

In addition to the online workshop, the document titled *18 Ways to Enhance the Clinical Learning Experience of ESL Nursing Students* (see Appendix A) has been made available on the Web and linked to the School of Nursing's home page, and staff report high use of the document.

RECOMMENDATIONS FROM THE INITIATIVE

As a result of feedback from students and the learning adviser's observations of the needs of students while supervising students on placement, it was recommended that two workshops be delivered each semester. The first workshop was mainly targeted at first- and second-year students and covered: (a) interviewing techniques to take a health history and (b) common colloquial expressions in the health context. The second workshop was targeted at second- and third-year students and covered: (a) communication strategies for phone conversations and (b) participating in team meetings.

These workshops were delivered until 2003 when the high number of ESL nursing students enrolled at the university made them unviable. Material from these face-to-face workshops was then incorporated into further online versions. Online workshops provide an accessible and enduring form of support for students' learning, which gives the students control over the development and management of their communication skills. However, it was recognised that there was still a need for some students to see a learning adviser individually for specific language problems, and one-to-one consultations continued.

AFTER THE COMMUNICATION WORKSHOPS

Since 2003, the number of international, as opposed to immigrant, ESL nursing students enrolled at Australian universities has been steadily increasing, and our university is no exception. The number of international students enrolled in nursing programs at the University of Southern Australia went from 17 in 2003 to 249 in 2007 (compared to the number of domestic ESL students that has been declining over the past few years, from 45 in 2003 to 36 in 2006 to 12 in 2007). The increase in international students is mainly due to the nursing shortage in Australia, which has led to the recruitment of large numbers of students from Asian countries, including China and India. The small-group communication workshops that had previously been provided were not really possible with larger numbers of students and no commensurate increase in support staff. Furthermore, nursing staff began to identify the need for more academic writing support for this emerging population of students.

In 2004 and 2005, various forms of learning support were provided to international students. This involved targeting one or two language-rich courses at each year level and providing voluntary workshops around the written assessment tasks in those courses. This integrated form of learning development was successful to some extent, but it meant that the only choice for students with oral communication difficulties was to meet with a learning adviser individually. However, this process relied on the students first perceiving that they had a difficulty and then judging that it was serious enough to address in addition to all their regular studies. They then had to access one or more of a finite number of consultations with a learning adviser, in competition with all other students.

In 2006, a new Service Agreement between Learning Connection and the School of Nursing and Midwifery was negotiated. Under this agreement, the learning adviser, in consultation with the nursing lecturers, designed a 10-week program of supplementary English Language and Communication for Nursing classes (see Appendix C). These were two-hour classes with the first hour on Academic English taught by the learning adviser. This hour was devoted to reading and writing in the context of the assessment requirements of a language-rich core nursing course that all the students were studying. The classes comprised some teacher input, followed by discussion and then some written work done by the students, which was collected and later marked by the learning adviser.

The second hour of the class was Vocational English and was team-taught by the learning adviser and two nursing lecturers who had volunteered to be rostered on for the session. This second hour focused on speaking and listening in the nursing practice context and began with the nursing lecturers presenting a 10-minute scenario-based role-play that they had prepared. This was followed by a class discussion of the model role-play where the nursing lecturers commented on the nursing content, and the learning adviser focused on important aspects of language use. The students then performed role-plays of the same scenarios in pairs while the three staff members circulated to listen and give feedback to the pairs. Finally, the staff members gave feedback to the whole class, and the students had the chance to ask further questions.

This program was quite resource-intensive, and so, in 2007, it was maintained but in a streamlined form. The Academic English component was cut down to eight one-hour classes delivered on a weekly basis by a learning adviser. The Vocational English component was delivered in a 2-day intensive format during a teaching break. It was team-taught by another learning adviser and six nursing lecturers, who were scheduled for different modules over the 2 days.

While the recent cohorts of international students have generally been successful in their nursing programs, there have always been some students who have been required to repeat particular courses or to do an extended clinical placement in a teaching break in order to complete their programs.

FUTURE RESEARCH AREAS

The mastery of a new discourse is closely allied to forming a new identity and a positive sense of self within a new role. In the clinical practicum, students are laying the groundwork for their new identities as health professionals who will need to negotiate their own working conditions and to advocate on behalf of their patients. To do this, the ESL students need a critical awareness of language and how it is used as well as an understanding of the "multiliteracies" in the clinical practicum as "social practices that are complex, multifaceted and ideologically loaded" (Baynham, 1995, p. 8).

Through focusing on their own language performance in workshops that focus on the clinical context, students are in part learning lifelong skills of ethnographic analysis, which will prepare them for their future working lives. As Swales (1990) expresses it: "in learning to analyse participant roles and sociorhetorical conventions they are preparing to survive the *rites of passage* of new discourse communities" (p. 218).

However, anecdotal evidence from both students and clinical instructors reveals the need for further research into how language is used in interactions in clinical settings. In particular, work with staff and students in clinical settings highlights areas of cross-cultural communication, such as "implicitness" and the expression of assertion, which need further research if placement outcomes for ESL students are to be improved. Students have to deal with varying degrees of implicitness, for example, the sophisticated forms of modality embedded in the kind of "hedging" that takes place in the giving of instructions in the clinical context. Possible research questions in this area are: *How is implicitness expressed in interactions in the clinical area? How can implicitness be unpacked by nonnative speakers and responded to?*

Another important research area is the need for the identification and exploration of degrees of assertion within cross-cultural role and power relationships. Clinical instructors complain that students "don't take initiative"; for example, they do not speak up for themselves or participate actively in team meetings. At the same time, students express frustration and uncertainty about *how* to contribute what they do in fact *know* about their patients. Of course, the expression of assertiveness is also related to how power is expressed in language and to culturally based expectations and perceptions of the student's role. As Kress (1988) points out: "the processes of communication always take place in a specific social and cultural setting . . . and the structures of power, of authority, as well as the structures of solidarity, exert their influence on the participants" (p. 5).

It is certainly the case that in this cross-cultural context the clinical instructor is a "gate-keeper" (Fairclough, 1989, p. 47) in a position of power, who decides whether or not a student gets a positive clinical assessment. On the other hand, students do not always have the cultural knowledge about expectations of role-relationships, as well as the language skills that are required to exercise any personal power, even at the level of asking a supervisor for formative feedback. Therefore, important research questions in relation to assertion include the following: *How is assertion expressed in cross-cultural relationships in the clinical area?* and *What is the impact of culture and of power on the expression of assertiveness in these relationships?*

RECOMMENDATIONS FOR NURSE EDUCATORS

Currently there is a shortage of health professionals, particularly nurses, in most Western English-speaking countries. This has led to the recruitment of large numbers of students from countries such as China, India, and Malaysia into university programs in English-speaking countries, including Australia. There are no signs that this trend is changing; indeed, some commentators predict that in 10 years' time, one in every four nurses in Australia will come from a non-English speaking country. Nurse educators play an important role in creating a culture of inclusion for ESL students who will be tomorrow's nurses. To create this inclusive culture, it is recommended that educators:

1. Use ESL students as resources and presenters in courses about cross-cultural family and health practices. The opportunity to

contribute knowledge about family and health practices in their own cultures will serve to validate this knowledge and will hopefully lead to more holistic nursing practice, particularly for the high numbers of non-English speaking background migrants who make up the multicultural population of our countries. Cross-cultural discussion will also teach ESL students more about practices in the dominant Anglo culture.

2. Set cross-cultural interviews about health practices as an assessment task. Interviews between English-speaking and non–English-speaking background students can be effective learning tools for both groups, and using them as assessment tasks serves to legitimize different sources of cultural knowledge.
3. Consider ESL students' language learning and communication needs, and negotiate with ESL specialist lecturers to provide adjunct workshops or supplementary classes. These classes should include opportunities for role-plays in the clinical context, including scenarios designed to address issues of direct or indirect racism. Decisions about the format of these sessions will need to be made by taking into account student needs, the number of students, the resources available, and the time students have available in their study schedules.
4. Give ESL students extra opportunities for structured oral communication coaching, such as practice handovers and phone calls before and during their clinical placements. This will increase their confidence before they have to perform in a public sphere.
5. Collaborate with ESL specialists or applied linguists on joint research projects that focus on areas of cross-cultural communication. The findings about how ESL students and their interlocutors use language in interactions in clinical settings can then be incorporated into teaching to improve students' clinical placement outcomes.

QUESTIONS FOR DIALOGUE

1. What ideas or concepts did you find most meaningful in this chapter? Identify your insights and questions to bring to a dialogue with your colleagues.
2. What kind of collaboration is there between nursing educators in your program and ESL faculty at your institution to assist

ESL nursing students reach their goal of becoming nurses? If none, dialogue with colleagues about the role ESL instructors could play in developing curriculum to prepare students for the language challenges of the clinical experience.

3. Dialogue with colleagues about how you could incorporate role-plays to assist students like Priyani to understand and apply the rules of sociolinguistic behaviour in clinical interactions with patients and colleagues.
4. Priyani was taught in a nurturing way how to interrupt politely, yet assertively. Recall how Yang (see chapter 5) was criticized for not being assertive enough. Discuss the cultural and ethical implications of asking or not asking students to learn how to communicate in ways that are contrary to their cultural upbringing.
5. In the beginning of this chapter, Hussin argues that "students often need overt instruction in areas of sociolinguistics, such as 'unpacking' implicit instructions to actually make them explicit." Identify instructions in your teaching that need unpacking—that need to be made explicit. Dialogue with colleagues about ways to critically examine your teaching for embedded cultural assumptions.
6. In her first and second recommendations for nurse educators, Hussin proposes interaction for mutual learning between ESL and native English-speaking students. Dialogue with colleagues about the dynamics to which you would attend to ensure that these are successful learning experiences.

APPENDIX A

FOR CLINICAL SUPERVISORS

18 Ways to Enhance the Clinical Learning Experience of ESL Nursing Students

1. Allocate *one preceptor* to the student for the duration of their placement in order to establish continuity and rapport.
2. Make students *feel welcome* by showing interest in their cultural backgrounds.
3. Seek opportunities for students to *contribute their knowledge* about health practices in their cultures and to work with patients with the same first language if appropriate.
4. Try to be aware of how the students' *culturally based beliefs and attitudes* can shape their attitude and behaviour; for example, a

Malaysian student was horrified when she saw relatives of her patient bringing in Frangipani because in Malaysia it's a flower reserved for the dead.

5. *Allow time* for students to become accustomed to Australian speech patterns and to develop language skills.
6. Speak *clearly* and *face* the students when giving explanations or instructions so that they can observe *nonverbal clues* to the meaning, for example, your lips moving and your body language.
7. Simplify the structure of your sentences by:
   - using *short* sentences with *pauses*
   - avoiding *negatives,* for example, *change* "Don't use the equipment if it hasn't been checked" to "Check the equipment before you use it."
   - avoiding *tag* questions, for example, *change* "You haven't done her dressing, have you?" to "Have you done her dressing?"
8. Check if your message has been received. *Avoid* asking *general questions* such as "Do you understand?" and instead ask the student to explain in his or her own words what has been said.
9. *Paraphrase* if the student has not understood an instruction. By *repeating* the *key information* in a different way, the student will have further opportunity to understand.
10. Give students a *handout* of the *abbreviations* that are acceptable in your hospital.
11. *Refer* students to the drug guide, nursing procedures manuals, and ward and equipment manuals, and give them *time to read* and *copy details. Written information* provides a good backup for effective learning.
12. Make your expectations for *documentation clear* to the student by:
    - providing *model copies* of documentation
    - providing *specific feedback* on their documentation, outlining their strengths and where and how they need to improve.
13. Allow students to do *practice documentation* until they gain confidence; for example, write progress notes on paper that you then check before they write them in the patient's file.
14. Allow students to do *practice handovers* with you before they have to perform in front of the whole team.
15. Give students *practice phone call exercises* to increase their confidence in coping with the real thing.

16. Recognise that students may not understand the kinds of *informal interactions* that take place in the staff room, especially *jokes* or *satire*, for example, this comment using emphasis and a sarcastic tone: "Don't you just *love* his bedside manner?"
17. Explain *commonly used idioms* to the students, for example, "He's a bit off today," and don't assume that students will understand *shortenings of words*, for example, "She's having a 'choly' " and "Check her 'peri.' "
18. Avoid *unnecessary colloquialisms* that may lead to a literal interpretation, for example, "She spat the dummy" and "It's no skin off his nose."

APPENDIX B

FOR NURSING STUDENTS

15 Hot Tips for Your Clinical Placement

- Try to visit the venue *before* your placement begins, so that you feel more relaxed in the setting and have more of an idea about what to expect once the placement begins.
- Make sure you know what sorts of *tasks* you are expected to do in the placement and how you will be assessed.
- Ask your clinical facilitator for feedback on your progress, including your communication skills, *early* in the placement, so that there will be time to work on improving them if there are any difficulties.
- Ask for *help* as soon as you think you may be having communication difficulties in the placement.
- Don't sit by yourself at breaks! *Talk* with the staff about your family, your study, or your favourite pastimes and ask them about theirs.
- Tell staff members that you want to *learn* more about "Australian culture." Ask them to explain colloquial language, slang terms, and jokes! Be prepared to inform them about aspects of your cultural background.
- Take a pocket Nurses' Dictionary with you and always carry a *notepad* and pencil in your pocket for jotting down unfamiliar vocabulary, which you can look up the meaning for later.
- Ask for a handout of common *abbreviations* that are used in the venue and become familiar with them.
- Borrow ward *manuals* overnight, so that you have the time to read and take notes from them.

- Always *face* the person who is speaking to you, so that you can observe nonverbal clues such as facial expressions and gestures. (If maintaining eye contact is not considered respectful in your culture, explain this to your supervisor.)
- Tell staff members that you sometimes need more *time* to understand what is being said to you and that you will probably need to ask for repetition sometimes.
- If a staff member asks: "Do you understand?" don't just say "yes" or nod your head. Instead, *show* that you do understand by repeating key words, paraphrasing, adding on information, or asking a follow-up question.
- If you do not understand something that is said to you, always ask for *clarification*.
- Practise *relaxation* techniques, deep breathing, and positive self-talk, so that you can use them if you make mistakes with your communication and start to get flustered.
- If you do make a mistake with your communication, discuss it with your clinical facilitator and try and view it as a positive *learning* experience, so that you maintain your confidence in yourself.

APPENDIX C

TIMETABLE FOR SUPPLEMENTARY CLASSES

Table 16.1

WEEKLY OUTLINE OF 2006 SUPPLEMENTARY *ENGLISH LANGUAGE AND COMMUNICATION FOR NURSING* CLASSES FOR BACHELOR OF NURSING AND BACHELOR OF MIDWIFERY INTERNATIONAL STUDENTS

	ACADEMIC ENGLISH READING AND WRITING–LEARNING ADVISER 4–5 P.M.	VOCATIONAL ENGLISH LISTENING AND SPEAKING NURSING LECTURERS AND LEARNING ADVISER 5–6 P.M.	UNDERPINNING SKILLS FOR VOCATIONAL ENGLISH CLASS
1.	Expectations of academic writing in various genres in nursing courses	Pronunciation of medical terminology and stress and intonation exercises	Using medical terminology
2.	Analysing questions for nursing assignments	Pronunciation of medical terminology in handover exercises	Giving information

(*Continued*)

Table 16.1 *Continued*

	ACADEMIC ENGLISH READING AND WRITING–LEARNING ADVISER 4–5 P.M.	VOCATIONAL ENGLISH LISTENING AND SPEAKING NURSING LECTURERS AND LEARNING ADVISER 5–6 P.M.	UNDERPINNING SKILLS FOR VOCATIONAL ENGLISH CLASS
3.	Critical reading of a nursing text	Communicating with patients. Role-play scenario: Taking vital signs	– Explaining procedures – Giving instructions – Requesting cooperation – Offering reassurance
4.	Noting and summarising a nursing text	Communicating with patients. Role-play scenario: Removing a drain and teaching client how to self-test blood sugar levels	– Seeking permission – Giving feedback – Comprehending colloquial language
5.	Avoiding plagiarism and paraphrasing in your own words	Interview techniques: open and closed questions; focused questions. Role-play scenario: Taking a nursing history (female client with acute illness)	– Interpreting nonverbal cues – Using attending behaviours – Using nonverbal communication
6.	Writing cohesive paragraphs for assignments	Interview techniques: Paraphrasing and clarifying information. Role-play scenario: Taking a nursing history (male client with chronic illness)	– Using reflective listening techniques – Using clarification devices – Using paraphrasing responses
7.	Critical analysis in written assignments	Communicating with colleagues. Role-play scenario: Understanding instructions.	– Comprehending verbal information – Asking for repetition and clarification – Demonstrating understanding
8.	Integrating sources into your text	Communicating with colleagues. Role-play scenario: Giving explanations	– Staging verbal information – Using appropriate medical terminology

(*Continued*)

Table 16.1 *Continued*

	ACADEMIC ENGLISH READING AND WRITING–LEARNING ADVISER 4–5 P.M.	VOCATIONAL ENGLISH LISTENING AND SPEAKING NURSING LECTURERS AND LEARNING ADVISER 5–6 P.M.	UNDERPINNING SKILLS FOR VOCATIONAL ENGLISH CLASS
9.	Referencing conventions	Communicating with family. Role-play scenario: Explaining illness states and treatments in accessible language	– Expressing empathy – Comprehending colloquial language
10.	Review of grammar: – sentence structure – noun–verb agreement – use of articles – use of the passive voice – perfect vs. past perfect	Communicating with family. Role-play scenario: Giving and receiving telephone messages	– Conventions for answering and placing telephone calls – Comprehending colloquial language – Understanding cultural conventions and taboos

REFERENCES

Baynham, M. (1995). *Literacy practices: Investigating literacy in social contexts.* New York: Longman.

Brinton, D., Snow, M., & Wesche, M. (1989). *Content-based second language instruction.* New York: Newbury House.

Brown, V. (1996). Nursing SPEAK Program. In *Advancing international perspectives.* Proceedings of 1997 HERDSA Conference, Adelaide.

Cope, B. (2000). The "how" of a pedagogy of multiliteracies. In B. Cope & M. Kalantzis (Eds.), *Multiliteracies: Literacy learning and the design of social futures* (pp. 30–37). Melbourne: Macmillan.

Faerch, C., & Kasper, G. (1983). On identifying communication strategies in interlanguage production. In C. Faerch & G. Kasper (Eds.), *Strategies in interlanguage communication* (pp. 210–237). London: Longman.

Fairclough, N. (1989). *Language and power.* London: Longman.

Gee, J. P. (1996). *Social linguistics and literacies: Ideology in discourses* (2nd ed.). London: Taylor & Francis.

Gonda, J., Blackman, I., Hussin, V., & Gaston, J. (1995). Migrant nurses: Their unique value. In G. Gray & R. Pratt (Eds.), *Issues in Australian nursing 4* (pp. 129–144). Melbourne: Churchill Livingstone.

Hussin, V. (2002). An ESP program for students of nursing. In T. Orr (Ed.), *English for specific purposes* (pp. 25–40). Alexandria, VA: TESOL.

Kress, G. (1988). *Communication and culture: An introduction.* Kensington: New South Wales University Press.

Ladyshewsky, R. (1996). East meets West: The influence of language and culture in clinical education. *Australian Physiotherapy, 42*(4), 287–294.

Stewart, M., McAllister, L., Rosenthal, J., & Chan, J. (1996). International students in the clinical practicum: Problems with English language proficiency, cross-cultural communication and racism. Paper presented at *ISANA 7th Annual Conference: Waves of Change,* Adelaide.

Swales, J. (1990). *Genre analysis—English in academic and research settings.* New York: Longman.

Tarone, E. (1983). Some thoughts on the notion of "communication strategy." In C. Faerch & G. Kasper (Eds.), *Strategies in interlanguage communication* (pp. 61–74). London: Longman.

17

Workforce Improvement With International Nurses (WIN): Immigrant Nurses WIN Road to Licensure

WILLIAM W. FRANK, JUDITH A. ANDERSEN, AND KATRINA NORVELL

When the millennium arrived, Bindu was practicing as a new nurse at some of the best hospitals in Liberia—John F. Kennedy Medical Center in Monrovia and United Methodist Hospital in Ganta. She was excited and proud to be working in medical/surgical, pediatric, and orthopedic units. Unfortunately, the civil war reerupted and quickly dashed her dreams of a peaceful life. She decided to emigrate to the United States to make a better life for herself and her family. Fortunately, Bindu was granted a visa as an asylee and moved half a world away to live with the cousin of a family friend in Portland, Oregon. It was very difficult for Bindu to leave her entire family behind and come to a strange land where she knew no one. Even though her brothers and sister have tried to get visas, they have all been denied. During each Christmas and New Year holiday, Bindu chooses to work so she does not have to spend tearful time alone at home. Her colleagues and patients have become her new family.

Initially, Bindu was not able to work as a nurse in Oregon because the state board would not recognize her foreign nursing license. She was very discouraged. Many people told her to get a job as a Certified Nursing Assistant (CNA), but even this meant she would have to go back to school, and she simply didn't have the money. Eventually, Bindu took a job at a nursing home making beds for minimum wage. It was humiliating, but her mother told her to keep her head up, work very hard, and remember that the United States was not her real home.

Bindu was one of over 200 internationally educated nurses who expressed interest in a pilot program called Workforce Improvement With International Nurses (WIN) in the fall of 2003. She was one of the few chosen to participate in the first cohort of WIN. While many of those interested in WIN needed extra help in English, Bindu had learned to speak English as a child, even though her native dialect is Kpelleh. This advantage, however, was offset by other significant challenges.

Participating in the WIN program was very challenging for Bindu. For over six months, she went to school four evenings a week while working 12–16 hour shifts on the weekends to make up for the lost days at work. Bindu graduated from the WIN program on January 13, 2005, and took the NCLEX-RN two weeks later—and passed. "It was one of the happiest days of my life," she said. "This is the land of opportunity—where you can grow from being nothing to something."

The story of Bindu's struggle is not unusual. The United States still inspires hope for many outside her borders who are motivated by aspiration or desperation. But the dream of a prosperous and promising life in America is not often the reality. Difficult choices, formidable sacrifices, and unexpected hurdles face most of those who arrive. In addition, few training programs have been designed specifically to help immigrant health care professionals return to meaningful work that pays a living wage.

> Adults who have limited English skills, usually immigrants or refugees, often face poor labor market prospects. The number of such individuals in the U.S. workforce has grown dramatically over the past decade—accounting for nearly half of all workforce growth—yet the workforce development implications of this growth have received scant attention. Current resources for language and job training services are dwarfed by the need. Moreover, few programs focus on providing the nexus of language, cultural and specific job skills that are key to helping low-income adults with limited English skills increase their wages. (Wrigley, Richter, Martinson, & Strawn, 2003, p. 1)

PROGRAM BACKGROUND AND PURPOSE

Each year, more than 1,700 new refugees and immigrants make their home in the State of Oregon. This state is the eleventh-largest refugee resettlement state in the nation (Immigrant and Refugee Community Organization, 2006). Among these refugees are health professionals, including people with training reasonably comparable to nurses in the United States, who could potentially relieve the current and predicted dearth of nurses in the region and help address the health care needs of the state's rising non–English-speaking populations. Workforce Improvement With International Nurses (WIN) at Clackamas Community College (CCC), a pilot program funded by a 4-year grant from the Northwest Health Foundation (NWHF), offers a viable solution to meet these needs.

In the state of Oregon, as in many places, the looming nursing shortage and the scarcity of minority and bilingual nurses are intersecting and overlapping issues. The nursing shortage is predicated on several key factors and trends, including the exodus of retiring nurses, the expected growth in population (especially one that is aging and culturally diverse), and the insufficient number of health care educational programs necessary to train new nurses. Currently, one-half of registered nurses (RNs) in Oregon are 50 years of age or older. Over the next 20 years, it is anticipated that 41% of currently licensed RNs in the state will retire. Still, the demand for RNs is expected to grow steadily. By 2020, an additional 15,700 nurse job openings are anticipated. At the same time, health care facilities throughout Oregon report difficulty in hiring qualified minority or bilingual nurses (Northwest Health Foundation, 2001).

The shortage of nurses comes at a time when Oregon population demographics will radically change. In the next generation, the number of Oregonians 65 or older will account for nearly 25% of all residents (Burton, Morris, & Campbell, 2005). As Oregonians live longer, their need for complex care will also grow. Furthermore, nearly 15% of the state's annual average population growth since 2000 has been due to an influx of foreign-born individuals according to the Federation for American Immigration Reform (2006). These trends set the scene for a health care challenge in Oregon that will likely be mirrored across the nation. As Guhde (2003) suggests, "Colleges and universities will need to develop innovative programs to attract these non-traditional students and support programs to help them complete the nursing curriculum" (p. 1). This statement is just as relevant to internationally educated nurses who are interested in entering the U.S. nursing workforce as it is to minority nursing students who are new to nursing.

The WIN program was developed to identify and select internationally educated nurses who are interested and are qualified to become licensed in the State of Oregon. Nurses who are credentialed in other countries need transitional educational opportunities to qualify for positions in the United States because they come from countries that may have different nursing standards and practices, nursing requirements, medical equipment, norms of communication, and cultural models of sickness and health. The challenge and the opportunity of the WIN program was to bring the English language skills of the group up to a level where they would be able to pass a state-required English assessment and to help them develop the skills and understanding of nursing standards and protocol in the United States.

The original proposal was submitted in summer of 2003. It was designed to be implemented within a 2-year period until the fall of 2005 and called for two cohorts of 12 students to begin English as a Second Language (ESL) instruction in January 2004. The first cohort would be at a more advanced level as determined by English assessments and interview performance and would participate in ESL for six months until June 2004, at which point these participants would take a state-required English assessment. Those who passed the assessment would move into the Nursing Transition Program (NTP) for 15 weeks during the summer. The second cohort would remain in ESL for an additional year and prepare to enter the NTP in the following summer of 2005. After students successfully completed the NTP and passed the national nursing licensing exam (NCLEX-RN), internships from the partner hospitals would be provided. After the internships, nurses would presumably be offered positions in local health care facilities. Not surprisingly, the original plan began to change almost as soon as the proposal was accepted.

The current WIN program has changed from its original vision. The program now lasts just under a year and is comprised of two major parts. The first six months focus on communication courses including *Medical Terminology* and *Professional Communication.* While these classes are being held, students complete the often complicated and time-consuming credential evaluation process of their nursing education and license. The NTP follows successful completion of the communication classes for another six months and prepares the students for the NCLEX-RN. After students successfully pass the NCLEX, they engage in preceptored clinical instruction that presumably leads to employment (see Appendix).

> We have a nursing shortage already, and it's growing. There's a clear need for programs like this. We have a wealth of nurses who've already acquired

nursing experience, and already moved to this country. We would be foolish if we didn't help them take the last steps necessary for a nursing career in America.

—Comment from an Oregon hospital recruiter, 2005

PROGRAM STRUCTURE AND DEVELOPMENT

The Early Days of WIN

The WIN program is located within Clackamas Community College (CCC) and utilizes several key departments. Two instructional departments were involved at the onset: the English as a Second Language department and the Health Sciences department. As the program progressed, the Speech and Theater Arts department and Education and Human Services department also became involved. Additionally, the Workforce Development Program of the college was involved.

The WIN Operations Team is comprised of the Project Coordinator; the Nursing Program Director; the Cultural Advocacy Coordinator, a new position that has played a critically important role in WIN; key faculty members from the ESL department; and support staff. The WIN Operations Team meets formally on a monthly basis to address operational issues, but its members also engage in ongoing communication related to student and program issues. It is this close collaboration that keeps each staff person able to address and support the many program challenges.

The Project Coordinator is from the Customized Training & Development Services department (CTDS). The role of the Project Coordinator is managing the project and its budget, facilitating interdepartmental resources for program development, hiring instructors and support personnel, and coordinating and evaluating the various components of the program. The WIN Nursing Program Director designs, implements, revises, and evaluates the educational program and its students based on the registered nursing scope of practice and competencies. She works closely with the Educational Consultant at the Oregon State Board of Nursing (OSBN) and with its licensing staff. The Cultural Advocacy Coordinator (CAC) provides case management for individual WIN students and is the key support person during the complex credential evaluation, application, and licensing processes. The CAC also maintains close working relationships with staff at the OSBN, staff members at agencies that evaluate foreign nursing credentials, financial assistance resources, and the WIN program staff.

Partners for Success

Collaborative partnerships with a number of stakeholder groups have contributed to the WIN program's success. Representatives from local health care facilities were present as key partners during the original proposal and continue to play an important role as the program has evolved. Cosigners of the original grant proposal included three health care partners, two representing local acute care hospitals and one representing long-term care. Another community partner was the Consulate of Mexico, a strong advocate for the WIN Program and a key link to the Hispanic community, the largest nonnative population in the Portland area. According to the 2000 Census, Mexicans constitute 39% of the foreign-born in Oregon (FAIR, 2006). The consulate has also been helpful in providing vital problem-solving insight related to the complexities of immigration issues that other WIN students face. Additionally, the Immigrant and Refugee Community Organization (IRCO) in Portland has been a helpful program resource. Its network reaches out to the entire immigrant community and has been helpful in spreading the word about WIN. Their Language Bank and translation services helped WIN's recruitment efforts by translating informational flyers into various languages and have also been used by WIN students to translate their educational and professional documents.

Other partners who assisted as program consultants were from the Chicago Bilingual Nurse Consortium, part of Saint Xavier University School of Nursing in Chicago, Illinois. This program was one of the first programs in the nation to focus on helping internationally educated immigrant nurses, originally Polish-educated nurses who resided in the Chicago area, to become licensed. Another key program consultant was from the Programa Internacional de Enfermería (PIDE) in Dallas, Texas, whose main focus is on helping Hispanic immigrant nurses with nursing degrees from Latin American countries.

Essential to the success of the WIN program was a collaborative relationship with the Oregon State Board of Nursing (OSBN). Their input regarding application, credentialing, and licensure procedures for internationally educated nurses has been tremendously helpful. Reciprocally, the WIN program has provided input and perspective to the board when policy and rule questions surface related to internationally educated nurses.

All of these strategic partnerships have helped generate support in the community and within the college since the program's inception. The synergy these partners bring has helped to find creative and workable solutions when problems have surfaced. The partners act in an advisory capacity and meet quarterly to receive program updates and, more importantly, to engage in problem solving. Members have also participated in selection screening interviews of WIN applicants, and health care partners have assisted in providing instructional resources, guest lecturers, job shadowing, field trips, and clinical placements. The importance of sound community partnerships, which bring continued contributions and support, cannot be overstated. Their active involvement is a key success factor for WIN.

THE WORKFORCE INVESTMENT ACT (WIA) CONNECTION

While the WIN program provided, free of charge, all instructional costs including textbooks, WIN students were initially expected to cover the costs of credential review, translation services, NCLEX-RN test fees, and OSBN application fees. To help defray the cost burden to these often underemployed students, the WIN program linked with the Workforce Development Program at CCC. Through the Workforce Investment Act of 1998, a national workforce preparation and employment system, this program has helped offset many of the costs associated with WIN, such as childcare expenses, textbooks, nursing scrubs and shoes, licensure and application fees, and even, on occasion, gas vouchers.

Recruitment and Selection Activities

Finding Immigrant Nurses in the Community

During the start-up phase, WIN promotional flyers were created and translated into Spanish and Russian. These materials were distributed to hospitals, churches, IRCO, schools, and state employment agencies. Press releases appeared in the local newspaper, newspapers serving the Asian and Latino communities, and other community communication outlets including radio, announcing a General Information Meeting to occur in late October 2003. A structured telephone interview protocol was created for the intake process and to pre-assess individual qualifications for the program when people called for information. Letters of invitation to the evening meeting were sent to all individuals who expressed interest in the program. Childcare was provided for those who came with their families.

The WIN staff expected 50 to 75 attendees. Surprisingly, nearly 200 people representing 33 countries arrived at the meeting. The purpose of the meeting was to provide an overview of the WIN program, to explain the costs and commitments of the program, and to gather detailed information about interested candidates. The keynote speaker was a former immigrant nurse who had completed the Chicago program. She shared her perspective of becoming a licensed nurse in the United States. Her talk was inspirational and practical. While she encouraged the audience not to give up on their dreams, she warned them that the road was very difficult and required a strong individual commitment, as well as support from the immigrant nurses' families.

Selecting Candidates for the First WIN Cohort

At the conclusion of the meeting, attendees who believed they met the entrance requirements were given a self-assessment. The self-assessment requested information about nursing education, licensure, and work experience in the country of origin, as well as an English language self-assessment. This information was collected from all interested participants to assist in the screening process and became part of a detailed database of all interested individuals. People were considered potential candidates for the WIN program if they reported three key pieces of information: (a) acceptable documentation to work, such as a permanent resident card or "green card," U.S. citizenship, or work authorization without sponsorship; (b) licensure as a nurse in their country of origin; and (c) a language self-assessment with "high" (5–7) ratings.

After their self-assessments were reviewed, selected candidates participated in formal ESL pretesting. The ESL screening consisted of the BEST test, COMPASS Reading, Grammar and Listening assessments, and the Holistically Scored Writing Assessment (HSWA). After the ESL testing results were reviewed, the highest scorers were invited for face-to-face interviews. Fifty-two candidates were interviewed using a structured group interview process. The interview committee consisted of: the WIN Nursing Director (representing the academic perspective of the WIN program), two health care partners (representing health care workforce recruitment), and a representative of the Consulate of Mexico (knowledgeable about immigration issues). Relevant documentation, test scores, and work experience were thoroughly reviewed. Finally, 38 individuals received a written invitation to participate in the first WIN program scheduled to begin in January 2004. The names of those individuals not invited to participate in the program at that time were kept in the WIN database for future opportunities.

The WIN program is the first in the nation designed to accommodate a multinational contingent of foreign-trained nurses. To date, 60 countries are named in the WIN database of 395 interested applicants. Many of the former nurses of these countries have found their way to the United States as refugees and asylum seekers, escaping persecution and violence. Some have arrived by marriage to U.S. citizens, while others have won the immigration lottery. In all cases, these former nurses have had to leave their homes and families, as well as their health care professions. Many have arrived with little or no English language skills and no job recommendations. Most arrived with only a faint dream to work once again in their profession.

In the four cohorts of students who have participated since 2004 in WIN NTP (N = 51), 23 countries have been represented, in the following descending order of representation: the Philippines (7 students), Romania (6), Russia (5), Nigeria (4), Bosnia (3), Germany (3), Japan (3), Cuba (2), Czech Republic (2), Kenya (2), Ukraine (2), and one student each from Latvia, Brazil, China, El Salvador, Ethiopia, Iran, India, Liberia, Norway, Peru, Togo, and Vietnam. The program has been described as a "United Nations" of nurses.

THE ENGLISH LANGUAGE COMPONENTS OF WIN

The First Six Months of English

The WIN Program was approved for funding by the NWHF in October 2003. Language classes were due to begin in early January 2004. The ESL department chair helped select a trio of ESL instructors to begin identifying curriculum and building the first WIN language courses. Curriculum searches for English for Special Purposes (ESP) materials related to nursing were conducted using Web searches, including listservs; however, little curriculum was found dealing specifically with health care or nurses. As a result, the instructors assembled a variety of traditional ESL texts and materials and worked to tailor the curriculum to the group.

The OSBN requires internationally educated nurses to demonstrate a high level of English proficiency in order to practice. It allows these nurses three choices for a standardized English language assessment: (a) Test of English for International Communication (TOEIC), (b) Test of English as a Foreign Language (TOEFL), and (c) International English Language Testing System (IELTS). (*Note:* Many states accept only one assessment.) The TOEFL is the most common English proficiency examination used in the United States by state boards of nursing (O'Neill, 2004). However, the TOEIC was selected for the WIN program because of its focus on workplace communication (Educational Testing Services, 2006). The OSBN requires a score of at least 780 on the TOEIC. Current OSBN rules, like most state boards, allow those who were educated in English, including English language textbooks and English-speaking clinical practice, to be exempted from the English assessment requirement. (The Philippines and certain countries in Africa fall into this category.) The task for the WIN ESL instructors was to build a curriculum focused on health care workplace communication that would assist students to meet the TOEIC language testing requirement.

Originally the WIN proposal planned to schedule ESL classes for 20 hours per week during the daytime. However, based on experience working with other adult learners, many of whom worked full-time and had families, ESL classes were ultimately scheduled for 6:00–9:00 P.M., Monday through Thursday. The new accommodation resulted in 12 hours of language and communication instruction per week.

The first ESL courses for WIN included TOEIC Preparation and English for Immigrant Nurses, which included pronunciation, oral communication (speaking and listening), grammar, and reading/writing. Medical English and Customer Service components were added during the second term. Each class session wove health-related subject matter, vocabulary, professional journals, and Web sites into the curriculum along with periodic assessments of student's abilities in speaking, grammar, vocabulary, and reading comprehension. Instruction began with a classroom of 38 students from 22 countries, with length of residency in the United States ranging from 3 to 15 years.

After several weeks, due to the large class size and the wide range of proficiency in English, the group was divided into two smaller groups based on their proficiency, as determined by a TOEIC sample examination. The first group consisted of 18 individuals who received scores above 845 on the TOEIC pre-assessment, already higher than the minimum score of 780 required by the OSBN. Five others who had not been required to take an English assessment (from the Philippines and some African nations) joined them for a total of 23 in the first group. With guidance from an ESL instructor, students in this higher-level group created

Individual Education Plans (IEPs) and worked independently to develop their language skills and prepare for the TOEIC. The second group consisted of 15 students who continued in the traditional ESL classes; they had TOEIC pre-assessment scores that ranged from 510 to 805. Both groups continued to attend the pronunciation component once a week.

The sorting technique used was a satisfactory predictor of TOEIC success. Everyone in the first group passed the test, with scores ranging from 780 (the minimum criteria accepted by the state board) to 980 (990 is the highest score possible). On the other hand, just one student from the second group was able to pass the TOEIC within the first six months, just in time to be included as one of the fifteen students in the first NTP cohort.

From Pronunciation to Accent Differentiation

A common complaint of patients and coworkers regarding foreign-born health care workers is the difficulty in understanding and communicating with them in the often fast-paced and stressful health care workplace. This supports the assertion that "acquiring good pronunciation is the most difficult part of learning a new language" (Orion, 1988, pp. xxiii–iv). To address this issue, nearly the entire original group of 38 attended pronunciation class one evening a week. The class was divided into two smaller groups, one of students from Eastern European countries with similar phonemic challenges, and the other of students from various language backgrounds. Unfortunately, over the course of the 10-week term, neither group made significant improvement in their pronunciation. Yet, WIN program managers still had a desire to address the communication problems associated with strong accents.

To further address this situation, WIN staff attempted a creative solution that utilized two departments at the college that routinely do not work together. The Speech and Theater Arts department was approached about meeting with members of the ESL department to craft a course that would focus on reducing pronunciation difficulties. The rationale was that if particular accents and dialects can be taught to actors, perhaps the "American" accent could also be taught to the WIN nurses. The course was eventually termed *Accent Differentiation*. It used techniques from Theater Arts to teach students to speak *with* an American accent, as well as how to project confidence.

While the model seemed to be sound, implementation was challenging, and the results were mixed. In practice, ESL faculty spent several weeks conducting in-depth analyses of each individual's pronunciation, using a standardized phonemic assessment, to identify difficult sounds for individual students and then teaching the mechanics of creating each challenging sound. Short health care monologues, which could be modified to integrate and emphasize the individual's phonemic challenges, and other more lengthy speeches were read multiple times by students with feedback provided that emphasized loudness, rate, pitch, and quality. Audio and videotaping occurred but with only limited opportunity for students to replay and reflect on their performances.

According to both instructors, after 10 one-hour sessions, most students made "good" progress. One student from Iran, whose native language was Farsi, commented how prior to the sessions she could not hear the sounds that she was making that were difficult for others to understand. She remarked, "Now, finally, I am aware of what I am doing." Another, a Spanish-speaking student from Cuba, said that he was having fewer problems with people misunderstanding him. Nevertheless, radical improvement was not achieved.

A lesson learned from the Accent Differentiation course was that accents are fossilized into an individual's speech pattern and are very difficult to change. Intensive attention by a highly motivated learner and tailored coaching for a significant period of time are required to affect long-lasting change. The expense of one-on-one coaching prevented its integration into the WIN language course. However, the college is exploring ways to continue with the Accent Differentiation model, such as by having Speech Pathology students from Portland State University tutor ESL students, including those in the WIN program. This initiative would both utilize the skills of Speech Pathology students and meet their need for clinical opportunities.

New Language Criteria for Selection

A considerable change to the original model of language instruction was initiated after 18 months of experience. By this time, 13 of the original 38 students still remained in ESL courses (not including pronunciation). The most immediate goal for this group was to pass the TOEIC assessment. Unfortunately, just two individuals from this group were able to meet the OSBN language proficiency requirement within 18 months. Their early pre-assessment TOEIC scores ranged from 690 to 805. These two individuals went on to be part of the 10 individuals who made up the second NTP cohort. The early assumption that 18 months of ESL instruction could bring the prescreened, internationally educated nurses up to the minimum language requirement was overly optimistic.

Table 17.1 shows the relationship between actual English assessment scores and the NCLEX-RN pass rates for the first two cohorts of WIN NTP students. The data suggest that for students who successfully complete the WIN program, TOEIC scores above 805 and TOEFL scores at or above 220 are positively related to passing the NCLEX-RN. On the other hand, the relationship is unclear for those with lower TOEIC scores (780–805) even if they pass the WIN program. The data also suggest that those WIN students who are exempted by OSBN from taking an English assessment also have a good chance of not passing the NCLEX-RN. There appears to be a correlation between performance on a standardized English assessment and passing the NCLEX-RN. (*Note:* Two WIN students from the second cohort passed the NCLEX-PN, one of whom had not been required by the state board to take an English assessment; the other had a lower TOEIC score of 805.)

The data in Table 17.1 is from a very small population, so further research would be necessary to confirm these interpretations. However, new admission requirements were implemented with the third and fourth cohorts. Beginning with the third cohort in 2006, all WIN candidates must now meet the minimum language requirement of the OSBN prior to being considered for entry into the WIN program. Currently, OSBN-minimum English assessment scores are 780 on the TOEIC, 220 on the computer version of the TOEFL, 83 on the Internet version of the TOEFL, or an overall score of 6.5 on the IELTS. A WIN selection rubric grants more weight to those who score higher on the English

Table 17.1

COMPARISON OF ENGLISH ASSESSMENT SCORES AND NCLEX-RN RESULTS FOR WIN NTP COHORTS ONE AND TWO (N = 25)

	TOEIC SCORE ABOVE 805	TOEIC SCORE 780–805	TOEFL SCORE 220 & ABOVE	NOT REQUIRED TO TEST BY OSBN
Passed NCLEX-RN	9	3	3	2
Did Not Pass NCLEX-RN	0	3	0	5

assessment. Furthermore, *all* nurses entering the WIN program must meet this requirement *even if they are exempted by the OSBN.* These new, more rigorous requirements have reduced the number of internationally educated nurses who are eligible for entry into WIN, but the program continues to attract enough qualified applicants who are more likely to succeed in the WIN program and ultimately in the workplace.

Based on these experiences, it seems that ESL courses focusing on grammar, listening, reading, and writing and targeted to meet a minimum language assessment requirement do not necessarily lead to success on the TOEIC, given the linguistic complexity and technical vocabulary of workplace communication. Such courses, however, can be an important beginning if combined with intensive practice outside of the classroom in the workplace setting.

From English as a Second Language to Advanced Communication

Health care facilities have been clear to state that the most significant problem with internationally educated nurses is their ability to communicate effectively. In addition to accent, another barrier is their unfamiliarity with U.S. expectations around workplace communication. For example, nurses in the United States are considered leaders in the organizations in which they work. They are often supervisors and important partners in the overall team that provides patient care. They are critical thinkers and problem solvers. Often, these are new expectations for internationally educated nurses. Meeting the state board's minimum language requirement is not a guarantee of effective workplace communication. Foreign nurses must learn to assert themselves appropriately and communicate effectively to work as part of the whole team of health care professionals.

Guhde (2003) has suggested several innovative strategies for building verbal and written skills for ESL nursing students. Building on these strategies, a new course was developed for WIN students to strengthen their workplace communication skills and leadership. Titled Advanced Communication for Healthcare Workers, this course replaced the initial ESL and pronunciation courses and spans two terms. The goal of the course is to build awareness and skill in communicating effectively in the U.S. health care environment, not on teaching nursing theory. The first-term course focuses on exploring personal preferences and communication styles, identified using the Myers Briggs Type Indicator (MBTI);

practicing assertive communication, listening, and questioning skills; and providing feedback to others. In addition, written communication is woven into the program by requiring a student research project on a nursing subject. Students write a two- to three-page research paper. They receive feedback on grammar and clarity of expression (rather than on content) at the mid-term and submit their final paper at the end of the term. In addition, the students are required to present their paper to the class in a 10-minute videotaped presentation using at least one visual aid, such as PowerPoint slides, flipchart graphics, or handouts. A DVD is made of everyone's presentation and given to each student so they can review the subject matter as well as the presentation styles of themselves and their classmates. The second term of Advanced Communication emphasizes listening and communication skills in challenging health care situations (such as speaking with surgical masks and working with taped shift reports), managing workplace conflict, customer service principles in health care, quality assurance and process improvement, and stress and change management. A second research paper and presentation is also required with a focus on psychology and mental health issues, a subject of particular importance to the widely diverse students in the WIN program, as cultural differences in attitudes and perceptions of mental health are common.

REQUIREMENTS AND DEADLINES

Credential Equivalency—A Stumbling Block for Some

The credential review process set by the National Council of State Boards of Nursing (NCSBN), in which equivalency of a student's credentials to the U.S. nursing curriculum is certified, is one of the most critical and, at the same time, one of the most complicated requirements for WIN students. Most students report spending three to nine months engaged in this important step, although in one unusual case a student, who had begun the credential review process prior to learning of the WIN program, spent a total of 3 1/2 years before her credential equivalency was completed. There are complicated instructions to understand, certified translations to be acquired, and universities to be contacted all over the world. In some cases, war or fire has destroyed records. Schools of medicine and nursing in some countries share parts of the same curriculum, further complicating the credential review process. Some foreign schools and national licensing organizations may be less than cooperative because of ethnic or religious conflict, creating significant challenges. The difficulty for some students in obtaining the necessary credentialing documentation is nearly insurmountable without assistance. These challenges underscore the importance of the role of the WIN Cultural Advocacy Coordinator, who shepherds the WIN students over these substantial hurdles.

In the state of Oregon, the OSBN recognizes three independent credential evaluation services for foreign nurses. (*Note:* Some states recognize only one.) During the initial planning of the WIN program, the planning committee decided to learn as much as possible about each of the credential evaluation organizations recognized by Oregon. At the time, two services were approved by OSBN: the Commission on Graduates of Foreign Nursing Schools (CGFNS) and the International Education Research Foundation (IERF). [*Note:* A third credential evaluation service, Educational Records Evaluation Service (ERES), was added to the approved provider list by the OSBN in 2005.] Although these organizations all abide by the same national standards, IERF worked closely with WIN to devise a "batch" system for processing credentialing information and designated a single point of contact for WIN nurses, an approach that has helped expedite the credential review process.

In the first two cohorts of students in the NTP (N = 25), 64% had credentials equivalent to an Associate Degree in Nursing (ADN), 20% had education equivalent to a Bachelor of Science in Nursing (BSN), and 16% had education equivalent to Diploma nurses.

Unfortunately, the credential review process has been a roadblock to other WIN students. Several students learned that their educational credentials were equivalent to Physicians Assistant or Medical Doctor. These students were required to exit the program, almost always before the beginning of the NTP, because there was no way they could become a Registered Nurse in the state of Oregon. Because only a very few WIN applicants arrive with completed credential evaluations, students are informed during the admission process that if their credential evaluation, when it arrives, is not equivalent to an RN, they would have to leave the program.

With the beginning of the third cohort (N = 12) in the fall of 2005, the WIN program agreed to allow students who had been admitted to the program but who had received a credential evaluation of Practical

Nurse (PN) to continue with the program. These students prepare for the NCLEX-PN and entry into the U.S. workforce as LPNs.

State Board Application Begins a Ticking Clock

Every state's board of nursing has its own policies, rules, interpretations, and processes that abide by the requirements established by the NCSBN. Two rules of the OSBN in particular have impacted WIN students. The first sets limits for the number of years that can elapse between a foreign nurse's practice and return to nursing practice in the United States. An internationally educated nurse who has practiced 960 hours (approximately six months of full-time work) within the last 5 years is only required to pass the NCLEX-RN before they can return to nursing. Internationally educated nurses who have worked 960 hours between 5 and 15 years ago must complete a state-approved education program, called a reentry program. If a nurse (U.S. or internationally educated) cannot meet the practice requirement within 15 years, he or she must complete a full nursing program again.

The second rule sets a timeframe for passing the NCLEX-RN once an application for licensure has been submitted to the OSBN. According to the OSBN, a foreign nurse applicant must meet all the requirements for licensure, including the language requirement, credential review, and passing the NCLEX-RN within 3 years of the application date. In the past, some internationally educated nurses, eager to begin the process, had applied as soon as possible, but then ran out of time before they were able to meet all of the requirements. To overcome this problem, the WIN program, with the help of the Cultural Advocacy Coordinator, developed individual application timelines based on each nurse's current level of English proficiency and dates of most recent nursing work experience. Those nurses whose English skills needed substantial development were counseled to delay applying to the OSBN unless they were near the end of the 15-year practice requirement. In those cases, applicants were informed of the possible consequences of applying and not meeting the OSBN requirements within the 3-year period. As of 2006, this rule has been reinterpreted by OSBN so that once an application has expired, the applicant may reapply as long as they are still within the 15-year limitation. As other states develop similar programs for internationally educated nurse populations, close scrutiny of changing state regulations is necessary to ensure that internationally educated nurses do not inadvertently lose their eligibility to reenter the nursing field in the United States.

THE WIN NURSING TRANSITION PROGRAM

NTP Curriculum Development

Originally, the nursing theory component of WIN (called the Nursing Transition Program or NTP) was to follow the ESL component and last for 15 weeks, based on WIN students attending classes 20 hours per week. As with the ESL classes, NTP scheduling was reconfigured to accommodate working adults. Students in the NTP now meet 3 days per week from 4:30 to 8:00 P.M. In addition, a series of all-day "Saturday Academies" are held once a month for eight months, focusing on current health care issues and featuring guest speakers.

The didactic portion of the NTP reviews the major content areas of nursing, emphasizing U.S. approaches to therapies and practice through the use of case studies and group process. It focuses sharply on developing critical thinking and evidence-based practice. As Donley (2005) states, "Faculty and students cannot address everything about nursing, regardless of the length of programs . . . However, faculty can create curricula to help students enhance their cognitive skills, methods of reflection, critical thinking, problem solving, analysis, synthesis and ability to evaluate structure, process and outcomes" (p. 14).

Focusing on critical thinking and evidence-based practice is particularly important for internationally educated nurses because, with few exceptions, WIN students were previously educated in a formal lecture style with a focus on memorizing facts and carrying out physician orders. The WIN NTP emphasis on problem solving, prioritization, and accountability for one's own actions, designed to prepare internationally educated nurses to be active members of the health care team while also preparing them for the nursing licensing examination, has been a new and compelling challenge for many internationally educated nurses.

Another important component of the NTP has been training to increase competence in technical skills, physical assessment, and recognition of patients' responses to drug and other therapies. Weekly sessions in the clinical lab closely follow, whenever possible, the didactic information presented in class and give WIN students an opportunity to practice with mannequins, equipment, and other materials in simulated experiences. These sessions are supplemented by visits to local health care facilities for demonstrations of equipment that is not available in the campus lab. The experiences gained through simulation most closely approximate those that WIN students will be exposed to as they transition to a preceptored clinical experience and ultimately to a position as a newly hired U.S. nurse.

Because of the vastly increasing and changing body of knowledge in health care generally, and nursing specifically, internationally educated nurses need exposure to the latest and most accurate information available. With an emphasis on evidence-based practice, they must learn how to access information quickly, not only in textbooks, reference books, and professional journals, but also via electronic means. The WIN students are required to have e-mail and Internet access and receive much of their information electronically. This preparation is critical in an age when hospitals are converting to electronic charts, orders, and data retrieval.

For similar reasons, exposure to instructors and advanced practice nurses with specialties in various aspects of nursing is also important. The WIN NTP program has a lead instructor who provides the majority of instruction but who also supplements the teaching with experts in areas such as psychiatric/mental health, pediatrics, diabetes, stroke recovery, head injuries, burns, wound care, and critical care. Another major component of the NTP is preparation for the NCLEX-RN, using *Saunders Comprehensive Review for NCLEX-RN* (Silvesteri, 2002). Initially, the intent was that this book, which includes summaries of major nursing topics as well as numerous review questions, would serve as the sole text for the NTP. However, it was quickly determined that the nurses needed to have access to a basic library of nursing information that they could use for class preparation and review. Furthermore, due to their demanding work schedules and distance from the college and each other, it was necessary to provide individual copies of the primary texts for use at home. Many of the needed texts were donated or lent to the students by nursing faculty when they did not need the books themselves (e.g., during the summer months). A few copies were purchased with the intention of using them for group work. Still others were generously donated by the publisher. As nursing practice and related technology continually and rapidly evolve, textbooks will need to be updated often. As a result, the purchase of new texts will continue to be an ongoing expense.

Finally, several three-hour nurse-shadowing experiences were instituted for students in the WIN program because it became apparent early on in classroom discussion that students were relying upon their previous knowledge and practice and, despite reading about U.S. practice, had little or no knowledge of the daily routine and responsibilities of the registered nurse in the United States. Arrangements were made with several hospitals to permit the NTP students to have three-hour "nurse-shadowing" observations at the start of a shift to view first-hand how a nurse receives report from the previous shift and organizes, prioritizes, assesses, and delivers care. Because the students could not legally assist in providing care, even in the role of student, their new knowledge was derived entirely from observation and comparing what they observed from the shadowing experience to examples of practice presented in their textbooks. Feedback from the health care facility staff was very positive, and several students received permission to remain on the units until the end of the shift.

Simulation—The Payoff for Partnership

Northwest Health Foundation (NWHF) periodically provides opportunities for grant recipients to gather together to learn about other programs and to seek input from others regarding current program challenges. During one of these conferences, the WIN program described the problem associated with the prohibition of patient contact and the dire need for clinical practice *before* the nurse is licensed. A neighboring community college had recently been awarded NWHF funding to develop a Simulation Manikin (SIM) Laboratory for its nursing students. After some discussion, the two programs, WIN and SIM, decided to team-up. A simulation specialist from the neighboring college and the WIN Nursing Director developed simulation scenarios for the WIN nurses. In order to promote optimum learning, the scenarios focused on assessment and communication skills in a postoperative environment. Cardiopulmonary issues, pain management, and effective communication of information between shifts at work were emphasized in an effort to stimulate sound problem solving and to build self-confidence in clinical performance. Student debriefing of each scenario allowed the WIN student to receive feedback from peers and instructors and reflect on his or her experience.

In the near future, CCC will have its own SIM laboratory, and the WIN program will be well-prepared to take full advantage of it. The WIN students will be able to build on their personal experience, reinforce their classroom discussions, and engage in even more simulated clinical training—the "next best thing" to actual patient contact.

Student Assessment in the NTP

Many of the WIN students are not familiar with multiple-choice testing because in their countries testing was done orally, by short answer, or by essay. Therefore, considerable time in the NTP is devoted to multiple-choice test-taking strategies and to understanding the structure and intent of NCLEX test items. Students are encouraged to answer several thousand practice questions prior to taking the NCLEX in order to familiarize themselves with the style of questioning, as well as with computer adaptive testing, which is also a new concept for many WIN nurses. Their review book contains 3,500 practice questions, and additional questions are presented and analyzed in class each week. Finally, each content area is assessed with a proctored, computer-based standardized exam. Prior to each of these tests, students have access to a nonproctored, computerized exam that can be taken at home. The intent of frequent testing is to provide familiarity with the style and format of NCLEX test items, as well as to assess students' grasp of content, prior to taking the NCLEX.

In addition to NCLEX preparation, students are tested on their knowledge of theory and are required to demonstrate their nursing and assessment skills during small group role-plays. In order to pass the WIN program, students are required to pass a comprehensive test of theory, a skills assessment, and a dosage calculation test with 100% accuracy.

The Saturday Academy Seminars

A special part of the WIN program is the eight monthly, day-long Saturday Academy seminars. These sessions bring guest speakers into the WIN classroom for instruction and discussion of timely nursing-related subject matter. The primary purpose of the seminars is to provide in-depth exploration of important subjects not addressed in the nursing theory course. The WIN Nursing Director selects these topics based on relevant or emerging health care issues, standards, requirements, or technologies. Example topics include: pain management, HIV/AIDS, legal and ethical issues in health care, abuse and neglect, and an overview of the Oregon Nurse Practice Act. Field trips have been arranged to a long-term health care facility for a review of geriatric care and to an acute-care facility for seminars on wound and ostomy care. In these settings, the WIN students have another opportunity to see the equipment and procedures common to long-term and acute care in the United

States and to meet health care professionals in their own workplace milieu. Following a session on vacuum-assisted wound closure and IV pumps, one student noted that in her native country, "We had to count the IV drops one by one."

The Wisdom of Teams in WIN

Part of the purpose of educating in cohorts is to tap the learning potential within a group. As individuals begin to learn from and support each other, they simulate the real-world collaborative efforts of a health care team. It is not uncommon to see students researching topics and sharing Web sites with everyone else in class via e-mail or gathering before class to study or practice assessment skills on each other. When a student passes the NCLEX-RN, congratulations flow; when one does not pass, words of encouragement help assuage the disappointment or shame.

Effective teams are built not only by working together but also by celebrating together. During the WIN program several opportunities exist to step back from the classroom and focus on building stronger relationships with colleagues. The International Day of the Nurse provides a unique opportunity to celebrate the "United Nations" that is WIN. During this springtime celebration of Florence Nightingale's birthday and amid a flurry of balloons, the WIN nursing class is interrupted while the students are given small gifts and goodies from the partner hospitals and WIN staff. Everyone joins the students in hearing the story of Florence Nightingale, and each reflects on what it means to be a nurse and what it will mean to become one again in the United States. International potlucks are also held periodically during the NTP. At these events, one might find a curried stew from Africa, stuffed cabbage rolls from Russia, or Chinese dumplings. Food nurtures relationships. Nurses from all cohorts are invited to attend these gatherings. When multiple cohorts of WIN students join together at these events, it is evident that the family of WIN has clearly grown, as has the menu.

The WIN NTP program culminates with a special graduation ceremony. Here the WIN graduates are recognized for completing the difficult road of coursework and adjustment to the U.S. culture of patient care. Candles are lit, speeches of thanks are given, photographs retell the previous year, and tears flow from family members, coworkers, and the supportive employers who have been invited. It is a time of reflection, celebration, and recognition of individual accomplishment.

> We left our home countries for different reasons, because of wars, political systems we disagreed with, discrimination, love and marriages, trying to build a better future . . . We found ourselves in a great country, the United States of America, where dreams can become reality.
>
> —Excerpt from WIN Nurse graduation speech, 2005

WIN—A STATE-APPROVED REENTRY PROGRAM

As mentioned earlier, in the state of Oregon, any nurse who has not practiced more than 960 hours over the course of the previous 5 years is a candidate for reentry. These nurses are required by the OSBN to complete a state-approved reentry program that includes a set amount of nursing review (at least 80 hours of nursing theory and 30 hours of pharmacology) and a specified amount of supervised or preceptored clinical (a minimum of 160 hours, unpaid, in an acute care facility). Most WIN students fall into this category and are required to complete a reentry program. The WIN NTP was designed to meet (and exceed) these requirements.

The WIN program is now one of three recognized reentry programs in the state of Oregon. There are some significant differences, however, among the programs. Traditional reentry programs in Oregon were designed for licensed U.S. nurses who had left the field for a period of time and wished to return to practice. Essentially, these programs are U.S. nursing refresher courses and offer the didactic portion online or as a self-study. The required unpaid clinical hours of reentry are generally arranged with local acute-care facilities while the nurse is registered in a college nursing clinical course. For many internationally educated nurses, these requirements are not sufficient to ensure understanding of the U.S. nursing culture or protocols for safe practice. The OSBN is currently reviewing and revising its standards for reentry for all nurses, with particular focus on the special needs of internationally educated nurses. It is exploring the use of competency-based testing and individualized reentry based on the individual nurse's learning needs and goals. The WIN Nursing Director has served on the OSBN Re-Entry Task Force to explore these issues.

The Clinical Dilemma for Immigrant Nurses

Participants in the WIN program are prohibited from having any patient contact until they hold a limited license from the OSBN. This is one of the most significant challenges for WIN students and the WIN program. The WIN participants must complete the NTP and pass the NCLEX-RN before they are issued a limited license and qualified as a nurse. Internationally educated nurses are not considered nursing students; they are considered unlicensed nurses and, as such, are not allowed to have patient contact. Ironically, students in a traditional nursing program often begin supervised clinical experience, including taking blood pressure and listening to lung sounds, within weeks of beginning their nursing program. Supervised patient contact is central to traditional nursing student education. The prohibition of patient contact for WIN participants poses a significant barrier to clinical training and thus to a thorough and comprehensive educational experience.

To complicate the issue, if an internationally educated nurse has practiced recently (within 5 years), they are not required to complete a reentry program; they need only to pass the NCLEX-RN. Consequently, these individuals are not required to perform unpaid supervised clinical (preceptored) experience. This essentially means that a participant in WIN who has worked within the last 5 years in a foreign country and who passes the NCLEX (without necessarily passing the WIN program) may accept a nursing position without having had any supervised clinical experience in the United States. Experience with the first WIN NTP cohort underscored the risk of having graduates become employed without having had any supervised clinical experience in the United States.

As a result, the WIN program now requires *all* WIN graduates who successfully pass the NCLEX to complete 160 hours of preceptored clinical experience in an acute care facility. The desire to return to employment as a nurse and the practical demand for an increase in income weigh heavily on many WIN graduates by this time. These unpaid hours are a hardship for some, but the experience is invaluable and can mean the difference between a successful transition into the workplace and a trying one.

A great challenge for the program has been to locate clinical sites and preceptors for WIN graduates following the NCLEX-RN. Other nursing schools in the region also require clinical sites for their students, resulting in a scarcity of available preceptors and sites. This demand means that WIN graduates may be required to wait until a site or preceptor becomes available—a delay that can add precious time to the already long journey to become a U.S. registered nurse. Another problem is that the staff at many clinical sites prefers to schedule students far in advance. Such scheduling is not always possible because WIN participants may take the

NCLEX-RN more than once or choose to wait until they believe they are ready to take it for the first time. Some have waited up to 18 months after completing the program to sit for the NCLEX-RN. To expedite the clinical placements for WIN students, the program has collaborated with the college's nursing department to create new affiliation agreements for clinical sites and to provide liability insurance for WIN nurses. Participating health care facilities are pleased with the arrangement, as are WIN nurses, who are anxious to start their clinical training and find employment. To date, most WIN graduates are offered employment as soon as their preceptored clinical is completed. As one WIN nurse reported after a long wait, "It is like a fish being placed back in the water."

Unfortunately, not all placements are successful. The right match between nurse and preceptor is an important consideration. For this reason, the WIN Nursing Director meets with each preceptor prior to placement to explain the program and to discuss the background, skills, and general impression she has of the WIN nurse. The WIN nurse is not like a U.S. nurse returning to the field. He or she is probably unfamiliar with many of the protocols and technological advances of patient care. For some, the learning curve will be slower than for others, even when compared to new graduates of traditional nursing programs. Yet, one preceptor has reported that the maturity and breadth of background that the WIN nurse brings to patient care is of great value. Of the 51 students who have participated in the WIN NTP program, 41% have had from 2 to 5 years of foreign nursing experience, 33% have had from 5 to 10 years, 8% have had from 10 to 15 years, and 10% more than 15 years. (*Note:* 8% had less than 2 years of experience.)

The Role of Donations and Volunteers in WIN

The strategy to solicit and encourage donations and volunteers has had a two-fold impact on WIN's success. First, the donations of equipment, such as stethoscopes from the equipment manufacturer and *RN-Notes,* a handy nurse's clinical pocket guide from the publisher, as well as nursing textbooks from CCC nursing faculty, former nursing students, and others, have been welcome learning tools for the WIN nurses. In addition, a WIN library of nursing textbooks has been created, available for check-out to WIN nurses. These donated volumes supplement the textbooks purchased by grant dollars in the library. Similarly, the use of volunteer speakers during certain sessions of the Saturday Academy or the NTP brings a change of pace and expertise to the sessions.

Secondly, the use of donations and volunteers has increased the visibility of WIN in the health care community. The increased visibility means new inroads for recruiting future students and helps spread the word about the WIN program to potential employers in the area. The danger of relying on volunteerism and donations to run a program, however, is that ultimately, like "soft" money funding, it cannot be projected too far into the future.

WINNING RESULTS

The WIN Program Is Working

As of December 2007, 48 students from 20 countries in four cohorts have successfully completed the WIN NTP. The first clear measure of success of the WIN program is the NCLEX pass rate, and the results have been promising. Table 17.2 shows success rates for the WIN cohorts. Fifteen students in the first cohort began the NTP in June 2004, 12 passed the WIN NTP program, and of these, 11, or 93%, have passed the NCLEX-RN. These 11 are all currently employed as registered nurses at regional health care facilities. Ten nurses began the second WIN cohort in March 2005; eight passed the WIN NTP, seven passed the NCLEX-RN, and two passed the NCLEX-PN, for a pass rate of 100%. Seven are currently licensed as RNs and two as PNs. One who did not pass the NTP program was able to successfully pass the NCLEX-PN. All who have passed the NCLEX are working in the field.

The second cohort provided a unique opportunity to compare the performance of those who were selected for WIN using the initial language standards to those using the later, more stringent, standards. Half of cohort two (5) began as part of the original WIN group of 38. Each completed 15 months of ESL education prior to admittance into the second cohort. Two were not required by the state board to meet the minimum English assessment requirements. For the others, their TOEIC scores hovered near the lower end of acceptability. During the NTP, one from this group dropped the program. Two completed the NTP but were unable to pass the NCLEX-RN and went on to pass the PN examination instead. The remaining two students completed the NTP and passed the NCLEX-RN but only after delaying for almost 2 years. In contrast, the other five members of cohort two, all who had excellent English language skills, passed the NCLEX-RN soon after completing the NTP. In sum, although the eventual pass rate of this cohort was 100%, the

Table 17.2

NCLEX PASS RATE OF WIN NTP COHORTS

	PASS WIN NTP	DID NOT PASS	DROP FROM WIN	PASS NCLEX RN	PASS NCLEX PN	NCLEX-RN PASS RATE	TOTAL NCLEX (RN + PN) PASS RATE
Cohort One: 2004 (N = 15)	12	2	1	11	0	93%	93%
Cohort Two: 2005 (N = 10)	8	1	1	7	2	88%	100%
Cohort Three: 2006 (N = 12)	11	1	0	6	4	55%	91%
Cohort Four: 2007 (N = 14)	11	0	3	5	1	45% (as of May 2008)	55% (as of May 2008)

difficulty and the delay that students with lower proficiency test scores encountered in passing the NCLEX-RN suggest the importance of language proficiency for passing the NCLEX-RN.

A third cohort of 12 met the more rigorous WIN language requirement and completed two terms of Advanced Communication and one term of Medical Terminology. The cohort completed the WIN NTP in the fall of 2006. Eleven passed the WIN NTP. As of December 2007, six (55%) had passed the NCLEX-RN, and four had passed the NCLEX-PN (for a pass rate of 91%) and are licensed as either an RN or a PN. All who have passed the NCLEX are now employed as nurses. The third cohort provides an example of how the credential evaluation process impacts results. Two members of the cohort received credential evaluations equivalent to PN; therefore, they were excluded from attempting the NCLEX-RN. These two students passed the PN examination and are currently employed at that level of licensure.

A fourth cohort of 14 began WIN in the fall of 2006. One student was dropped from Advanced Communication because she was unable to meet the language requirement for WIN, even though she was not required to meet it for the state board. One other dropped from the program at the beginning of the second term of Advanced Communication but was able to pass the NCLEX-PN on her own and is now currently employed as a PN. A third student dropped to return to her country of origin with her family. Of the remaining 11 students and as of this writing, all have passed the WIN NTP. Five have passed the NCLEX-RN, one has passed the NCLEX-PN, and the remainder are scheduled to test in the near future.

THE FUTURE OF WIN

Sustaining WIN

Sustaining this program beyond its pilot funding is a primary goal of the WIN program. It will be important to eventually transition from a grant-funded program that has received verbal support from college leadership to a self-supporting program nested within the Health Sciences Division and Nursing programs of CCC. This may mean assimilating certain WIN roles (e.g., the Cultural Advocacy Coordinator, Project Coordinator, and support staff) into the job descriptions of existing college and nursing department staff. Fortunately, the college is in the process of developing a long-term health care training and education initiative in partnership with local health care providers, regional universities, and health care product manufacturers. The WIN program is an example of an innovative program that fits well into this new initiative. Nevertheless, a significant challenge faced by the WIN program at the end of the NWHF grant is the procurement of funds for sustainability. Nursing programs, in general, are costly because of the small teacher/student ratios needed to ensure safe practice, as well as the technology, equipment, and reference materials required. The WIN students, because of their often low-income status and limited resources, are less able than many generic nursing students to afford program tuition and costs. While a traditional tuition or fee-based program integrated into the college system is the goal, in the short term, various alternatives are being explored.

Individual and corporate sponsorships as well as additional grants are now being explored. Course realignment to enable students to carry sufficient credit hours for eligibility for full student loans may offer another option. Workforce Investment Act assistance may continue to be an option for some individual students. As of this writing, the post-grant funding challenge is being addressed creatively and enthusiastically by stakeholders at the college and in the community. All partners espouse the value of the WIN program and are actively seeking strategies for its long-term financial sustainability. Several sizeable financial contributions have been made. As a result, a fifth cohort (N = 16) funded with residual general fund and partner dollars, began in January 2008. This is a strong demonstration of the willingness to integrate WIN into the college and the community.

The Right Staff—Cultural Sensitivity and Intercultural Experience

Expanding the number of nursing instructional staff and volunteer content experts is critical to effectively cover the wide breadth of subject matter that WIN students require during the NTP and Saturday Academy. These staff members should be well versed in working with a culturally diverse population such as the WIN nurses. Experience educating or working with other cultures or non-English speakers is of great value. Being able to speak another language, even without fluency, is a great advantage even though English is exclusively spoken in all WIN courses. Having struggled with learning another language provides the educator with an appreciation of the great accomplishment the WIN students have achieved to transition into such a complex linguistic workplace environment as health care. The WIN program has benefited from a bilingual, foreign-born Cultural Advocacy Coordinator and nurse educators who are either bilingual or foreign-educated. Even the experience of foreign travel can be of value working with the WIN population. These skills and experiences assist in establishing rapport with the WIN students and provide a background of personal stories that can be integrated into the classroom.

The need for professionals skilled at working with a culturally diverse population extends outside the classroom into the post–NCLEX-RN clinical sites. Matching WIN graduates with clinical preceptors who appreciate the special needs and the special gifts of internationally educated nurses, especially when working with an increasingly diverse patient population, is important to the success of the WIN nurse. Identifying these clinical sites and preceptors that can accommodate internationally educated WIN nurses is essential to sustaining WIN.

Continued Targeted Recruitment

An important factor yet to be determined is whether or not there is a population of adequately credentialed internationally educated nurses sufficient to sustain the WIN program into the future. The program has been modeled on a 10- to 16-candidate capacity per year. This seems to be a realistic number, considering the fact that broad-based community marketing has not yet been employed. Ironically, despite the high percentage of Hispanics in the region and despite over 22% of those with an expressed interest in WIN stating they were educated in Mexico, the WIN program has yet to admit one nurse who was educated in Mexico. Reasons for this dilemma include: problems with permanent resident status, inadequate English language skills, and/or lack of credentials deemed equivalent to a U.S. registered nurse. There is little that can be done to overcome the residency requirement or credential issues.

Regarding language barriers, however, the WIN program has encouraged interested individuals to continue to develop their English skills by attending ESL classes at the college or elsewhere in the community, routinely practicing speaking and reading English, and obtaining employment as a certified nursing assistant. Most are potential WIN candidates once they have improved their language skills. Furthermore, beginning Spring Term 2006, CCC recognizing the importance of strengthening the pathway into health care for all nonnative speakers and, building on the success of the WIN Program, has developed a promising new project that will prepare immigrants and refugees for employment as nursing assistants. The Nursing Assistant Pathway for English Language Learners (NAPELL) will provide advanced-level ESL instruction that will lead into nursing assistant classes, skills lab, and clinical practicum in a long-term care facility in the community. Several "pre-WIN" internationally educated nurses, who have not yet met the WIN language requirements, are taking advantage of this opportunity.

Success Factors Bring a Positive Conclusion

Four factors have contributed to WIN's current level of success: sound partnerships, a supportive college, a dedicated and creative staff, and motivated students. All factors are essential and interwoven. At the core of WIN's success, however, is the synergistic relationship between two unmet needs. The first need is to return the pool of talented and motivated internationally educated nursing professionals to their field of choice. The second need is to fill the region's looming nursing shortage with qualified nurses who are equipped to work with diverse populations. The WIN program is positioned at the nexus of these two needs. The WIN students are a special and exceptional group of motivated and talented individuals who have, in some cases, overcome incredible hardship to come to the United States. The WIN program, with the help of many partners, is extending a hand to those whose dream is to once again help heal others.

RECOMMENDATIONS FOR NURSE ADMINISTRATORS

Nurse administrators are in a unique and important position to support or undermine the success WIN nurses experience in the field. The following recommendations are offered to help nurse administrators ensure a successful clinical experience for internationally educated nurses (IENs):

1. Orient nurse administrators, preceptors, and staff to the WIN reentry program's objectives and course content as well as to the IEN's prior background in nursing.
2. Expect preceptorships for IENs to take longer than for traditional new nursing graduates or U.S. reentry nurses. Most IENs have been prevented from any clinical contact during their reentry education.
3. During preceptorship, pair IENs with preceptors who are culturally competent. An excellent and experienced preceptor is not always the best choice for an IEN. Simply because a preceptor has worked with many traditional nursing students in the past does not mean he or she is the best fit for an IEN. In fact, preconceived ideas of how a generic nursing student should perform often do not fit the IEN.
4. Avoid randomly assigning the IEN to any unit that has an opening. Better success can be achieved by identifying several nurses who can work well with the IEN and assigning the WIN graduate to those nurses or their unit.
5. Include several days of shadowing the assigned nurse preceptor during orientation to the nursing unit to observe management of patient case load and other unit responsibilities. Allow the IEN nurse to participate in patient care as they are able.
6. Following several days of observation, assign the IEN to the care of one patient to permit the nurse to integrate the parts of care that have been observed.
7. Establish daily goals with the IEN and preceptor, as well as provide honest feedback and evaluation regarding progress. Assignments can be advanced as appropriate.

8. Consult regularly with the IEN's nursing director to identify specific strengths and weaknesses that the IEN brings to the workplace and to monitor the IEN's progress. Adjust assignments, as needed.
9. Take advantage of the expertise the IEN brings. Their nursing experience, skills, and stories can be educational and inspirational to others.

The WIN program is a career pathway for internationally educated nurses who are often stymied in their efforts to return to their chosen profession. Currently, within many larger communities across the United States is a pool of talented and motivated health care professionals who are eager to help address the nursing shortage. The WIN model provides a proven template for effectively assimilating this nursing talent into the health care workforce.

QUESTIONS FOR DIALOGUE

1. What ideas or concepts did you find most meaningful in this chapter? Identify your insights and questions to bring to a dialogue with your colleagues.
2. Review the story of Bindu. Identify the challenges and barriers Bindu faced in trying to reenter the professional nursing workforce. What barriers do immigrant nurses encounter in your community when they seek to reenter the profession at the same level at which they were educated in their home country?
3. What is the need in your community for reentry programs for immigrant nurses? What are the potential benefits for the community? Given the experience of the WIN program, what characteristics are essential to a successful outcome of such a program?
4. Discuss the implications of the decision to replace the ESL component of the WIN program with Advanced Communication.
5. Compare and contrast the benefits and costs of using a test such as the TOEIC, which is not specific to language used in clinical nursing practice, versus a test such as CELBAN (see chapter 12), which is specific to nursing practice, as a criterion for program entry.
6. What considerations might be given to internationally educated nurses during the postlicensure clinical component of reentry in order to facilitate a successful transition into the U.S. health care workforce? Discuss the rationale for not allowing internationally

educated nurses to have patient contact until fully licensed, in contrast to traditional nursing students who have supervised patient contact soon after beginning their nursing education. How might clinical sites be evaluated for readiness prior to placement of the internationally educated nurse?

APPENDIX

WIN PROGRAM FLOWCHART

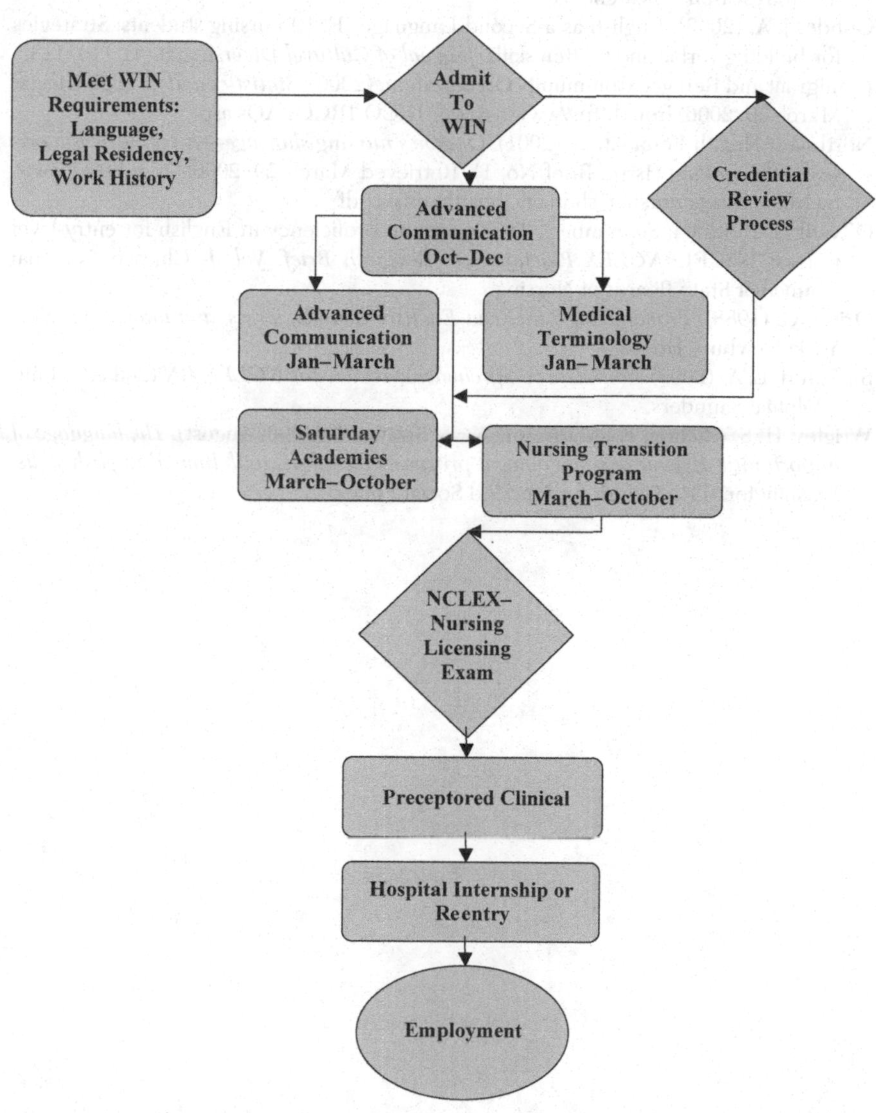

REFERENCES

Burton, D. A., Morris, B. A., & Campbell, K. K. (2005). *When, not if . . . A report on Oregon's registered nurse workforce.* Portland: The Oregon Center for Nursing.

Donley, R. (2005). Challenges for nursing in the 21st century. *Nursing Economics, 23*(6), 312–318.

Educational Testing Services. (2006). *Comparing TOEIC to TOEFL.* Retrieved April 3, 2006, from http://www.ets.org/portal/site/ets.menuitem

Federation for American Immigration Reform (FAIR). (2006). *City fact sheet: Portland Oregon.* Retrieved March 29, 2006, from http://www.fairus.org/site/PageServer?pagename=research_researchd0a6

Guhde, J. A. (2003). English-as-a-Second Language (ESL) nursing students: Strategies for building verbal and written skills. *Journal of Cultural Diversity, 10*(4), 113–118.

Immigrant and Refugee Community Organization. (2006). *Statistics and facts.* Retrieved March 29, 2006, from http://www.irco.org/IRCO/IRCOFAQs.asp

Northwest Health Foundation. (2001). *Oregon's nursing shortage—A public health crisis in the making* (Issue Brief No. 1). Retrieved March 29, 2006, from http://www.nwhf.org/assets/nursing_shortage_health_crisis.pdf

O'Neill, T. R. (2004, September). The minimum proficiency in English for entry-level nurses: TOEFL. *NCLEX Psychometric Research Brief, Vol. 1.* Chicago: National Council of State Boards of Nursing.

Orion, G. (1988). *Pronouncing American English: Sounds, stress, and intonation.* New York: Newbury House.

Silvesteri, L. A. (2002). *Saunders comprehensive review for NCLEX-RN* (2nd ed.). Philadelphia: Saunders.

Wrigley, H. S., Richter, E., Martinson, K., & Strawn, J. (2003, August). *The language of opportunity: Expanding employment prospects for adults with limited English skills.* Washington, DC: Center for Law and Social Policy.

Index